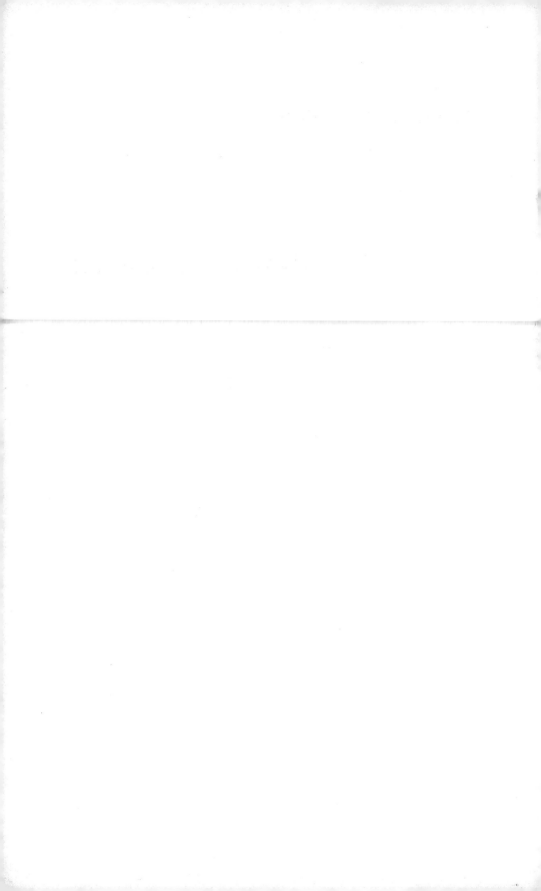

Cardiovascular MR Manual

Sven Plein • John Greenwood
John P. Ridgway
Editors

Cardiovascular MR Manual

Second Edition

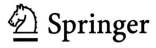 Springer

Editors
Sven Plein
Leeds Institute for Cardiovascular
and Metabolic Imaging
University of Leeds
Leeds
UK

John P. Ridgway
Department of Medical Physics
and Engineering
Leeds Teaching Hospitals NHS Trust
Leeds
UK

John Greenwood
Leeds Institute for Cardiovascular
and Metabolic Imaging
University of Leeds
Leeds
UK

ISBN 978-3-319-20939-5   ISBN 978-3-319-20940-1   (eBook)
DOI 10.1007/978-3-319-20940-1

Library of Congress Control Number: 2015951451

Springer Cham Heidelberg New York Dordrecht London

Printed on acid-free paper

Springer International Publishing AG Switzerland is part of Springer Science+Business Media
(www.springer.com)

Contents

Contributors

Mark Ainslie, MBChB (Hons), BSc (Hons), MRCP Department of Cardiology, University Hospital of South Manchester, Manchester, UK

Amedeo Chiribiri, MBBS, CCST in Cardiology, PhD Department of Cardiovascular Imaging, King's College London/St Thomas's Hospital, London, UK

Andrew M. Crean, BSc, BM, MRCP MSc, MPhil, FRCR Department of Cardiology, University of Cincinnati Medical Center and Cincinnati Children's Hospital, Cincinnati, OH, USA

Timothy Fairbairn, MBChB, PhD Department of Cardiology, Liverpool Heart and Chest Hospital, Liverpool, UK

Pankaj Garg, MD Leeds Institute of Cardiovascular and Metabolic Medicine (LICAMM), University of Leeds, Leeds, UK

John P. Greenwood, MBChB, PhD, FRCP Division of Biomedical Imaging, Leeds Institute of Cardiovascular and Metabolic Medicine, University of Leeds and Leeds Teaching Hospitals, Clarendon Way, Leeds, UK

Department of Cardiology, Leeds Teaching Hospitals NHS Trust, Leeds, UK

Gerald F. Greil, MD, PhD Pediatric Cardiology, University of Texas Southwestern/Children's Medical Center Dallas, Dallas, TX, USA

Bernhard A. Herzog, MD Cardiac Imaging, University Hospital Zurich, Zurich, Switzerland

Tarique M. Hussain, MBBCHir, PhD Division of Imaging Sciences, King's College London, St Thomas' Hospital, Guy's & St Thomas' NHS Trust, London, UK

Neil Maredia, MB ChB, MRCP (UK), MD Department of Cardiology, James Cook University Hospital, Middlesbrough, UK

Adam N. Mather, MBBS, MD, MRCP Department of Cardiology, Castle Hill Hospital, Hull and East Yorkshire Hospitals NHS Trust, Hull, East Yorkshire, UK

Daniel R. Messroghli, MD Internal Medicine – Cardiology, Deutsches Herzzentrum Berlin, Berlin, Germany

Christopher A. Miller, BSc(Hons), MBChB(Hons), MRCP, PhD Cardiac MRI Unit, University Hospitals of South Manchester NHS Foundation Trust, North West Heart Centre, Manchester, UK

Manish Motwani, MB ChB Division of Cardiovascular and Diabetes Research, Leeds Institute of Cardiovascular and Metabolic Medicine, Multidisciplinary Cardiovascular Research Centre, University of Leeds, Leeds, UK

Charles Peebles, MBBS, MRCP, FRCR Department of Cardiothoracic Radiology, University Hospital Southampton, Southampton, Hampshire, UK

Sven Plein, MD, PhD Division of Biomedical Imaging, Leeds Institute of Cardiovascular and Metabolic Medicine, University of Leeds and Leeds Teaching Hospitals, Leeds, UK

Kawal Rhode, PhD Biomedical Engineering, Guy's & St. Thomas' Hospitals, London, UK

David P. Ripley, BSc (Hons), MBChB, MRCP Division of Biomedical Imaging, Leeds Institute of Cardiovascular and Metabolic Medicine, University of Leeds and Leeds Teaching Hospitals, Clarendon Way, Leeds, UK

John P. Ridgway, PhD Department of Medical Physics and Engineering, Leeds Teaching Hospitals NHS Trust, St James's University Hospital, Leeds, UK

Matthias Schmitt, MD, PhD Cross-Sectional Cardiac Imaging Unit, Cardiovascular Division, University Hospital of South Manchester, Manchester, UK

Part I

How Does CMR Work?

What's Inside the Magnet and Why? 1

John P. Ridgway

Abstract

Three types of magnetic field are used to generate images for magnetic resonance imaging, (MRI):

A strong, constant magnetic field, a gradient magnetic field that can be rapidly switched on and off and a radiofrequency (RF) magnetic field. A typical MRI system therefore consists of three main components that generate these three fields; the main magnet, the gradient coil assembly and the integral rf body transmitter coil. The most common main magnet configurations are superconducting, with a horizontal patient bore. The magnet coils generate a highly uniform magnetic field at the centre of the patient bore which is brought to within a specified limit of homogeneity by a process known as shimming. Three cylindrical copper windings (gradient coils) positioned inside the inner bore of the cryostat each generates a magnetic field gradient which varies the resonant frequency, enabling the MR signal to be encoded in three dimensions. This provides the unique ability to directly acquire cross sectional images in any orthogonal or oblique plane. The integral RF body transmitter coil generates a much smaller magnetic field that oscillates at the resonant (Larmor) frequency, causing the hydrogen nuclei in the patient's tissue to resonate and then to re-emit the energy, also in the form of an oscillating rf magnetic field. This MR Signal is detected by a RF receiver coil. For Cardiac MRI this is usually a dedicated receiver coil or coil array.

Keywords

Magnetic field • Gradient magnetic field • Gradient coils • Radiofrequency magnetic field • RF • Patient bore • Superconducting • Cryostat • Liquid helium • Passive shimming • Dynamic shimming • Resonant frequency • Larmor frequency • Specific absorption rate • SAR • Transmitter coil • Receiver coil

J.P. Ridgway, PhD
Department of Medical Physics and Engineering, Leeds Teaching Hospitals NHS Trust, St James's University Hospital, 1st Floor, Bexley Wing, Leeds LS2 9TJ, UK
e-mail: j.p.ridgway@leeds.ac.uk

© Springer International Publishing 2015
S. Plein et al. (eds.), *Cardiovascular MR Manual*,
DOI 10.1007/978-3-319-20940-1_1

The use of Magnetic Resonance (MR) in medicine involves the interaction of magnetic fields with biological tissue. For magnetic resonance imaging, (MRI), three types of magnetic field are used to generate images.

- A *strong, constant magnetic field*. This has the symbol B_0 and defines the nominal operating field strength of a particular MRI system. This is measured in units of Tesla, (T) with 1 T equal to approximately 20,000 times the earth's magnetic field.
- A *gradient magnetic field* that can be rapidly switched on and off. This magnetic field has a strength that increases with position along a chosen direction and is measured in units of milliTesla per metre (mT/m).
- A *radiofrequency (RF) magnetic field* that oscillates at a characteristic frequency in the Megahertz range, the exact value of which is determined by the nominal field strength of the main magnet. This is given the symbol B_1.

A typical MRI system therefore consists of three main components that generate these three fields, the main magnet, the gradient coil assembly and the integral radiofrequency body transmitter coil. These are described in the sections that follow which will use the convention of Cartesian axes (x, y, and z) in the directions as shown in Fig. 1.1.

The Main Magnet

The most common main magnet configurations are *Superconducting*, with a *Horizontal Patient Bore* with field strengths of 1.0 T, 1.5 T, 3.0 T.

Superconducting magnets consist of several circular magnet coils each consisting of many turns of wire (windings) carrying a high electrical current. This generates a *strong, constant magnetic field, B_0*, in a horizontal direction through the centre of the coils (parallel to the z axis as shown in Fig. 1.1a).

The windings are made of a material that becomes superconducting when cooled to liquid helium temperatures (approx. 4 K or −269 °C). They are immersed in liquid helium contained within a vessel (the *'Cryostat'*) surrounded by two vacuum layers to reduce the boil-off rate of the liquid Helium (Fig. 1.1b). The Cryostat has a central bore open at both ends of the magnet (the *patient bore*).

The magnet coils are positioned to generate a highly uniform magnetic field at the centre of the patient bore typically over a spherical region between 45 and 50 cm in diameter, known as the homogeneous volume. The extent of this region determines the maximum field of view that can be imaged at one time.

The magnetic field is brought to within a specified limit of homogeneity by a process known as shimming. At the time of installation, small pieces of steel are placed around the inside of the magnet bore to modify the magnetic field so that it has the best uniformity within the homogenous volume. This process is known as

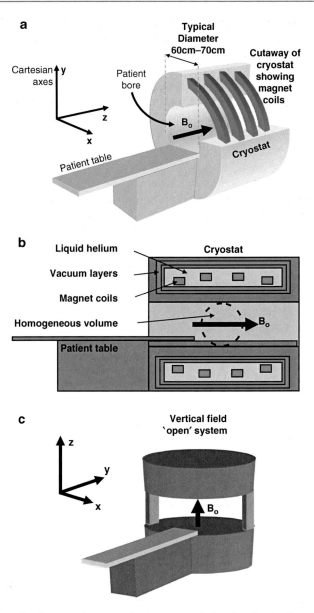

Fig. 1.1 (**a**) The Key features of superconducting magnet design showing the Cartesian axes with the horizontal z-axis, the static B$_o$ field direction, the patient bore and magnet coils. (**b**) Internal construction of magnet cryostat. The spherical homogenous volume is indicated by the dotted line. (**c**) A vertical field, open magnet configuration. The z-axis is vertical for this configuration

passive shimming and it takes into account the effect that any steel within the building structure might have. It is also possible to perform *active Shimming* of the magnetic field by using small magnetic fields generated by additional electromagnetic coils to correct any remaining variations in the magnetic field. This may be done by using either the *gradient coils* (see next section) or dedicated *shim coils*. A standard shim is determined at installation to provide the best uniformity over the whole imaging volume. *dynamic shimming* may also be performed on a scan by scan basis in order to provide the best magnetic field homogeneity over a particular region for specific applications.

Once the magnet has been energised after installation, it *remains on at all times.* Superconductivity is maintained by minimising the boil-off rate of liquid helium using a cooling system and periodically topping it up. Current systems can maintain sufficient levels of helium for several years before topping up.

Safety Point

As the magnet remains on all the time, (even outside normal working hours), the strong magnetic field presents a constant hazard and safety measures must therefore be applied at all times (See Chap. 2).

Vertical field 'open' MR systems are also commercially available, currently having field strengths of up to 1.0 T (Fig. 1.1c). Open MR systems often use magnet designs that are based on permanent magnets or iron cored resistive magnets but these have lower field strengths than superconducting systems.

The Gradient Coil Assembly

This consists of a set of three cylindrical copper windings (*gradient coils*) positioned inside the inner bore of the cryostat (Fig. 1.2). Each gradient coil generates a *magnetic field gradient* This is a field applied in the same direction as the main

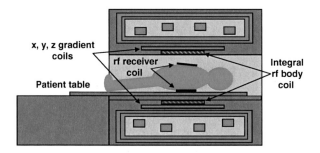

Fig. 1.2 The relative locations of the gradient coils, integral RF body coil and RF receiver coils

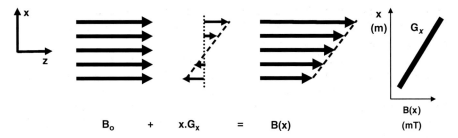

Fig. 1.3 This diagram shows how gradient field of slope G_x is superimposed onto the main magnetic field, B_o to produce a total field that varies in the x direction, $B(x)$. The strength of the magnetic field is represented by the length of the arrows in each case. The direction of each magnetic field is along the z axis but the direction of the gradient (change in strength) is along the x axis

magnetic field that either adds or subtracts in such a way as to create a net total field that varies in strength with position along each of the *x, y* and *z* directions (Fig. 1.3). This also varies the resonant frequency and enables the MR signals subsequently emitted to be related to particular locations (see Chap. 6). The use of the three gradients enables the signal to be encoded in three dimensions and provides the unique ability to directly acquire cross sectional images in any orthogonal or oblique plane. The gradient magnetic fields can be independently switched on or off rapidly in less than a millisecond and may be kept on for a few milliseconds at a time. As the fields are switched rapidly within the main magnetic field they cause the gradient coils to vibrate creating the familiar loud banging noise that is associated with MRI systems.

Safety Point
The rapidly switched gradient magnetic fields are only active during image acquisition however they present two additional hazards:

- The rapidly changing electromagnetic field (often denoted **dB/dt**) can cause peripheral nerve stimulation of patients.
- The banging noise is sufficiently loud to warrant the use of hearing protection by patients and carers that remain in the examination room.

The Integral Radiofrequency (RF) Body Transmitter Coil

This consists of a cylindrical copper antenna mounted inside the gradient coil assembly (Fig. 1.2). It generates a much smaller magnetic field, B_1 that oscillates in a direction at right angles to the main magnetic field along the x or y axes. The frequency of oscillation (known as the *resonant frequency* or *Larmor frequency*), corresponds to the nominal operating frequency of the MRI system which in turn is

Table 1.1 Resonant frequencies for the three most common field strengths used for CMR

Field strength	Resonant frequency
1.0 T	42.6 MHz
1.5 T	63.9 MHz
3.0 T	127.8 MHz

determined by the nominal field strength of the main magnetic field. The operating frequency is typically in the Megahertz range (as used by short wave radios) and hence $\mathbf{B_1}$ is known as the *radiofrequency (RF)* magnetic field. The resonant frequencies for the most common nominal field strengths are given in (Table 1.1):

The RF magnetic field produced by the integral body coil is used to transmit energy into the patient. It is normally delivered in the form of a short pulse, known as a RF pulse (see Chap. 4). When applied at the resonant frequency this causes the hydrogen nuclei in the patient's tissue to absorb the energy, to resonate and then to re-emit the energy, also in the form of an oscillating RF magnetic field.

Safety Point

The radiofrequency field creates a further hazard as it has the potential to cause heating of body tissue. The rate of energy deposition is characterised by the *specific absorption rate (SAR)* with units Watts per Kilogram of tissue (W/Kg) and is carefully monitored and controlled.

The Receiver Coil

The oscillating magnetic field (MR Signal) emitted is detected by a RF receiver coil. For cardiac MRI this is usually a dedicated *receiver coil* or *coil array*, whose design is tailored to maximise signal detection around the heart and to minimise the detection of 'noise' from elsewhere in the body and surrounding environment (see Fig. 1.2). The MR signal is small; the voltage induced in the receiver coil is typically measured in microvolts and so it is very sensitive to interference from external sources of electrical noise. The integral body transmitter can also be used as a receiver coil. Although it is less sensitive than a dedicated receiver coil, it can provide a more uniform detection field which is sometimes advantageous.

Summary
- Cardiac Magnetic Resonance Imaging uses three types of magnetic field to generate images:
  - A strong constant magnetic field is generated by the main magnet
  - A rapidly switched gradient magnetic field is generated by an assembly of three gradient coils (one for each direction, x, y and z) mounted inside the main magnet
  - A radiofrequency (RF) magnetic field is generated by the integral rf body transmitter coil mounted inside the gradient coil.
- A separate RF receiver coil that is tailored to maximise signal from the heart is normally used to detect the emitted MR signal.

GE www.gehealthcare.com
Philips www.medical.philips.com
Siemens www.healthcare.siemens.com
Toshiba www.toshibamedicalsystems.com

Further Reading

McRobbie DW, Moore EA, Graves MJ, Prince MR. Let's talk technical: MR equipment. In: MRI from picture to proton. 2nd ed. Cambridge: Cambridge University Press; 2007. p. 167–91.

The MRI Environment

2

John P. Ridgway

Abstract

The examination room which contains the magnet assembly and patient table is enclosed within a RF shield (or Faraday cage) to prevent environmental electrical noise from interfering with the MR signal. The main magnet also generates a magnetic fringe field that is always present and extends well beyond the outside the magnet. This can create an extremely hazardous environment unless control measures are put in place. The general public are excluded from entering the fringe field above the 0.5 mT threshold as values above this may adversely affect the operation of cardiac pacemakers. A controlled area is defined to fully enclose the 0.5 mT magnetic fringe field contour. Access to this area is restricted to authorised staff with appropriate training. Patients and visitors should not enter unless they have first been screened for the presence of pacemakers and other contraindicated implants. Access is also restricted to prevent accidents caused by ferromagnetic objects being attracted by the magnet and becoming projectiles. Specific items should be identified as being safe, unsafe or conditional using an international labelling system. Most commercially available magnets use active shielding to reduce the extent of the fringe field. Additionally the examination room may be passively shielded using steel plate to prevent the fringe field from extending outside the controlled area.

Keywords

Examination room • RF shield • Faraday cage • Fringe field • Controlled area • Cardiac pacemakers • 0.5 mT fringe field contour • Projectiles • Active shielding • Passive shielding • Safety guidelines • ASTM labelling • MR safe • MR conditional • MR unsafe

J.P. Ridgway, PhD
Department of Medical Physics and Engineering, Leeds Teaching Hospitals NHS Trust,
St James's University Hospital, 1st Floor, Bexley Wing, Leeds LS2 9TJ, UK
e-mail: j.p.ridgway@leeds.ac.uk

© Springer International Publishing 2015
S. Plein et al. (eds.), *Cardiovascular MR Manual*,
DOI 10.1007/978-3-319-20940-1_2

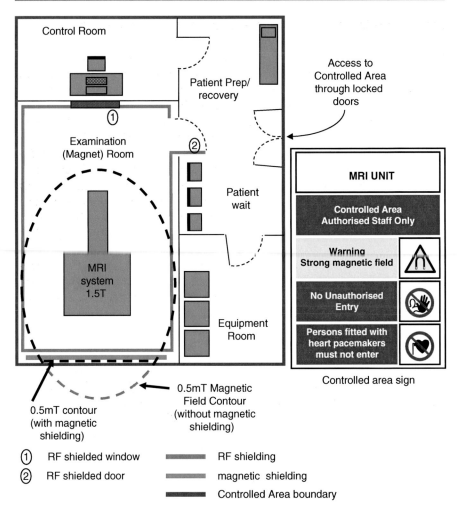

Fig. 2.1 Typical layout of an MRI unit showing the examination (magnet) room, control room, equipment room and ancillary rooms. The boundary of the controlled area is shown red. Steel sheet shielding has been used to prevent the 0.5 mT fringe field from extending outside the controlled area. The examination room is completely enclosed by a copper RF shield (RF cabin). An example sign for the controlled area access doors is shown

The Examination Room and RF Shielding

The examination room contains the magnet assembly and patient table (Fig. 2.1). To prevent environmental electrical noise from interfering with the MR signal, this room is enclosed within a *RF shield* (or *Faraday cage*) made of copper or aluminium sheet. The door into the examination room forms part of this shield and must always be closed during the MR examination. The observation window also forms part of this shield.

The Magnetic Fringe Field Hazard and the Controlled Area

The main magnet generates the strongest magnetic field at its centre but also has a *fringe field* that is always present and extends well beyond the outside the magnet, decreasing with distance from the magnet. This can create an extremely hazardous environment unless control measures are put in place. For this reason the general public must be excluded from entering the fringe field above a certain threshold. Currently this threshold is set at 0.5 mT, as magnetic fields above this value have been shown to adversely affect the operation of *cardiac pacemakers*. A *controlled area* is therefore defined to include the examination room and any adjacent rooms necessary to fully enclose the *0.5 mT fringe field contour* (Fig. 2.1). Access to this area is restricted to authorised staff with appropriate training. Patients and visitors should not enter unless they have first been screened for the presence of pacemakers and other contraindicated implants (see Chap. 20 for a list of other MR contraindications).

A second very important reason to restrict access to the controlled area is to prevent accidents caused by ferromagnetic objects being attracted by the magnet and becoming *projectiles*. All equipment or other items that are taken into the examination room must first be carefully checked to ensure they are not ferromagnetic.

> **Safety Point**
> Specific items should be identified as being safe, unsafe or conditional (Fig. 2.2) using the labelling system introduced by the ASTM [4] (ASTM International, Standard practice for marking medical devices and other items for safety in magnetic resonance environments, F2503–05).
>
> Items such as watches, credit cards and mobile phones may also be damaged by the magnetic field and should not be taken into the magnet room.

 MR Unsafe: Not safe in the magnet room.

 MR Conditional: Only safe within the conditions described on a notice fixed to the equipment.

 MR Safe: Safe in the magnet room.

NO LABEL   Assume unsafe unless you know otherwise.

ASTM Labelling System

Fig. 2.2 Labelling system developed by the ASTM to identify ancillary equipment as MR safe, Conditional or Unsafe

Though there is the potential to cause serious harm due to the above hazards there are relatively few deaths recorded due to MR equipment. Most recorded fatalities have been caused by pacemaker malfunction with one fatality caused by a gas cylinder becoming a projectile. If the above control measures are strictly adhered to, the MR environment can be managed relatively safely.

Active and Passive Magnetic Shielding

Most commercially available magnets have *active shielding* (additional windings within the cryostat located just outside the main magnet coils) that produces a counteracting field that in turn reduces the extent of the fringe field. This reduces the requirement for the controlled area and enables magnet systems to be installed in relatively small departments. Magnetic shielding using steel plate is often additionally used (known as *passive shielding*) to further reduce the extent of the fringe field to prevent it from extending outside the controlled area (Fig. 2.1). For example, magnetic shielding is commonly used in multi-storey buildings to prevent the fringe field from extending into areas in the floors above and below the magnetic location.

Summary

- The examination room is enclosed within a RF shield (Faraday cage) made of copper or aluminium to prevent external RF 'noise' from interfering with the MR signal
- The main magnet generates a fringe field that can both adversely affect the operation of pacemakers and other implants *and* cause ferromagnetic items to accelerate towards the magnet causing a projectile hazard
- A controlled area must be defined that encloses the 0.5 mT fringe field contour (pacemaker line)
- Access to the controlled area is restricted to authorised staff and patients that have been screened for pacemakers and other contraindicated implants
- Items of equipment must not be taken into the MR examination room unless they are clearly identified to be safe in the MR environment.
- Magnetic shielding can be used to restrict the extent of the fringe field.

Further Reading
National and international guidance is published for the safe installation and operation of magnetic resonance imaging systems. Useful information and links can be found in the following:

- MHRA Safety Guidelines for Magnetic Resonance Imaging Equipment in Clinical Use. https://www.gov.uk/government/publications/safety-guidelines-for-magnetic-resonance-imaging-equipment-in-clinical-use

- Expert Panel on MR Safety, Kanal E, Barkovich AJ, Bell C, Borgstede JP, Bradley WG Jr, Froelich JW, Gimbel JR, Gosbee JW, Kuhni-Kaminski E, Larson PA, Lester JW Jr, Nyenhuis J, Schaefer DJ, Sebek EA, Weinreb J, Wilkoff BL, Woods TO, Lucey L, Hernandez D. ACR Guidance Document on MR Safe Practices:2013. J Magn Reson Imaging. 2013;37:501–30. doi:10.1002/jmri.24011

References

ASTM Standard F2503–13. Standard practice for marking medical devices and other items for safety in magnetic resonance environments. ASTM International, West Conshohocken, PA. 2013. doi:10.1520/F2503, www.astm.org.

Protons and Spins: The Origin of the MR Signal

3

John P. Ridgway

Abstract

The MR signal originates from hydrogen nuclei within water and fat within the patient's tissue. Hydrogen nuclei, (protons) possess an intrinsic property known as Nuclear Spin. This combined with the proton's positive charge gives rise to a small magnetic field, known as a magnetic moment. In the presence of the externally applied B_0 field, the magnetic moments tend to align either with or against the externally applied magnetic field. An equilibrium state is quickly attained where there is a small excess aligned with the field, generating a net magnetisation. The greater the applied magnetic field strength, the greater is the size of the Net Magnetisation. The value of the Net Magnetisation determines the maximum available MR signal.

Keywords

MR signal • Hydrogen nuclei • Protons • Water • Fat • Free water • Lipid molecules • Nuclear spin • Magnetic moment • Equilibrium • Net magnetisation • Field strength

J.P. Ridgway, PhD
Department of Medical Physics and Engineering, Leeds Teaching Hospitals NHS Trust,
St James's University Hospital, 1st Floor, Bexley Wing, Leeds LS2 9TJ, UK
e-mail: j.p.ridgway@leeds.ac.uk

© Springer International Publishing 2015
S. Plein et al. (eds.), *Cardiovascular MR Manual*,
DOI 10.1007/978-3-319-20940-1_3

Fig. 3.1 Transverse section through the thorax. Visible signal originates from either water based tissue such as muscle or from lipid molecules within fat

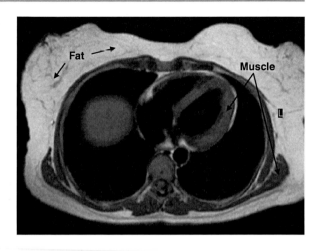

MR Images: What Are We Looking at?

The primary origin of the MR signal is from water and fat within the patient's tissue; specifically it is from the *hydrogen nuclei* (consisting of a single proton) contained within *free water* and *lipid molecules* (Fig. 3.1). Hydrogen is one of a number of elements whose nuclei exhibit magnetic resonance properties but the high intrinsic sensitivity and natural abundance in the form of water and lipid molecules makes it particularly favourable for imaging. Other nuclei of potential interest for cardiac applications in the future may include ^{31}P, ^{23}Na, ^{13}C but their sensitivity for imaging is low as they are only normally present in the body in trace amounts.

Proton Spin and Net Magnetisation

Hydrogen nuclei, (protons) possess an intrinsic property known as *nuclear spin.* This combined with their positive charge gives rise to a small magnetic field for each proton, known as a *magnetic moment.* Normally the magnetic moments (spins) are randomly oriented but in the presence of the externally applied B_0 field, they tend to align either with or against the externally applied magnetic field. An *equilibrium* state is quickly attained where there is a small excess aligned with the field (typically just a few spins per million) as this is the more favourable direction of alignment. A more accurate description of this process relies on statistical quantum mechanics. It becomes easier, however, to develop a simpler picture by considering a population of billions of protons. In this model (known as the classical model) the excess of proton magnetic moments combines to form a net magnetic field or *net magnetisation* (Fig. 3.2). This is often given the symbol **M** and at equilibrium it is aligned along the +ve z axis (along B_0) and has its maximum value, $\mathbf{M_0}$. It is often shown as an arrow or vector.

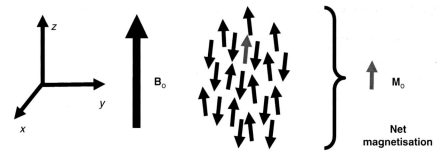

Fig. 3.2 Proton magnetic moments, represented by arrows align either with or against the direction of the magnetic field, B_o (i.e., along the z-axis). In this example there is an excess of just one proton (shown in red) aligned with the field out of a population of 21, giving rise to the Net Magnetisation M_o

What Determines the Size of the Net Magnetisation?

The size of this net magnetisation is one of the key determinants of the maximum signal intensity that can be generated and used to form images. The exact proportion of excess spins the gives rise to the net magnetisation at equilibrium is described by the *Boltzmann distribution* which shows that it depends on both the temperature (37 °C for in vivo imaging) and the applied magnetic field strength, B_o as determined by the main magnet (see box). The greater the field strength, the greater is the size of the net magnetisation (i.e., the greater the excess of protons aligned with the magnetic field).

> **Point of Interest**
> The Boltzmann distribution tells us that the excess of protons aligned with the field at equilibrium is determined by the temperature and the applied magnetic field strength. Assuming body temperature:
>
> At 1.5 T, the excess is about *4 protons* per million
> At 3.0 T the excess is *7 protons* per million.
>
> Therefore the *higher* the field strength, the *greater* the available signal.

The presence of the net magnetisation aligned with the magnetic field at equilibrium is not measurable as an MR signal. The next chapter shows that in order to produce a signal, energy must first be delivered to the system of protons in a very specific form.

Summary
- The origin of the MR signal is from hydrogen nuclei (single protons) contained within free water and lipid molecules.
- Hydrogen nuclei (protons) possess a property known as nuclear spin that gives rise to a small magnetic field known as a magnetic moment
- When a large magnetic field is applied, a small proportion of the magnetic moments of a large population of hydrogen nuclei combine to form a Net Magnetisation aligned in the same direction as the applied magnetic field.
- The greater the strength of the applied magnetic field, the greater the value of the Net Magnetisation.
- The value of the Net Magnetisation determines the maximum available MR signal.

Further Reading

Balaban RS, Peters DC. Basic principles of cardiovascular magnetic resonance. In: Manning WJ, Pennell DJ, editors. Cardiovascular magnetic resonance. 2nd ed. Philadelphia: Saunders; 2010. p. 3–18.

McRobbie DW, Moore EA, Graves MJ, Prince MR. Getting in tune: resonance & relaxation. In: MRI from picture to proton. 2nd ed. Cambridge: Cambridge University Press; 2007. p. 137–41.

Ridgway JP. Cardiac magnetic resonance physics for clinicians: part I. J Cardiovasc Magn Reson. 2010;12(1):71. doi:10.1186/1532-429X-12-71.

Generating a Signal: RF Pulses and Echoes

4

John P. Ridgway

Abstract

In order to generate an MR signal from the net magnetisation, the RF oscillating magnetic field is used to deliver energy into the population of protons at the Larmor Frequency. The Larmor frequency (resonant frequency) is proportional to the strength of the magnetic field and is typically in the Megahertz range. The RF field is normally applied as a short pulse, known as an rf pulse. When it is applied, the proton magnetic moments start to rotate together about the main magnetic field, causing the net magnetisation to move away from its alignment with the main magnetic field and to rotate around it. The greater the amount of energy applied by the RF pulse, the greater the angle that the net magnetisation makes with the B_0 field. This angle that the net magnetisation is rotated through by the RF pulse is known as the flip angle. Commonly used RF pulses for imaging are a low flip angle RF pulse, a 90° RF pulse, 180° RF refocusing pulse and a 180° RF inversion pulse. The low flip angle and 90 RF pulses are used as excitation pulses and generate a transverse component of magnetisation which rotates about the main magnetic field direction, generating an oscillating magnetic field that is detected by the RF receiver coil as an MR signal. The MR signal generated by a single RF pulse gradually decays and is known as a free induction decay or (FID).

Keywords

Larmor frequency • Resonant frequency • Gyromagnetic ratio • Multi-nuclear imaging • Net magnetisation • Coherence • Precession • Flip angle • Longitudinal magnetisation • Transverse magnetisation • Excitation pulse • Low flip angle • 90° RF pulse • 180° RF pulse • Saturated • Saturation pulse • Refocusing pulse • Inversion pulse • Inversion recovery • Free induction decay • FID

J.P. Ridgway, PhD
Department of Medical Physics and Engineering, Leeds Teaching Hospitals NHS Trust, St James's University Hospital, 1st Floor, Bexley Wing, Leeds LS2 9TJ, UK
e-mail: j.p.ridgway@leeds.ac.uk

© Springer International Publishing 2015
S. Plein et al. (eds.), *Cardiovascular MR Manual*,
DOI 10.1007/978-3-319-20940-1_4

How Do We Generate a Signal?

In order to generate a signal from the net magnetisation that is detectable, the radio-frequency (RF) magnetic field described in Chap. 1 is generated by the RF transmitter coil (the integral body coil) and used to deliver energy into the population of protons. This field must be applied at a particular frequency, known as the *Larmor Frequency,* that is determined by the strength of the magnetic field (see Table 1.1 in Chap. 1) such that:

$$\text{Larmor frequency} = \text{constant} \times B_0$$

This equation is known as the *Larmor equation.* The Larmor frequency is proportional to the strength of the magnetic field and is typically in the Megahertz range, e.g., for 1.5 T, the Larmor frequency is 63 MHz. This is also known as the r*esonant frequency,* as the protons only absorb energy (or resonate) at this characteristic frequency. The constant in the Larmor equation is known as the *gyromagnetic ratio* and has a value that is characteristic for a particular nucleus (42.6 MHz/T for the proton). The RF field is normally applied as a short pulse, known as an *RF pulse.*

Is the Larmor Frequency the Same for Other Nuclei?
As we saw in Chap. 3, magnetic resonance imaging is normally performed using hydrogen nuclei, however, there are other MR-active nuclei such as the most common isotopes of phosphorus (^{31}P) and sodium (^{23}Na), as well as a much less common of carbon (^{13}C). In each case the constant in the Larmor equation is different, leading to different resonant frequencies for each nucleus for a particular magnetic field strength. MR systems that have *multi-nuclear imaging* capability can perform imaging and spectroscopy of these and other nuclei.

What Does the RF Pulse Do to the Magnetisation?

Before the RF pulse is switched on, the proton population, and therefore the net magnetisation, M_0, is at *equilibrium,* aligned along the z-axis (Fig. 4.1a). When the RF pulse is switched on, the proton magnetic moments start to rotate together about the main magnetic field. This causes the *net magnetisation* to move away from its alignment with the z-axis and to rotate around it (Fig. 4.1b). Remember that the Net Magnetisation is the result of the sum of the individual magnetic moments. So long as they rotate together (a condition known as coherence) they will produce a Net Magnetisation that is rotating. The speed of this rotational motion, known as *precession,* is also at the Larmor frequency (The Larmor frequency is therefore also sometimes referred to as the as the frequency of precession). The greater the amount of energy applied by the RF pulse, the greater the angle that the net magnetisation makes with the B_0 field (or the z-axis). If the RF pulse were to remain on (i.e., a continuous RF

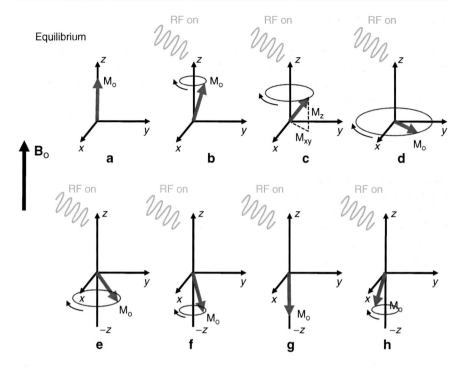

Fig. 4.1 Initially, Mo is at equilibrium (**a**). As the RF field is applied, M_o makes an increasing angle with the z-axis (**b**) and rotates in the direction of the curved arrow. For as long as the RF field is applied, the angle with the z axis continues to increase (**b–f**) until M_o lies along the –ve z-axis (**g**). If the RF field continues to be applied the angle will Increase beyond 180°, driving the magnetisation back toward the +ve z axis once more (**h**). At any instant the magnetisation can be split into two components, M_z and M_{xy}, (**c**). The rotating M_{xy} component generates the detectable MR signal once the applied RF field is switched off. The maximum detectable signal amplitude occurs when M_o lies entirely in the plane of the x and y axes (**d**) as this gives the largest M_{xy} component

field, constantly delivering energy), the net magnetisation will continue to move away from the z-axis, pass through the plane of the x and y axes (Fig. 4.1d) and eventually become aligned along the –ve z axis (Fig. 4.1g), and then continue to rotate back up towards the +ve z-axis and so on. In practice the RF field is delivered as a short pulse that is switched off once the angle of precession has reached a prescribed value, usually somewhere between 0° and 180° (Figs. 4.1b–g). This angle that the net magnetisation is rotated through by the RF pulse is known as the *flip angle.*

Longitudinal and Transverse Components of Magnetisation

Once the RF pulse has caused the Net Magnetisation to make an angle with the z-axis, it can be split into two components (Fig. 4.1c). One component is parallel to the z-axis. This is known as the z-component of the Magnetisation, *Mz,* also known as the *longitudinal component.* The other component lies at right angles to the z axis within the plane of the x and y axes and is known as the *x-y component* of the magnetisation, *Mxy,* or the *transverse component.* This rotates at the Larmor frequency within the *xy* plane and it is this transverse component of the Net Magnetisation that produces the detectable signal as it rotates by generating its own small, oscillating magnetic field which can be detected by an *RF receiver coil* once the transmitted RF pulse is switched off.

Flip Angle and Common RF Pulses

The *flip angle* of an RF pulse is determined by the energy delivered by the pulse which in turn depends upon both its amplitude and its duration. The greater the energy delivered, the greater the flip angle. RF pulses that generate an MR signal by delivering energy to the spin system, causing the magnetisation to move away from its equilibrium position are known as *excitation pulses,* Commonly used RF excitation pulses are identified by their flip angle as follows:

Low Flip Angle RF Excitation Pulse

In this case the net magnetisation is rotated through a pre-defined angle of less than 90° (often referred to as a *low flip angle,* often represented by the symbol α or assigned a specific value, e.g., 30°). Only a proportion of the net magnetisation is transferred from the *z*-axis into the *xy* plane, with some remaining along the *z*-axis (Fig. 4.2). While a *low flip angle* RF pulse produces an intrinsically lower signal than the 90° excitation pulse described next, it can be repeated more rapidly as it always leaves some of the magnetisation along the *z*-axis. This excitation pulse is used to generate the signal in gradient echo pulse sequences (see Chap. 11) to control the amount of magnetisation that is transferred between the *z*-axis and the *xy* plane for fast imaging applications.

90° RF Excitation Pulse

The *90° RF excitation pulse* delivers just enough energy to rotate the net magnetisation through 90° (Fig. 4.3). When the net magnetisation is at equilibrium, aligned along the *z*-axis, this transfers all of the net magnetisation from the *z*-axis into the *xy* (transverse) plane. This leaves no magnetisation along the *z*-axis immediately after the pulse and the system of protons is said to be *saturated.* The 90° RF pulse is sometimes referred to as a *saturation pulse.* When applied once, a 90° RF pulse produces the largest possible transverse magnetisation and MR signal and therefore provides better image quality than an RF pulse with a lower flip angle. It cannot be repeated as rapidly, however, as the *z*-component of the magnetisation needs time to recover. The 90° excitation pulse is used to initially generate the signal for spin echo-based pulse sequences (see Chap. 11).

The next most common RF pulse delivers enough energy to rotate the net magnetisation through 180°. This is used in one of two ways:

Fig. 4.2 Low flip angle (α) RF pulse

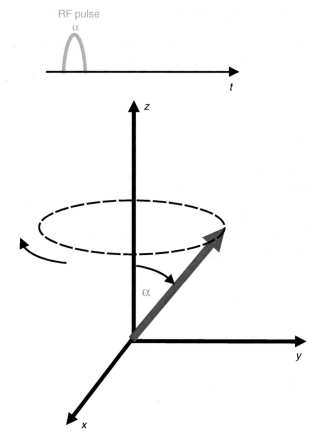

180° RF Pulse (Refocusing Pulse)

The *180° refocusing pulse* is used in spin echo pulse sequences after the 90° excitation pulse, where the net magnetisation has already been transferred into the *x-y* plane. It instantaneously swaps the direction of the magnetisation in the x-y plane through 180° (Fig. 4.4). This is used to reverse the loss of coherence caused by magnetic field inhomogeneities (see Chap. 5).

180° RF Pulse (Inversion Pulse)

The *180° inversion pulse* is normally used when the net magnetisation is at or close to equilibrium and will therefore rotate it from the positive to the negative *z*-axis (Fig. 4.5). It is known as an inversion pulse as it inverts the excess population of proton magnetic moments from being aligned to anti-aligned with the magnetic field. Because the resultant magnetisation lies only along the *z* -axis this pulse does not result in a detectable signal. It is used to prepare the *z*-magnetisation in *inversion recovery* pulse sequences

Fig. 4.3 90° RF pulse

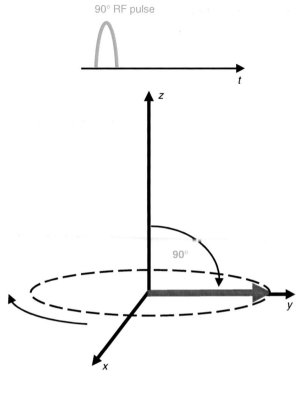

Fig. 4.4 180° RF refocusing
pulse

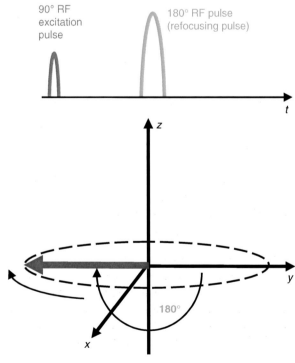

Fig. 4.5 180° RF inversion
pulse

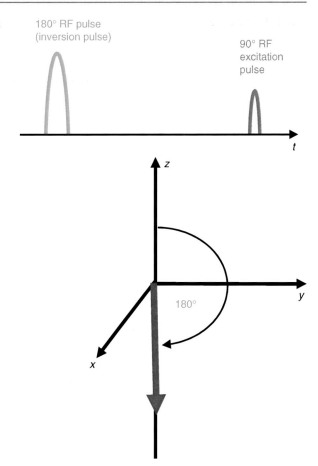

and in black blood preparation schemes (see Chaps. 12 and 16). This type of pulse is therefore also often referred to as a magnetisation preparation pulse.

What Does the MR Signal Look Like?

The simplest way of generating an MR signal is to apply a 90° RF excitation pulse to a spin system at equilibrium. This rotates all of the net magnetisation that is aligned long the z-axis, into the x-y plane. The resulting rotating transverse component of magnetisation produces an oscillating magnetic field that can be detected with a receiver coil (Fig. 4.6).

The signal that the receiver coil detects is seen as an oscillating magnetic field that gradually decays (known as a *free induction decay or FID*). The reason for the decay can be understood by remembering that the Net Magnetisation is the result of the sum of the magnetic moments (spins) of a whole population of protons. Immediately after the RF pulse they rotate together in a coherent fashion, i.e., as they rotate they point in the same direction within the *xy*-plane. This angle of the direction they point

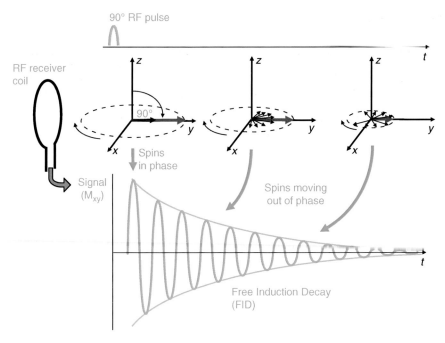

Fig. 4.6 The net transverse magnetisation (*red arrow*) generated by a 90 RF pulse generates an oscillating magnetic field as it rotates in the xy plane that can be detected by a RF receiver coil. Initially the signal has a maximum amplitude as the population of proton magnetic moments (spins) is in phase. The amplitude of the signal detected decays as the proton magnetic moments move out of phase with one another (shown by the small *black arrows*). The resultant decaying signal is known as the Free Induction Decay (FID)

at any instant is known as the phase angle and the spins are said at this initial stage to be 'in phase'. Over time, this coherence is gradually lost and the magnetic moments no longer rotate together. They are thus said to move 'out of phase'. The net sum of the magnetic moments is thus reduced, resulting in a reduction in the measured net (transverse) magnetisation which is observed as a decay of the signal strength.

Summary
- RF excitation pulses are used to generate an MR signal by flipping the Net Magnetisation away from its equilibrium position along the z-axis
- The flip angle of the RF pulse determines the angle that the Net magnetisation makes with the z-axis after the RF pulse
- After excitation by the RF pulse, the Net Magnetisation can be split into two components: One that remains along the z-axis (longitudinal component) and one that rotates at the Larmor frequency around the z-axis in the xy plane (transverse component).
- The rotating transverse component generates an oscillating magnetic field that can be detected by a RF receiver coil as an MR signal.
- The freely decaying MR signal is known as a free induction decay (FID)

Further Reading

Balaban RS, Peters DC. Basic principles of cardiovascular magnetic resonance. In: Manning WJ, Pennell DJ, editors. Cardiovascular magnetic resonance. 2nd ed. Philadelphia: Saunders; 2010. p. 3–18.

McRobbie DW, Moore EA, Graves MJ, Prince MR. Chapter 8, Getting in tune: resonance & relaxation. In: MRI from picture to proton. 2nd ed. Cambridge: Cambridge University Press; 2007. p. 137–43.

Ridgway JP. Cardiac magnetic resonance physics for clinicians: part I. J Cardiovasc Magn Reson. 2010;12(1):71. doi:10.1186/1532-429X-12-71.

Relaxation Times, Gradient Echoes and Spin Echoes

5

John P. Ridgway

Abstract

There are two distinct relaxation processes that relate to the two components of the net magnetisation. The first longitudinal relaxation process, commonly referred to as T1 relaxation is responsible for the re-growth of the z -component along the longitudinal (z) axis to its original value at equilibrium. The second transverse relaxation process is responsible for the decay of the xy component as it rotates about the z -axis and hence the observed decay of the MR signal. There are two types of transverse relaxation, known as T2 relaxation and T2* relaxation. T2 relaxation is caused by a loss of coherence of the rotating proton spins due to the interaction neighbouring magnetic moments (spin-spin interactions). This is an exponential process with a time constant, T2. Signal decay is also caused by a loss of coherence between rotating spins due to non-uniformities in the magnetic field This together with T2 relaxation leads to a more rapid decay known as T2* relaxation with a time constant, T2*. For MR imaging the MR signal generated and measured in the form of an echo. Gradient echoes are generated by switching the direction of a magnetic field gradient to first de-phase then re-phase the MR signal. Spin echoes are generated by applying a 180° RF refocusing pulse to reverse the decay caused by magnetic field inhomogeneities. The time from the RF pulse to the maximum amplitude of the echo is known as the echo time, TE.

Keywords

Relaxation • Longitudinal relaxation • Transverse relaxation • T1 relaxation • Saturation recovery • Molecular tumbling rate • Macromolecular content • T2 relaxation • T2* relaxation • Spin-spin relaxation • Magnetic field inhomogeneities • De-phasing • MR echoes • Gradient echoes • Spin echoes • Echo time • TE

J.P. Ridgway, PhD
Department of Medical Physics and Engineering, Leeds Teaching Hospitals NHS Trust, St James's University Hospital, 1st Floor, Bexley Wing, Leeds LS2 9TJ, UK
e-mail: j.p.ridgway@leeds.ac.uk

© Springer International Publishing 2015
S. Plein et al. (eds.), *Cardiovascular MR Manual*,
DOI 10.1007/978-3-319-20940-1_5

Relaxation: What Happens After the RF Excitation Pulse?

Immediately after the RF pulse the spin system starts to return back to its original state, i.e., equilibrium. This process is known as *relaxation*. In fact there are two distinct relaxation processes that relate to the two components of the net magnetisation, the longitudinal (z) and transverse (xy) components. The first *longitudinal relaxation* process, commonly referred to as *T1 relaxation* is responsible for the re-growth of the z component along the longitudinal (z) axis to its original value at equilibrium. This is explained more fully in the next section. The second *transverse relaxation* process is responsible for the decay of the xy component as it rotates about the z-axis and hence the observed decay of the MR signal. There are two types of transverse relaxation, known as *T2 relaxation* and *T2* relaxation* and these are explained more fully later in this chapter. Longitudinal and transverse relaxation both occur at the same time, however, transverse relaxation is typically a much faster process in human tissue, i.e., the signal decays away long before the spin system returns to equilibrium.

What is T1 Relaxation?

T1 relaxation describes the recovery of the z-component (M_z) of the magnetisation following an RF pulse as the population of protons returns to its equilibrium state. In the previous example of a 90° pulse (*saturation pulse*), the z-magnetisation is *saturated* (reduced to zero) immediately after the pulse, but then returns along the z-axis towards its equilibrium value initially rapidly, slowing down as it approaches its equilibrium value. The return of the M_z component along the z -axis is an exponential process with a time constant *T1* (Fig. 5.1). The shorter the T1 time constant is, the faster the relaxation process and the return to equilibrium. Recovery of the z-magnetisation after a 90° RF pulse is sometimes referred to as *saturation recovery*.

What's the Significance of the T1 Value?
T1 relaxation involves the release of energy from the proton spin population as it returns to its equilibrium state. The rate of relaxation is related to rate at which energy is released to the surrounding molecular structure. This in turn is related to the size of the molecule that contains the hydrogen nuclei and in particular the rate of molecular motion, known as the tumbling rate of the particular molecule. As molecules tumble or rotate they give rise to a fluctuating magnetic field which is experienced by protons in adjacent molecules. When this fluctuating magnetic field is close to the Larmor frequency, energy

exchange is encouraged. For example, lipid molecules are of a size that gives rise to a tumbling rate which is close to the Larmor frequency and therefore extremely favourable for energy exchange. Fat therefore has one of the fastest relaxation rates of all body tissues and therefore the shortest T1 relaxation time. Larger molecules have much slower tumbling rates that are unfavourable for energy exchange, giving rise to long relaxation times. For free water, its small molecules have much faster molecular tumbling rates which are also unfavourable for energy exchange and therefore it has a long T1 relaxation time. The tumbling rates of water molecules that are adjacent to large macromolecules can however be slowed down towards the Larmor frequency shortening the T1 value. Water-based tissues with a high macromolecular content (e.g., muscle) tend to have shorter T1 values. Conversely, when the water content is increased, for example by an inflammatory process, the T1 value also increases.

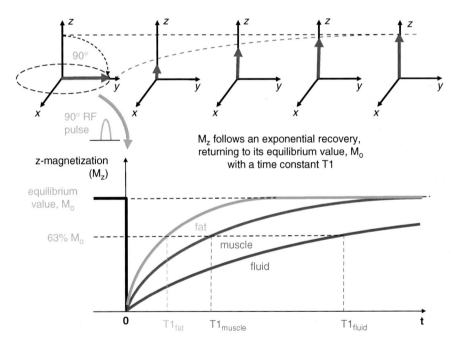

Fig. 5.1 Following a 90 RF pulse, the z component of the Net Magnetisation, M_z is reduced to zero, but then recovers gradually back to its equilibrium value if no further pulses are applied. The recovery of M_z is an exponential process with a time constant T1. This is the time at which the magnetization has recovered to 63 % of its original value. Different tissues have different T1 values. Fat has the shortest T1 value of all tissues (fat recovers the fastest) while fluid has the longest T1 value (fluid recovers the slowest)

Transverse Relaxation and MR Signal Decay

In Chap. 4 we saw that the decay of the MR signal (or free induction decay) is due to a loss of coherence as the magnetic moments (spins) of proton population move out of phase. The causes of this loss of coherence are twofold:

(i) The presence of interactions between neighbouring protons.
(ii) Local variations (inhomogeneities) in the applied magnetic field.

The transverse relaxation caused by (i) alone is known as *T2 relaxation*. The transverse relaxation actually observed in an FID is the combination of (i) and (ii) and is known as *T2* relaxation*.

What is T2 Relaxation?

The rate of precession for an individual proton depends on the applied magnetic field. It is however possible for the magnetic moment of one proton to slightly modify the magnetic field of a neighbouring proton (Fig. 5.2). As the protons are constituents of atoms within molecules, they are moving rapidly and randomly and so such effects are transient and random. The net effect is for the Larmor frequency of the individual protons to fluctuate in a random fashion, leading to a loss of coherence across the population of protons. i.e., the spins gradually acquire different phase angles, pointing in different directions to one another and are said to move out of phase with one another (this is often referred to as *de-phasing*).

The resultant decay of the transverse component of the magnetisation (M_{xy}) has an exponential form with a time constant, T2, hence this contribution to transverse relaxation is known as *T2 relaxation*. As it is caused by interactions between neighbouring proton spins it is also known as *spin-spin relaxation*. Due to the random nature of the spin-spin interactions, T2 relaxation is irreversible.

What's the Significance of T2 Value?
T2 relaxation is related to the amount of spin-spin interaction that take place. Free water are small molecules that are relatively far apart and moving rapidly and therefore spin-spin interactions are less frequent and T2 relaxation is slow (leading to long T2 relaxation times). Water molecules bound to large molecules are slowed down and more likely in interact, leading to faster T2 relaxation and shorter T2 relaxation times. Water- based tissues with a high macromolecular content (e.g., muscle) tend to have shorter T2 values. Conversely, when the water content is increased, for example by an inflammatory process, the T2 value also increases.

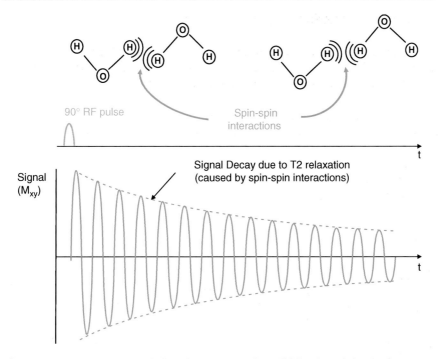

Fig. 5.2 The FID signal decays due to spin-spin interactions. This is where the magnetic moment of one proton moves transiently adjacent to another proton, slightly modifying the local magnetic field of its neighbour and therefore causing the Larmor frequency to briefly alter. This in turn leads to a loss of phase coherence (de-phasing). Due to the random nature of molecular motion, this process is irreversible

What is T2* Relaxation?

The second cause for the loss of coherence (de-phasing) relates to non-uniformities in the applied magnetic field, B_0. If this field varies with position, then so does the Larmor frequency (Fig. 5.3). Protons at different spatial locations will therefore rotate at different rates, causing further de-phasing and the signal to decay more rapidly. In this case, as the cause of the variation in Larmor frequency is fixed, the resultant de-phasing is potentially reversible.

The combined effect of T2 relaxation and the effect of magnetic field non-uniformities is referred to as *T2* relaxation* and this determines the actual rate of decay observed when measuring an FID signal.

MR Echoes

Whilst the FID can be detected as a MR signal, for MR imaging it is more common to generate and measure the MR signal in the form of an echo. This is because the magnetic field gradients that are used to localise and encode the MR signals in space

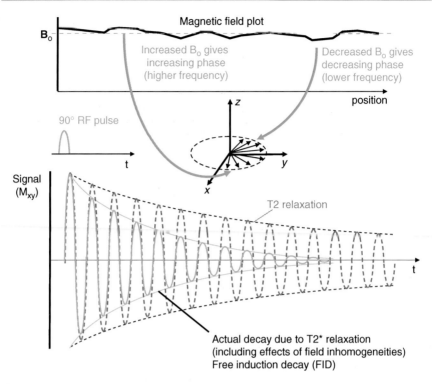

Fig. 5.3 A further cause of loss of phase coherence is that the applied magnetic field, B_o is not uniform. While the nominal magnetic field value is assumed to be uniform (shown by the dotted green line) the actual field value varies. Where the magnetic field is decreased, the Larmor frequency is decreased and the relative phase of the proton magnetic moments decreases over time relative to the proton magnetic moments at the nominal Larmor frequency. Where the field is increased in value, this results in a increasing phase. This causes additional de-phasing and accounts for the more rapid decay of the FID signal, known as T2* decay

(as we shall see in Chap. 6) cause additional de-phasing which disrupts the FID. The two most common types of echo used for MR imaging are *gradient echoes* and *spin echoes*. The following sections describe how these echoes are generated.

Gradient Echoes

Magnetic field gradients are used to produce a change in field strength and hence a corresponding change in Larmor frequency along a particular direction. When a magnetic field gradient is switched on it causes proton spins to lose coherence or de-phase rapidly along the direction of the gradient as they precess at different frequencies (Fig. 5.4). This de-phasing causes the amplitude of the FID signal to rapidly drop to zero.

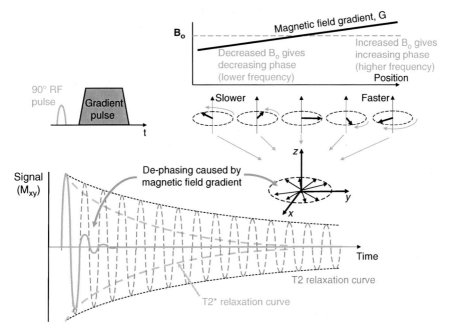

Fig. 5.4 This shows how the application of a magnetic field gradient causes loss of detectable MR signal. The range of frequencies along the direction of the gradient causes the spins to rapidly de-phase, resulting in a rapid reduction of the transverse magnetisation

The amount of de-phasing caused by one magnetic field gradient can however be reversed by applying a second magnetic field gradient along the same direction with equal amplitude but with the opposite slope (Fig. 5.5). If the second gradient is applied for the same amount of time as the first gradient, the de-phasing caused by the first gradient is cancelled and the FID re-appears. It reaches a maximum amplitude at the point at which the spins de-phased by the first gradient have moved back into phase, or 're-phased' (ignoring any effects of T2* relaxation).

If the second gradient then continues to be applied, the FID signal de-phases and disappears once more (Fig. 5.6). The signal that reappears (re-phases) through the switching of the gradient direction is known as a *gradient echo*.

The time from the point at which the transverse magnetisation (the FID) is generated by the RF pulse, to the point at which the gradient echo reaches its maximum amplitude is known as the *echo time* (abbreviated *TE*). If the echo time is chosen to be longer, more natural T2* de-phasing occurs and the maximum echo amplitude becomes smaller. In practice, the TE is set by the MR system operator (in milliseconds) as it determines, amongst other things, the influence of T2* on the image contrast.

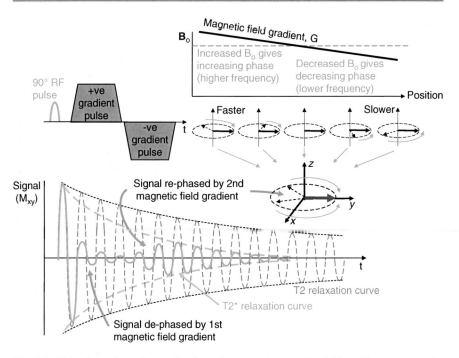

Fig. 5.5 This shows how the application of a second magnetic field gradient reverses the de-phasing caused by the first gradient pulse, resulting in recovery of the FID signal

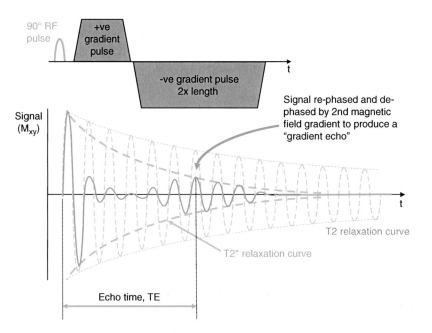

Fig. 5.6 Extension of the time duration of the second gradient to twice that of the first gradient causes the FID to first re-phase and then de-phase. The resultant transient signal is known as a gradient echo. The maximum amplitude of the echo depends on the T2* relaxation rate and the echo time TE

Spin Echoes

Earlier in this chapter we learned that while the de-phasing caused by T2 relaxation was a random, irreversible process, the additional de-phasing caused by the presence of magnetic field non-uniformities was potentially reversible. At a certain time after the initial generation of the FID signal, a proportion of the relative phase change for each proton spin will be related to the local value of the applied magnetic field. The application of a 180° refocusing pulse rotates the spins through 180°, effectively changing the sign of the relative phase change within the *xy* plane (Fig. 5.7). Where the previous relative phase change was positive due to a locally increased field, the 180° pulse causes it to become negative and visa versa. As the local field variations remain fixed, the spins still continue to have the same Larmor frequency, so a spin in an increased field continues to gain in phase, while a spin in a decrease field continues to lose phase. Because the sign of their phase shifts has been swapped halfway through by the 180° refocusing pulse, the spins all come back into phase causing the FID to increase in amplitude, reaching a maximum at the echo time, TE. For the spin de-phasing caused by the field non-uniformities to be completely reversed at time TE, the 180° pulse must be applied halfway through the echo time at time TE/2. The signal that appears (re-phases) through the application of the 180° RF refocusing pulse is known as a *spin echo* (Fig. 5.8). After reaching a maximum amplitude at time TE, the signal again de-phases due to the T2* relaxation process.

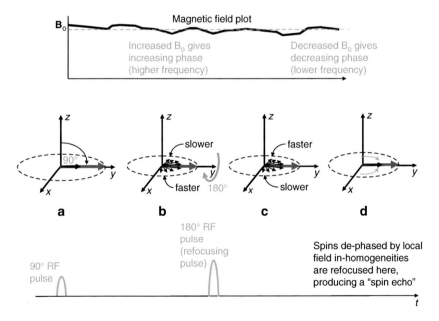

Fig. 5.7 The presence of magnetic field inhomogeneities cause the proton magnetic moments to de-phase (**a–b**). The application of a 180° RF pulse causes an instantaneous change in sign of the phase shifts by rotating the spins about the y axis (**b–c**). The proton magnetic moments the move back into phase, reversing the de-phasing effect of the magnetic field inhomogeneities (**c–d**)

For the purposes of imaging, a magnetic field gradient is also applied during both the de-phasing period and during the measurement of the spin echo (Fig. 5.9). In general, because of the 180° refocusing pulse, the amplitude of the spin echo signal

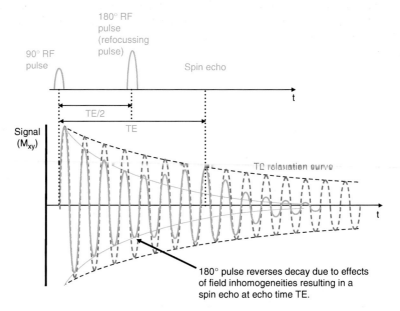

Fig. 5.8 The MR signal that is refocused by the 180° pulse is known as a spin echo. To produce an echo at time TE, the 180° pulse is applied at time TE/2

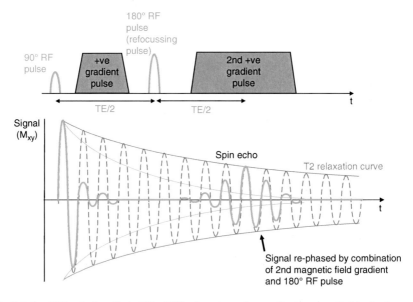

Fig. 5.9 In addition to the effect of the 180° refocusing pulse, gradients are applied to de-phase and re-phase the signal for imaging purposes (see Chap. 6). Note that the second gradient has the same sign as the first as the 180° pulse also changes the sign of the phase shifts caused by the first gradient

is greater than the gradient echo signal. Spin echo images are therefore generally of higher image quality. Imaging based on spin echo is also less affected by the presence of field inhomogeneities caused by metallic artefacts (e.g., sternal wires or metallic heart valves – see also Chap. 17). Gradient echo imaging is however more affected by the presence of magnetic field inhomogeneities caused by iron and so can be useful, for example, in the assessment of patients with increased iron deposition within the heart and liver.

Summary
- Following RF excitation, two relaxation processes occur as the spin system gradually returns back to its equilibrium state.
- As the spin system releases it energy the longitudinal component returns to its equilibrium value through longitudinal relaxation. This is an exponential process with time constant, T1 (also known as T1 relaxation).
- The rotating transverse component decays more rapidly than this due to transverse relaxation. This is also an exponential process and has two causes:
  - Loss of coherence of the rotating proton spins due to the interaction neighbouring magnetic moments (spin-spin interactions). This has a time constant, T2 and is known as T2 relaxation.
  - Loss of coherence between rotating spins due to magnetic field inhomogeneity. This together with T2 relaxation leads to a more rapid decay with a combined time constant, T2*.
- In practice, the FID signal is disrupted by the presence of the magnetic field gradients used to generate images.
- Instead signal echoes are generated and used for the formation of images.
- Gradient echoes are generated by switching the direction of a gradient to first de-phase then re-phase the MR signal
- Spin echoes are generated by applying a 180° RF refocusing pulse to reverse the decay caused by magnetic field inhomogeneities.
- The time from the RF pulse to the maximum amplitude of the echo is known as the echo time, TE.

Further Reading

Balaban RS, Peters DC. Basic principles of cardiovascular magnetic resonance. In: Manning WJ, Pennell DJ, editors. Cardiovascular magnetic resonance. 2nd ed. Philadelphia: Saunders; 2010. p. 3–18.

McRobbie DW, Moore EA, Graves MJ, Prince MR. Chapter 8, Getting in tune: resonance & relaxation. In: MRI from picture to proton. 2nd ed. Cambridge: Cambridge University Press; 2007. p. 144–60.

Ridgway JP. Cardiac magnetic resonance physics for clinicians: part I. J Cardiovasc Magn Reson. 2010;12(1):71. doi:10.1186/1532-429X-12-71.

Making an Image: Locating and Encoding Signals in Space

6

John P. Ridgway

Abstract

The MR signal from a patient is localised in three dimensions by using the magnetic field gradient coils to superimpose three gradient magnetic fields in sequence onto the static magnetic field in three orthogonal directions. Each gradient field varies the magnetic field, and therefore the Larmor frequency, along the direction in which it is applied. The slice selection gradient is applied at the same time as the RF pulse, causing resonance in a slice of tissue at right-angles to the gradient direction. The phase encoding gradient encodes the phase of the signal according to position along its direction. The frequency encoding gradient encodes the frequency of the signal according to position along its direction. The sequence of slice selection, phase encoding and frequency encoding is repeated many times, with a repetition interval, TR, each time with a different amount of phase encoding (known as a phase encoding step). The MR image is reconstructed using an algorithm, known as a two-dimensional (2D) Fourier transform. This is applied to the resultant signals to decode the contributions from different locations based on their frequency and the change in phase with each phase encoding step. The field of view is related to the receiver bandwidth selected and the frequency encoding gradient. The image acquisition time is related to the TR and the total number of phase encoding steps, which in turn depends on the selected image acquisition matrix.

Keywords

Slice selection • Slice selection gradient • Slice selection direction • Phase encoding • Phase encoding gradient • Phase encoding direction • Frequency encoding • Frequency encoding gradient • Frequency encoding direction • Field of view •

J.P. Ridgway, PhD
Department of Medical Physics and Engineering, Leeds Teaching Hospitals NHS Trust, St James's University Hospital, 1st Floor, Bexley Wing, Leeds LS2 9TJ, UK
e-mail: j.p.ridgway@leeds.ac.uk

© Springer International Publishing 2015
S. Plein et al. (eds.), *Cardiovascular MR Manual*,
DOI 10.1007/978-3-319-20940-1_6

Bandwidth • Receiver bandwidth • Slice orientation • Fourier transform • Demodulation • Nyquist theorem • De-phasing gradient • Re-phasing gradient • Repetition time • TR • Phase encoding step • Acquisition time • Aliasing

Single MR echoes produced by RF pulses alone cannot be used to produce an image as they do not contain any information about position. This information is introduced by using the gradient coils described in Chap. 1 to generate magnetic field gradients. When a gradient is applied in a particular direction, this causes the strength of the magnetic field and therefore the Larmor frequency to depend on position along that direction. MR echoes that are generated and measured in the presence of magnetic field gradients therefore contain spatial information that can be used to build up an image. The sections that follow describe the most commonly used method to build up a cross-sectional image (or image slice) using RF pulses and gradient magnetic fields.

Selecting an Image Slice

First, the resonance of protons is confined to a slice of tissue. This is done by applying a gradient magnetic field at the same time as the RF excitation pulse (Fig. 6.1). The frequency of the RF pulse corresponds to the Larmor frequency at a chosen point along the direction of the applied gradient. The result is for resonance to occur only for protons in a plane that cuts through that point at right angles to the gradient direction, effectively defining a slice of tissue. This process is known as *slice selection* and the gradient is known as the *slice selection gradient*, G_S. The orientation of the slice is determined by the direction of the applied gradient known as the slice selection direction (in the example of Fig. 6.1 this is the z –direction).

Rather than just a single frequency, the RF pulse is comprised of a small range of frequencies, known as the *bandwidth* of the RF pulse. This gives the slice a thickness. The thickness of the slice is determined by the combination of the RF pulse bandwidth and the steepness (or strength) of the gradient.

Encoding the MR Signal within the Slice

Once the slice selection process has created resonance within the slice of tissue, two further gradients are applied in sequence, this time within the plane of the image slice but at right angles to each other. The first of these two gradients is known as the *phase encoding gradient*, G_P, while the second is known as the *frequency encoding gradient*, G_F. Each of these gradients causes the protons to rotate at different frequencies according to their relative position along each gradient. Where the gradient increases the magnetic field, the protons acquire a higher frequency of precession; while where the gradient decreases the magnetic field the protons acquire a

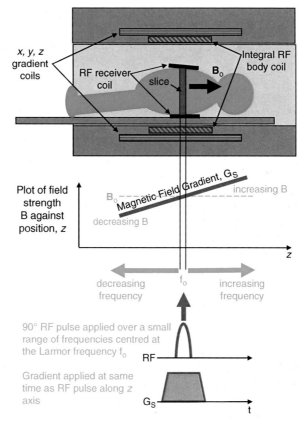

Fig. 6.1 Slice selection is achieved by applying a magnetic field gradient for the duration of the RF excitation pulse. The gradient causes the Larmor frequency to be dependent on location along the gradient (in this example in the z -direction). Resonance only occurs where the Larmor frequency matches the frequency of the RF pulse, defining a plane (slice) of tissue perpendicular to the z -axis. The RF pulse has a small range of frequencies, thus causing resonance over a small range of locations, defining the thickness of the slice

lower frequency of precession. The protons are therefore also constantly changing their relative phase according to their position along the gradient. One consequence of this is that the magnetic field gradients cause de-phasing in the direction along which the gradient is applied.

Phase Encoding

The phase encoding gradient, G_P, is applied only for a specified time, such that when it is switched off, the protons will have changed their relative phase by a prescribed amount depending on their position along the gradient (Fig. 6.2). This process is known as *phase encoding* and the direction of the applied gradient is known as the *phase encoding direction*. In the example in Fig. 6.2 the phase encoding direction is along the y -axis. This example also shows the effect of a phase encoding gradient with a particular amplitude and duration, such that the protons at the edges of a pre-defined *field of view* have acquired a phase change of $+180°$ and $-180°$ relative to the centre of the field of view.

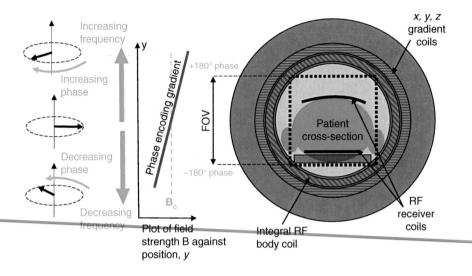

Fig. 6.2 Phase encoding is achieved by applying a gradient magnetic field (known as the phase encoding gradient, *GP*), in a direction along the selected image plane (in this case the phase encoding direction is along the y direction). The amplitude (steepness) and duration of the gradient are chosen to cause a range of phase shifts of the proton magnetic moments dependent on their position along the gradient. In this example the edges of a predefined field of view have acquired phase shifts of +180° and −180° relative to the centre of the field of view

Frequency Encoding

The *frequency encoding gradient*, G_F, is applied for longer, and at the same time the signal is measured or digitally sampled (Fig. 6.3). The signal is comprised of a range of frequencies (or bandwidth), corresponding to the Larmor frequencies of the proton magnetic moments at their different locations along the gradient (Fig. 6.4). This process is known as *frequency encoding*, the direction of the frequency encoding gradient defines the *frequency encoding direction*.

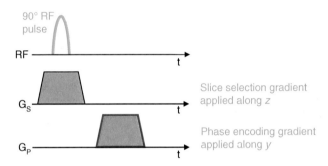

In summary, to localise the MR signal in three dimensions, three separate magnetic field gradients are applied.

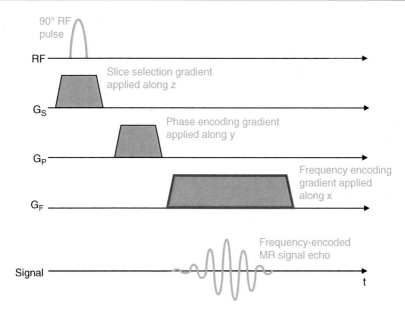

Fig. 6.3 Following the phase encoding gradient, the frequency encoding gradient, *GF*, is applied also in the plane of the selected slice but perpendicular to the phase encoding direction. The MR signal echo is measured during this period

For the examples shown in Figs. 6.1, 6.2, 6.3, and 6.4 these gradients are applied in sequence as follows:

Slice-section gradient, G_S applied along the z-axis
Phase-encoding gradient, G_P applied along the y-axis
Frequency-encoding Gradient, G_F applied along the x-axis

This defines a slice perpendicular to the z-axis i.e., a slice oriented in the transaxial plane. Other slice orientations can easily be obtained by re-assigning each of the gradients to a different axis as shown in Table 6.1. Note that for each orientation there are two possible combinations for the phase and frequency encoding directions with the second combination shown in parentheses. The choice of phase encoding direction is important as it influences the direction in which motion artefacts appear across the image.

It is also possible to obtain an angled slice by simply combining gradients along two or more axes to perform each of the localisation tasks. *The ability to define an arbitrary slice orientation is a key strength of magnetic resonance imaging.*

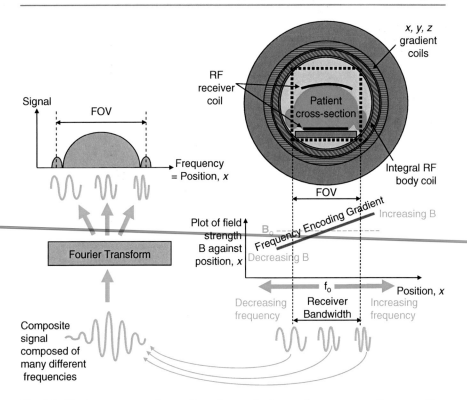

Fig. 6.4 The frequency encoding gradient changes the Larmor frequency according to position along its direction. The detected MR signal from a subject that extends in that direction is therefore comprised of many different frequencies. This signal is analysed by a Fourier Transform to determine the contribution of each of the frequency components, each corresponding to a unique location along the frequency encoding gradient. The field of view is predefined and matched to a specific range of frequencies (the receiver bandwidth)

Table 6.1 Assignment of the slice selection, phase encoding and frequency encoding functions to the appropriate magnetic field gradient axes allows the arbitrary definition of the image slice orientation

	Slice selection, G_S	Phase encoding, G_P	Frequency encoding, G_F
Transaxial	z	y (or x)	x (or y)
Coronal	y	x (or z)	z (or x)
Sagittal	x	y (or z)	z (or y)

How is the Frequency-Encoded Signal Decoded?

The frequency encoded signal is analysed using a *Fourier transform*. This is a mathematical tool that transforms the time-dependent MR signal into its different frequency components. The amplitude of each frequency component can be mapped onto a location along the frequency encoding gradient to determine the relative signal at each location. A *field of view* is also predefined in this direction, and the

Fig. 6.5 The field of view (FOV) in the frequency encoding direction is determined by the slope of the frequency encoding gradient and the selected receiver bandwidth. The MR signal originating from within this FOV contains frequencies in the range $\pm \Delta f$ (the receiver bandwidth) centred on the Larmor frequency, f_o. Before the signal is digitally sampled, it is demodulated, removing the high frequency content. The result is a signal with the same range of frequencies (same bandwidth) but centred around zero Hertz

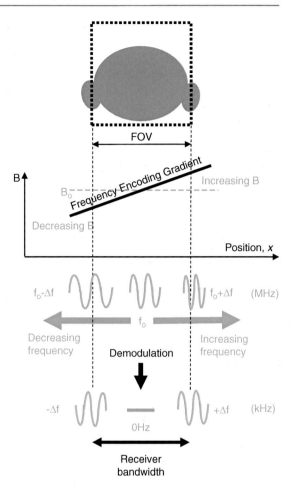

range of frequencies across this field of view is directly related to the frequency at which the signal is digitally sampled, known as the *receiver bandwidth.*

The field of view in the frequency encoding direction is defined by the operator in mm or cm. This, in combination with the choice of receiver bandwidth, determines the amplitude (or slope) require for the frequency encoding gradient (Fig. 6.4).

Before the signal is digitally sampled it commonly undergoes a process known as *demodulation* (Fig. 6.5). This process removes the high frequency content but preserves the range of frequencies, so that they are centred around zero Hertz, rather than the Larmor frequency. This makes the sampling process simpler (It is easier to digitally sample a signal in the kHz range than a signal in the MHz range although some MR systems now directly sample the high frequency signal).

The choice of receiver bandwidth also determines the rate (or frequency) at which the MR signal is digitally sampled as it is measured. A rule, known as Nyquist's theorem states that in order to faithfully detect a signal, it must be sampled at a frequency that is twice the maximum frequency contained within the signal. So if the signal contains the frequency range $\pm \Delta f$, then it must be sampled at a frequency $2\Delta f$.

If the sampling frequency is set at this value, signals with frequencies outside the range $\pm \Delta f$, (from outside the defined field of view) are not properly detected. In fact they appear to have the same frequency as a signal from a point within the defined field of view. If it is not dealt with, this would cause an artefact known as image aliasing, seen as 'wrap around' or 'folding-in' of features from outside the field of view into the image. In practice this is easily removed in the frequency encoding direction (see section on image aliasing in Chap. 17).

How Do We Make Sure That the Gradients We Apply for Imaging don't Destroy the Signal?

Pulse sequences must be designed to provide the maximum possible signal at the centre of the MR signal echo. This requires that any de-phasing caused by one of the imaging gradients must be reversed by another gradient along the same direction, but with opposite slope, so that the proton magnetic moments are brought back into phase. This is particularly important in the slice selection and frequency encoding gradient directions. The frequency encoding gradient is normally preceded by a *de-phasing gradient* (Fig. 6.6) so that when the frequency encoding gradient is applied, the de-phasing is reversed by the first half of the frequency encoding gradient and the signal echo reaches its maximum amplitude at the centre of the sampling period, (see Chap. 5 on *gradient echo*). For the same reason, the slice selection gradient is followed by a *re-phasing gradient*. This ensures that de-phasing that occurs along the slice selection gradient is reversed. The re-phasing gradient is only half the length of the slice selection gradient since the transverse magnetisation is only generated halfway through the applied rf pulse. De-phasing therefore only occurs during the second half of the slice selection gradient.

Why isn't a Single Phase and Frequency Encoded Signal Enough to Reconstruct an Image?

While analysis of this signal by the Fourier transform provides the frequency content of the signal, the phase changes imparted by the phase encoding gradient cannot be decoded by a similar process. The Fourier transform can only analyse a signal that changes over time. To enable this, a number of signal echoes must be generated and measured by repeating the above process (slice selection, phase encoding and frequency encoding), each time applying the same slice selection and frequency encoding gradient, but a different amount of phase encoding so that the resulting changes in phase over time can be analysed in a similar way (Fig. 6.7). In practice, the strength (or slope) of the phase encoding gradient is increased for each repetition in equal increments. The time interval between each repetition is known as the *repetition time*, abbreviated as *TR*. TR is another important parameter that can be set by the operator in milliseconds. As we will see in later sections it not only determines how fast MR images can be acquired (see Chap. 8), but also affects the image contrast (see Chap. 10).

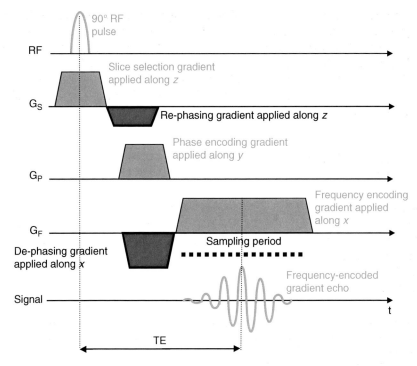

Fig. 6.6 Additional gradient pulses are required both immediately after the slice selection gradient and immediately before the frequency encoding gradient (shown in *red*). These additional pulses ensure that any de-phasing of the transverse magnetisation caused by the imaging gradients is cancelled once the echo time, TE, is reached. This results in the echo having its maximum possible signal at this point

Field of View in the Phase Encoding Direction

The amount that signal phase changes with each *phase encoding step*, increases with distance from the centre of the phase encoding gradient (Fig. 6.8). The edge of the field of view in the phase encoding direction is defined to be where the phase changes by 180° with each phase encoding step. Thus the phase of protons located at one extreme edge of the field of view will change in steps of +180° relative to those at the centre, while the phase of those protons located at the opposite edge of the field of view will change in steps of −180° relative to those at the centre. Protons located outside this field of view in the phase encoding direction appear to have the same behaviour as a point located within the field of view. This causes image *aliasing* (see section in Chap. 17 on image aliasing).

Phase Encoding, Image Matrix and Acquisition Time

For each repetition and therefore phase encoding step, the signal echo is measured and stored as an array of numbers or matrix (Fig. 6.9). Once all the signals for a prescribed number of phase encoding steps have been acquired, they are analysed

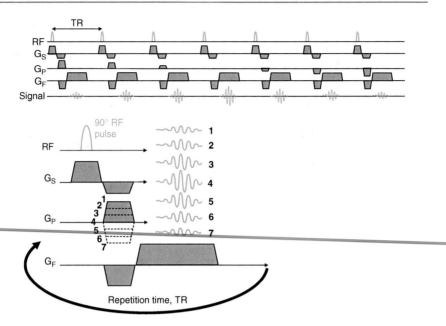

Fig. 6.7 To fulfil the phase encoding process, the pulse sequence must be repeated a number of times, with a different amplitude (slope) of phase encoding gradient being applied each time. In this example, 7 values of phase encoding gradient slope are used (shown by the dotted lines), causing different amounts of change in phase according to position along the direction of the gradient. Note that as the strength of the phase encoding gradient increases, this increases the amount of de-phasing along the gradient. When the strength (or slope) of the phase encoding gradient is zero (step 4), there is no de-phasing and the signal has its maximum possible amplitude

together as a group by a two-dimensional (2D) Fourier transform in order to decode both the frequency and the phase information. The number of pixels calculated by this process in the phase encoding direction is determined by the number of phase encoding steps used. The spatial resolution of the reconstructed image therefore depends on the number of phase encoding steps, and is hence often limited by the image *acquisition time* (see box).

Number of pixels in phase encoding direction is equal to the number of phase encoding steps, N_P.

Image acquisition time $= TR \times N_P$.

If a greater spatial resolution is required in the phase encoding direction (for a fixed field of view), the number of acquired pixels N_P (acquired image matrix size) must be increased and so must the number of phase encoding steps. This requires a greater number of repetitions, and therefore a longer image acquisition time.

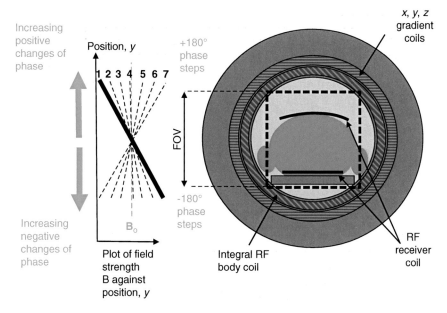

Fig. 6.8 The phase of the proton magnetic moments at a given location change with each phase encoding step according to their position along the phase encoding gradient. The field of view in this direction is defined such that the signal generated by proton magnetic moments at its edges have phase changes of +/− 180° relative to that generated at the centre of the field of view

Summary
- The MR signal is localised in three dimensions by using the three magnetic field gradient coils to superimpose three magnetic field gradients in sequence onto the static magnetic field in three different directions.
- Each gradient field varies the magnetic field, and therefore the Larmor frequency, along the direction in which it is applied.
- The slice selection gradient is applied at the same time as the RF pulse, causing resonance in a slice of tissue at right-angles to the gradient direction.
- The phase encoding gradient encodes the phase of the signal according to position along its direction.
- The frequency encoding gradient encodes the frequency of the signal according to position along its direction.
- The sequence of slice selection, phase encoding and frequency encoding is repeated many times, with a repetition interval, TR, each time with a different amount of phase encoding (known as a phase encoding step).
- The MR image is reconstructed using an algorithm, known as a two-dimensional (2D) Fourier transform.
- This is applied to the resultant signals to decode the contributions from different locations based on their frequency and the change in phase with each phase encoding step.

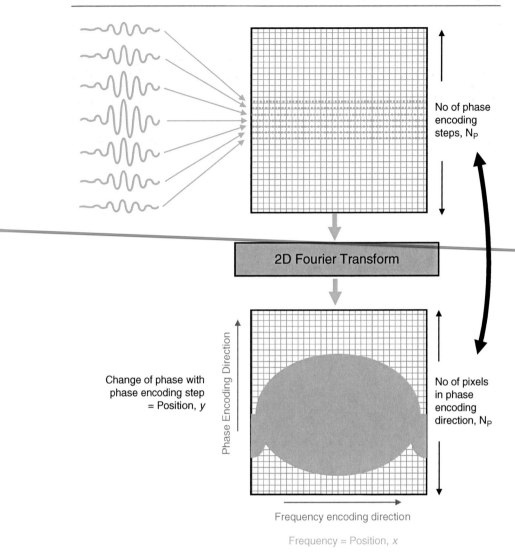

Fig. 6.9 The MR signals derived from each phase encoding step are stored in a matrix. Two dimensional Fourier transformation of this matrix results in the reconstruction of the image. The number of phase encoding steps determines the number of pixels in the image along the phase encoding direction. The location of MR signal contributions along the frequency encoding direction (x) is related to their frequency, while their location along the phase encoding direction (y) is related to their change in phase with each phase encoding step

Further Reading

Balaban RS, Peters DC. Basic principles of cardiovascular magnetic resonance. In: Manning WJ, Pennell DJ, editors. Cardiovascular magnetic resonance. 2nd ed. Philadelphia: Saunders; 2010. p. 3–18.

McRobbie DW, Moore EA, Graves MJ, Prince MR. Chapter 7, Spaced out: spatial encoding. In: MRI from picture to proton. 2nd ed. Cambridge: Cambridge University Press; 2007. p. 108–32.

Ridgway JP. Cardiac magnetic resonance physics for clinicians: part I. J Cardiovasc Magn Reson. 2010;12(1):71. doi:10.1186/1532-429X-12-71.

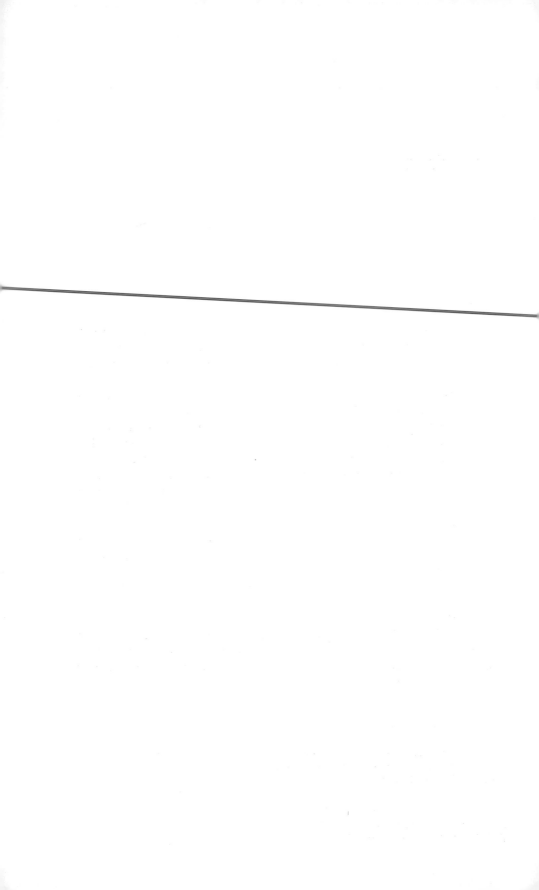

Image Space and k-Space

7

John P. Ridgway

Abstract

The way that the MR signals are generated and encoded by the use of magnetic field gradients gives rise to a particular relationship between the data points in the signal and those in the image. There is an inverse relationship between the image space and k-space. Whereas the coordinates of the image are spatial position (x, y) the coordinates of k-space are $1/x$ and $1/y$, sometimes referred to as spatial frequencies kx and ky. A low spatial frequency contributes mostly the signal content and contrast of the image. A high spatial frequency contributes fine detail or edges, effectively defining the spatial resolution of the image. To make an image that is a totally faithful representation of the imaged subject, the whole range of spatial frequencies must be acquired. For standard imaging this is done by filling k-space with equally spaced parallel lines of signal data, line by line, known as a Cartesian acquisition. Usually k-space is filled starting at one edge of k-space and finishing at the opposite edge known as a linear phase encoding order. An alternative approach, known as centric or low-high k-space order starts at the centre of k space and works outwards to the edges of k-space. This approach is particularly important in some dynamic applications such as angiography where it is important to acquire the contrast information at the beginning of the image acquisition.

Keywords

k-space • Special frequencies • Low spatial frequency • High spatial frequency • kx • ky • Contrast • Spatial resolution • Cartesian acquisition • Linear phase encoding order • Centric phase encoding order • Low-high phase encoding order • Radial k-space trajectory • Spiral k-space trajectory • Acquired image matrix

J.P. Ridgway, PhD
Department of Medical Physics and Engineering, Leeds Teaching Hospitals NHS Trust, St James's University Hospital, 1st Floor, Bexley Wing, Leeds LS2 9TJ, UK
e-mail: j.p.ridgway@leeds.ac.uk

© Springer International Publishing 2015
S. Plein et al. (eds.), *Cardiovascular MR Manual*,
DOI 10.1007/978-3-319-20940-1_7

The way that the MR signals are generated and encoded by the use of magnetic field gradients gives rise to a particular relationship between the data points in the signal and those in the image. A single data point in an MR signal contributes a particular attribute to the whole image. Conversely, a single pixel in the image may have contributions from all of the MR signals collected. Just as each pixel occupies a unique location in image space, each point of an MR signal echo belongs to a particular location in a related space known as *k-space* (Fig. 7.1).

There is an inverse relationship between the image space and k-space. Whereas the coordinates of the image are spatial position (*x, y*) the coordinates of k-space are *1/x* and *1/y*, sometimes referred to as *spatial frequencies kx* and *ky*. The value of each point in k-space therefore relates to how much of a particular spatial frequency is contained within the image.

A spatial frequency is difficult to picture. An image consisting of a single spatial frequency looks like a wave propagating across the image with bright and dark peaks and troughs (Fig. 7.2). A *low spatial frequency* (arising from a point near the centre of k-space) has peaks and troughs far apart and thus contributes mostly the signal content and *contrast* of the image. A *high spatial frequency* (arising from a point near the edge of k-space) has peaks and troughs close together and thus contributes fine detail or edges, effectively defining the *spatial resolution* of the image.

The location of a particular signal data point in k-space depends on the strength and duration of each gradient that has been applied from the time when the transverse magnetisation was first generated by the rf excitation pulse to when that particular point was measured. If no gradients are applied (or if the sum of the areas of the positive and negative gradients applied up to that point, when added together, completely cancel out) then the point collected is at the centre of k-space. As no gradients are applied, there is no de-phasing and the signal therefore has a high amplitude and contributes mainly signal content to the image.

As gradients are applied, they move the signal data point away from the centre of k-space. The stronger the gradients are and the longer that they are applied for, the

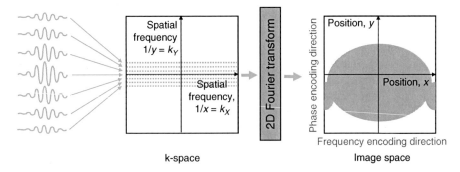

Fig. 7.1 k-space is related to the image space by the Fourier Transform. The coordinates of image space are the spatial coordinates x and y. The Coordinates of k-space are the spatial frequencies $k_x = 1/x$ and $k_y = 1/y$. The sampled data points from the MR signals therefore contribute different spatial frequencies to the image

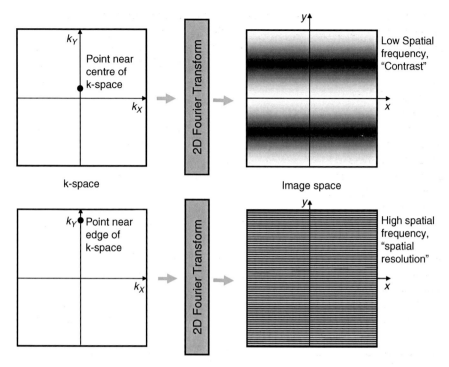

Fig. 7.2 A single spatial frequency (single point in k-space) can be represented as a wave in image space. A point close to the centre of k-space contributes a low spatial frequency, represented by a wave with broad peaks and troughs. This provides the signal content for large regions of uniform signal in the image. A point at the edge of k-space contributes a high spatial frequency and is represented by a fine 'toothcomb' wave. The highest spatial frequency content defines the spatial resolution of the image

further from the centre of k- space they move the data point. The phase encoding gradient moves the data points along ky, the frequency encoding gradient along kx. At the same time, the gradient de-phases the signal and so the amplitude of the signal decreases away from the centre of k-space.

To make an image that is a totally faithful representation of the imaged subject, it is important that the whole range of spatial frequencies is acquired (up to a maximum that defines the spatial resolution of the image), i.e., that the whole of k-space is covered. For standard imaging this is done by filling k-space with equally spaced parallel lines of signal data, line by line, along the kx direction. This is known as a *Cartesian acquisition* (Fig. 7.3).

As the data points from each signal echo are sampled, with the frequency encoding gradient applied, a line of k-space is filled from left to right of k-space (The de-phasing gradient moves the acquisition from the centre of k-space to the left of k-space ready for the signal to be sampled). The phase encoding gradient moves the acquisition either up or down in the ky direction by a prescribed distance. Usually the amplitude of the phase encoding gradient is incremented in steps such that the

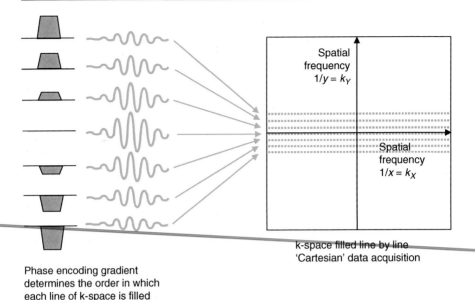

Phase encoding gradient
determines the order in which
each line of k-space is filled

Fig. 7.3 In a Cartesian data acquisition, the MR signals are sampled and the data points stored line by line along the k_x direction. The position along k_x depends on the time point during the application of the frequency encoding gradient. The location of each line of data points in the k_y direction is determined by the amplitude and duration of the phase encoding direction at each phase encoding step

next adjacent line in k-space is filled with each successive repetition, starting at one edge of k-space and finishing at the opposite edge (Fig. 7.4). This is known as a *linear phase encoding order*.

Choosing a different phase encoding step order is particularly important in some dynamic applications such as angiography. Here it is important to acquire the contrast information immediately once the contrast agent reaches a particular vessel segment. In this case, the phase encoding gradient is incremented from zero, but with alternating sign, starting at the centre of k space and working outwards to the edges of k-space (Fig. 7.4). This is known as *centric* or *low-high k-space order*.

Although the majority of cardiac applications use a Cartesian k-space acquisition scheme, it is possible to cover k-space using different schemes such as *radial* or *spiral k-space trajectories*. These have particular advantages as well as some potential technical drawbacks.

Once the data acquisition is complete and k-space is filled to a sufficient extent to obtain the desired image resolution, the two-dimensional Fourier transform is applied to all the data points in k-space, transforming the data from k-space into the image space.

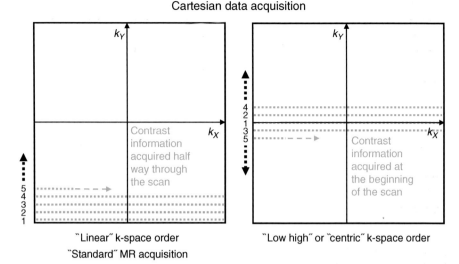

Fig. 7.4 For a standard Cartesian MR data acquisition, lines of k-space are filled starting at one edge of k-space, incrementing line by line until the opposite edge of k-space is reached. This is known as linear k-space order. For some fast imaging applications where it is important to acquire the contrast information first, lines of k-space are filled from the centre outward to both edges in an alternating fashion. This is known as 'centric' or 'low-high' k-space order

The number of acquired pixels in image space (the *acquired image matrix*) is equal to the number of data points acquired in k-space (Fig. 7.5). The number of lines of data points acquired in the *ky* direction is equal to the number of phase encoding steps (i.e., repetitions with different phase encoding gradient amplitudes). The number of data points along each line in the *kx* direction is equal to the number of samples taken of the MR signal echo as it is measured (see box). The number of sampled data points from each echo therefore determines the acquired image matrix size in the frequency encoding direction.

How Is a Data Point in k-Space Related to the MR Signal?
The MR signal is an oscillating magnetic field produced by the transverse component of the net magnetisation as it rotates. The RF receiver coil converts the signal into an electrical signal which is then digitally sampled to generate a series of numbers which are then stored as rows of data points in k-space.

Summary
- The MR signals are digitally sampled and stored as data points in a domain known as k-space.
- The information stored in k-space is related to the image via the Fourier Transform which forms the basis of the image reconstruction process.
- A single data point in k-space contributes to the whole image. The number of data points acquired in each direction k-space is the same as the number of data points in each direction of the image (the acquired image matrix)
- Data points near the centre of k-space provide most of the signal content and therefore the image contrast (low spatial frequency content).
- Data points near the edge of k-space provide fine detail, defining the spatial resolution of the image (high spatial frequency content).
- Cartesian data acquisition fills k-space with data points line by line. The order in which lines of k-space are filled can determine contrast properties for some fast imaging applications such as angiography.

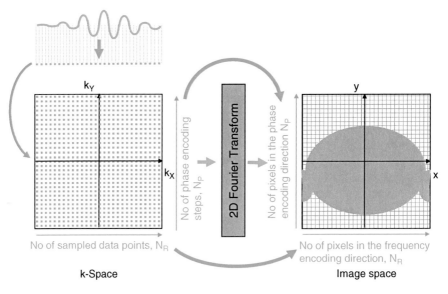

Fig. 7.5 The number of data points in k-space determines the number of pixels in the image following the two-dimensional Fourier Transform. The number of points along k_x is determined by the number of samples taken from the MR signal. The number of points along k_y is determined by the number of phase encoding steps

Further Reading

Balaban RS, Peters DC. Basic principles of cardiovascular magnetic resonance. In: Manning WJ, Pennell DJ, editors. Cardiovascular magnetic resonance. 2nd ed. Philadelphia: Saunders; 2010. p. 3–18.

McRobbie DW, Moore EA, Graves MJ, Prince MR. Chapter 7, Spaced out: spatial encoding. In: MRI from picture to proton. 2nd ed. Cambridge: Cambridge University Press; 2007. p. 108–36.

Mezrich R. A perspective on k-space. Radiology. 1995;195:297–315.

Paschal CB, Morris HD. K-space in the clinic. J Magn Reson Imaging. 2004;19(2):145–59. doi:10.1002/jmri.10451.

Ridgway JP. Cardiac magnetic resonance physics for clinicians: part I. J Cardiovasc Magn Reson. 2010;12(1):71. doi:10.1186/1532-429X-12-71.

Imaging Parameters and Image Attributes

8

John P. Ridgway

Abstract

The acquired matrix size, together with the field of view in each direction determines the pixel dimension in each direction and therefore the spatial resolution of the image. These parameters, together with the thickness of the selected 2D image slice, also determine the voxel dimensions. The voxel volume strongly influences the size of the signal. The signal to noise ratio (SNR) is a major determinant of image quality in MRI. There is an interdependence between SNR, spatial resolution (voxel volume), receiver bandwidth and image acquisition time. Increasing spatial resolution (same field of view) reduces SNR and increases image acquisition time. Increasing spatial resolution by decreasing field of view reduces SNR for same imaging time Reducing image acquisition time reduces spatial resolution or SNR or both. Signal averaging increases SNR but also increases image acquisition time. Increasing receiver bandwidth leads to faster echo sampling, shorter TE and TR hence shorter image acquisition time, but reduces SNR. In comparison to 2D imaging, 3D imaging allows thinner, contiguous slices to be acquired with improved SNR but with a longer acquisition time.

Keywords

Acquired matrix size • Field of view • Pixel dimension • Spatial resolution • Voxel volume • Image quality • Image acquisition time • Noise • Signal-to-noise ratio • SNR • Pixel intensity • Signal averaging • Receiver bandwidth • Low bandwidth • High bandwidth • Two-dimensional image acquisition • Three-dimensional image acquisition 2D imaging • 3D imaging • Slice encoding

J.P. Ridgway, PhD
Department of Medical Physics and Engineering, Leeds Teaching Hospitals NHS Trust,
St James's University Hospital, 1st Floor, Bexley Wing, Leeds LS2 9TJ, UK
e-mail: j.p.ridgway@leeds.ac.uk

© Springer International Publishing 2015
S. Plein et al. (eds.), *Cardiovascular MR Manual*,
DOI 10.1007/978-3-319-20940-1_8

65

Spatial Resolution and Image Acquisition Time

The *acquired matrix size*, together with the *field of view* in each direction determines the *pixel dimension* in each direction and therefore the nominal *spatial resolution* of the image. These parameters, together with the thickness of the selected 2D image slice, also determine the voxel dimensions and hence the *voxel volume* (Fig. 8.1). The voxel volume determines the number of protons that contribute to each pixel location. This strongly influences the size of the signal and is consequently a major determinant of *image quality*.

The acquired image matrix size also determines the image acquisition time. In the phase encoding direction, increasing the number of samples requires additional phase encoding steps, thus requiring additional repetitions of the MR signal acquisition. Thus the image acquisition time is very sensitive to the chosen spatial resolution in the phase encoding direction. In the simplest case, as we saw in Chap. 6,

$$\text{Image acquisition time} = \text{TR} \quad N_P$$

In the frequency encoding direction, however, increasing the number of samples, and hence the spatial resolution can be achieved without affecting the overall acquisition time. Although this increases overall sampling time of each echo, it only lengthens the TR if the shortest possible TR and TE are already selected.

If time were no object (unfortunately not the case for cardiac imaging!), then one could increase the number of digital samples and phase encoding steps so that the

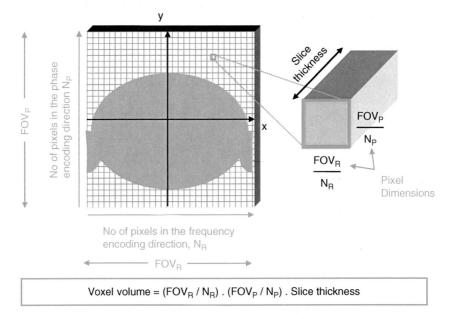

Voxel volume = (FOV$_R$ / N$_R$) . (FOV$_P$ / N$_P$) . Slice thickness

Fig. 8.1 The image matrix size and field of view in each direction determine the acquired pixel dimensions. These dimensions, together with the slice thickness determine the voxel volume

spatial resolution could be increased without limit. There is however a second major limiting factor. As the spatial resolution increases, the pixel dimensions become smaller, the voxel volume becomes smaller and the number of protons contributing to the signal in a voxel reduces and so the signal within the corresponding image pixel (the pixel intensity) diminishes proportionately. As the signal becomes smaller, the pixel intensity approaches the noise level and the image quality is severely degraded. It is this that ultimately limits the spatial resolution of the MR technique.

Noise and Signal-to-Noise Ratio

The 'noise' in MRI is electrical noise that is evenly spread across all frequencies. At higher field strengths (0.5 T and above) the main source of this noise is from the patient. The primary measure of image quality in MRI is the *signal-to-noise ratio* or *SNR*. It is measured as the ratio of the signal amplitude to the amplitude of the noise. In a typical image, noise can be seen as a salt-and-pepper pattern in background areas where there is little or no MR signal, for example outside the body or in the lung fields (Fig. 8.2).

Factors that Determine Image Quality

Intrinsic Signal Amplitude

Image quality strongly depends on the overall SNR of an image. Apart from the image noise level, SNR depends on the *pixel intensity* which is determined by the amplitude of the MR signal. This, in turn, depends on a multitude of factors as follows:

- The number of protons within a voxel, which depends on the proton density and the *voxel volume*.

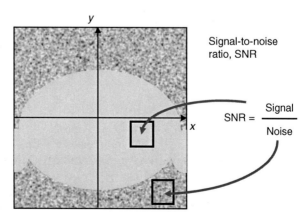

Fig. 8.2 Background noise is visible in areas of low signal, such as outside the body and in the lung fields. The signal-to-noise ratio for a particular tissue area can be calculated from the mean pixel value within a region of interest placed over that area, divided by the mean pixel value from a region of interest placed in the background noise

Signal-to-noise ratio, SNR

$$SNR = \frac{Signal}{Noise}$$

- The net magnetisation which is in turn dependent on the field strength (see Chap. 3). A higher static magnetic field strength (e.g., moving from 1.5 T to 3.0 T), increases the available signal.
- The tissue relaxation properties of the particular tissue, T1 and T2, in combination with the selected pulse sequence and timing parameters, such as TR and TE (see Chaps. 5 and 10).
- De-phasing of the net magnetisation due to the presence of magnetic field gradients e.g., caused by tissue susceptibility (T2*), or due to fluid motion or water diffusion along the imaging gradients.

Signal Averaging

As noise is random, averaging two or more signals together can have a beneficial effect upon the SNR. For example if two signals are averaged, the relative noise component is reduced by a factor $1/\sqrt{2}$ and so the SNR increases by a factor of about 41 %. This effect is manifested in a number of ways. First, as the signal is sampled many times, either through digital sampling of each signal echo, or by repeated sampling of the signal echo for different phase encoding steps, the SNR increases according to the square root of the total number of samples. Additionally, it is possible to repeat each phase encoding step a number of times in order to improve the SNR, a process known as *signal averaging* (Fig. 8.3).

The Nomenclature of Signal Averaging
Philips: Number of Signals Averaged, (NSA)
Siemens: Number of Acquisitions (ACQ)
GE: Number of Excitations, (NEX)

The drawback of the signal averaging approach is that the imaging time increases in proportion to the number of averages, whilst only gaining by the square root of the same factor in SNR. For techniques where speed is not of primary importance signal averaging is often used to improve image quality, whereas for cardiac imaging, the requirement for fast acquisition times limits its use.

SNR and Receiver Bandwidth

As noise is spread evenly across all frequencies, the level of noise in the image is extremely sensitive to the *receiver bandwidth* of the image acquisition (Fig. 8.4).

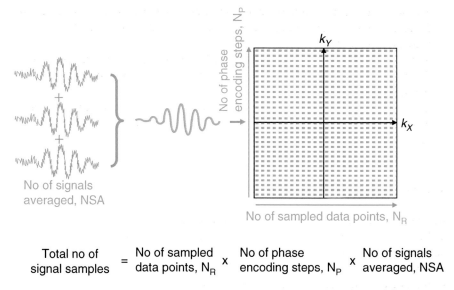

$$\begin{array}{c}\text{Total no of}\\\text{signal samples}\end{array}=\begin{array}{c}\text{No of sampled}\\\text{data points, } N_R\end{array}\times\begin{array}{c}\text{No of phase}\\\text{encoding steps, } N_P\end{array}\times\begin{array}{c}\text{No of signals}\\\text{averaged, NSA}\end{array}$$

Fig. 8.3 Image SNR ratio is related to the total number of times the MR signal is sampled. This is related to the number of times each signal is digitally sampled and the number of phase encoding steps. The MR signal acquisition at each phase encoding step is also sometimes repeated and averaged to increase the SNR. In this example, the number of signals averaged, NSA = 3

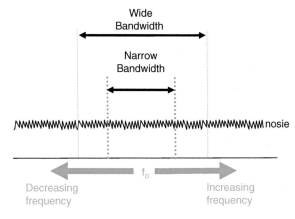

Fig. 8.4 Noise in MRI is spread evenly across all frequencies. A wide receiver bandwidth includes more noise, leading to a poorer SNR. A narrow receiver bandwidth reduces the amount of noise and therefore increases the image SNR

A *high (or wide) bandwidth* includes more of the noise spectrum, reducing the SNR. A *low (or narrow) bandwidth* only accepts noise from a narrow range of frequencies and therefore increases the SNR.

One might expect therefore to always use a narrow bandwidth to maximise the SNR. There are a number of reasons why not. First, chemical shift artefact in the frequency encoding direction becomes more pronounced at narrow bandwidths (see section on chemical shift artefact in Chap. 17). The low bandwidth usually also means that the frequency encoding gradient is not particularly steep, so that any intrinsic magnetic field distortion becomes more apparent, leading to geometric image distortion. Second, a narrow bandwidth necessitates slower digital sampling rates of the signal, resulting in an increased signal sampling time. This limits the minimum possible TE and TR and therefore the minimum image acquisition time. In practice there is usually a compromise, dependent upon the requirements of the particular pulse sequence and application, balancing the image quality (SNR) against the acquisition speed and artefact level. In some instances, artefacts are tolerated in order to reduce noise in the image. In other instances one is prepared to accept a noisy image in the exchange for imaging speed. In practice, altering the bandwidth of a given pulse sequence should be left to expert users as it can have a substantial, detrimental effect on image quality.

Imaging Parameters: Practical Examples

In summary, imaging parameters affect the three aspects of an MR acquisition, image acquisition time, spatial resolution and image quality (or SNR). An improvement in one of these aspects necessitates a reduction in at least one of the other two aspects. This is illustrated in the following examples:

Example 1
Two-fold increase in-plane spatial resolution (i.e., a decrease in the in-plane voxel dimensions by two-fold in each direction). See Fig. 8.5
There are at least two distinct ways of doing this:

(a) Keep the matrix size the same and reduce the field of view by half in both directions.
   - The image acquisition time stays the same (same number of phase encoding steps).
   - The voxel volume decreases four-fold
   - The SNR decreases four-fold.
   - There is an increased possibility of image aliasing as the subject may now be larger than the field of view (see section on aliasing in Chap. 17).
(b) Keep the Field of view the same and increase the image matrix size by two fold in each direction.
   - The number of phase encoding steps is increased two-fold. The total image acquisition time is doubled.
   - The number of digital samples for each signal is increased two-fold. If the bandwidth stays the same (signal sampling rate) the signal echo takes twice the time to sample (for all but the fastest techniques, this is probably not important).

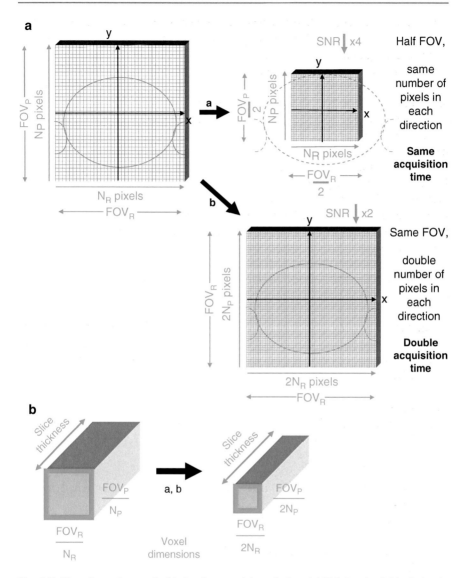

Fig. 8.5 Two alternatives to double in-plane spatial resolution. (**a**) Halving the field of view in both directions leads to a four-fold reduction in SNR with no change in imaging time. (**b**) Doubling the image matrix in both directions keeps the field of view the same but doubles the image acquisition time

- The four fold decrease in SNR due to the four-fold reduction in voxel volume is countered by the four-fold increase in the total number of signal samples, giving a two-fold ($\sqrt{4}$) increase in SNR. This leads overall to a net two-fold decrease in SNR.

In (a) the imaging time stays the same, but the image quality (SNR) is drastically reduced. In (b), the reduction in image quality (SNR) is less, but the image acquisition time is increased.

Example 2

Decrease image acquisition time by half (See Fig. 8.6)

There are again at least two distinct approaches:

(a) Half the image matrix dimension in the phase encoding direction, keeping the field of view constant in both directions.
   - The number of phase encoding steps is decreased by two fold leading to a two-fold reduction in image acquisition time.
   - The spatial resolution is reduced in the phase encoding direction by two fold.
   - The total number of signal samples is halved leading to a $\sqrt{2}$-fold reduction in SNR.
   - This is countered by a two-fold increase in the pixel dimension in the phase encoding direction, leading in turn to a two-fold increase in voxel volume and therefore a net increase in SNR by a factor of $\sqrt{2}$.
   - The field of view is preserved.
(b) Half both the image matrix dimension and the field of view in the phase encoding direction, keeping the pixel dimensions constant.
   - The number of phase encoding steps is decreased two-fold leading to a two-fold reduction in image acquisition time.
   - The spatial resolution is preserved.
   - The total number of signal samples is halved leading to a $\sqrt{2}$-fold reduction in SNR.
   - As the voxel volume is unchanged, this leads to a net $\sqrt{2}$-fold reduction in SNR.
   - As the field of view is reduced, there is a possibility of image aliasing as the subject may now be larger than the field of view (see section on aliasing in Chap. 17).

Summary of Factors Affecting Image Quality (SNR)

$$\text{SNR is proportional to} \frac{(\text{Voxel Volume}) \times \sqrt{(\text{No of signal samples})}}{\sqrt{\text{Bandwidth}}}$$

2D and 3D Imaging

For the major part of anatomical and functional Cardiac MR imaging, *two-dimensional (2D) image acquisition* techniques are used to acquire 2D slices through the heart (Fig. 8.7). Complete anatomical coverage is then achieved either by repeating the acquisition to acquire multiple parallel 2D slices, or by acquiring

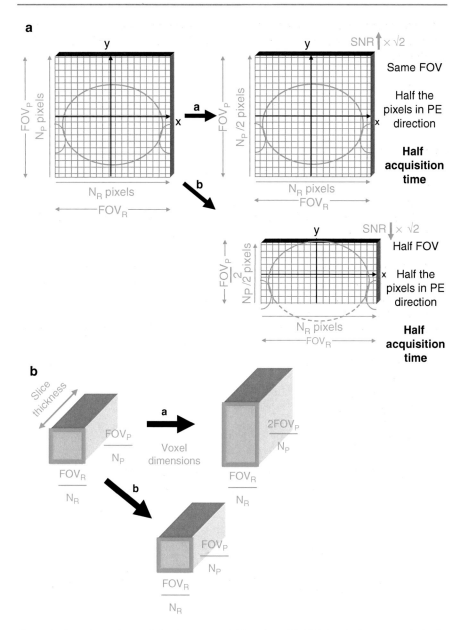

Fig. 8.6 Two alternatives to halve image acquisition time: (**a**) Halving the image matrix in the phase encoding steps leads to a two-fold reduction in spatial resolution in that direction, but a net increase in image quality (SNR). (**b**) Halving both the image matrix and the field of view in the phase encoding direction maintains the same spatial resolution but leads to a net ($\sqrt{2}$) decrease in image quality (SNR)

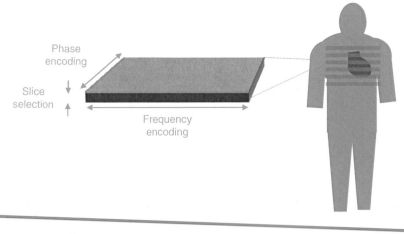

$$\text{Total acquisition time} = TR \times \text{No of phase encoding steps, } N_P \times \text{No of signals averaged, NSA}$$

Fig. 8.7 Two dimensional imaging is performed by slice selection and then using the MR signal frequency and phase to spatially encode the signal according to position within image plane in the two remaining directions. Volume coverage is achieved by repeating the acquisition at different slice locations

images in different image planes. For 2D imaging, the thickness of the slice is limited by the need to maintain adequate image quality (SNR). The acquisition time is related to the number of phase encoding steps (determined by the resolution in the phase encoding direction).

For selected techniques a *three-dimensional (3D) image acquisition* is more appropriate. In this case, a volume, rather than a slice of tissue is selected by the excitation pulse and subsequently encoded in three directions by applying frequency encoding in one direction, and phase encoding in the remaining two directions (Fig. 8.8). The phase encoding applied in the 'slice' direction effectively partitions in the volume into slices with the number of encoding steps being determined by the number of reconstructed slices required. For every phase encoding step in the 'slice' direction, the sequence must step through all the phase encoding steps in the 'in-plane' phase encoding direction. The imaging time is therefore related to the number of phase encode steps (in-plane encoding) multiplied by the number of phase encode steps (*slice encoding*).

Advantages of 3D Imaging
- Thinner slices can be achieved (resolution is closer to 'isotropic')
- Slices are contiguous (no gap).
- SNR is greater compared to the equivalent 2D technique by a factor equal to the square root of the number of encoded slices.

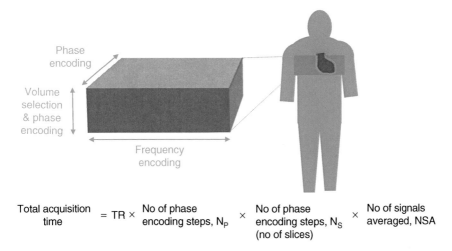

$$\text{Total acquisition time} = TR \times \text{No of phase encoding steps, } N_P \times \text{No of phase encoding steps, } N_S \text{ (no of slices)} \times \text{No of signals averaged, NSA}$$

Fig. 8.8 3D imaging is performed by selecting a volume, and then spatially encoding the signal in all three directions. The signal frequency is used to encode one direction and the signal phase is used for the other two directions. The image acquisition time is increased, relative to the 2D acquisition, by the number of phase encoding steps used to spatially encode the slice locations in the volume-selection direction

Summary
- Signal to noise ratio (SNR) is a major determinant of image quality in MRI.
- There is a interdependence between SNR, spatial resolution (voxel volume), receiver bandwidth and image acquisition time.
- Increasing spatial resolution (same field of view) reduces SNR and increases image acquisition time.
- Increasing spatial resolution by decreasing field of view reduces SNR for same imaging time
- Reducing image acquisition time reduces spatial resolution or SNR or both.
- Signal averaging increases SNR but also increases image acquisition time
- Increasing receiver bandwidth leads to faster echo sampling, shorter TE and TR hence shorter image acquisition time, but reduces SNR.
- In comparison to 2D imaging, 3D imaging allows thinner, contiguous slices to be acquired with improved SNR but with a longer acquisition time.

Further Reading

McRobbie DW, Moore EA, Graves MJ, Prince MR. The devil's in the detail: pixels, matrices and slices. In: MRI from picture to proton. 2nd ed. Cambridge: Cambridge University Press; 2007a. p. 47–64.
McRobbie DW, Moore EA, Graves MJ, Prince MR. What you set is what you get: basic image optimisation. In: MRI from picture to proton. 2nd ed. Cambridge: Cambridge University Press; 2007b. p. 65–78.

Improving SNR with Surface Coils and Array Coils

John P. Ridgway

Abstract

The choice of appropriate RF receiver coil is one of the most important factors in maximising image quality. Dedicated receiver coils improve SNR by being closer to the region of interest while receiving less noise from outside the region of interest. Appropriate coil selection is particularly important for paediatric applications. Array coils with multiple receiver elements provide improved SNR over a large field of view. Multi-element coils can also be used to provide information about the spatial distribution of the signal, reducing the number of phase encoding steps needed and therefore the image acquisition time (known as Parallel Imaging).

Keywords

Signal-to-noise ratio • SNR • RF coils • Receiver coil • Integral body coil • Surface coil • Paediatric CMR • Multi-element coil • Array coil • Parallel imaging

Perhaps the most important aspect of MR in optimising *signal-to-noise ratio*, (SNR) is the choice of *receiver coil*. The *integral body coil* has a large field of view (Fig. 9.1a), but for imaging a smaller region of interest, it is much more appropriate to use a smaller, more tailored, *surface coil* (Fig. 9.1b). This has two advantages:

1. It is closer to the origin of the signal from the region of interest.
2. It detects less of the noise originating from outside of the region of interest.

J.P. Ridgway, PhD
Department of Medical Physics and Engineering, Leeds Teaching Hospitals NHS Trust, St James's University Hospital, 1st Floor, Bexley Wing, Leeds LS2 9TJ, UK
e-mail: j.p.ridgway@leeds.ac.uk

© Springer International Publishing 2015
S. Plein et al. (eds.), *Cardiovascular MR Manual*,
DOI 10.1007/978-3-319-20940-1_9

Fig. 9.1 The integral body coil (**a**) has a large, uniform field of view coverage but receives more noise from a larger part of the body, resulting in a reduced SNR. Surface coils (**b**) have a smaller field of view but receive noise from a smaller part of the body, resulting in a higher SNR. As the sensitivity of the coil falls rapidly with distance from the coil, the image uniformity of the surface coil is poorer. This can partially be compensated by using two surface coils on either side of the body as shown

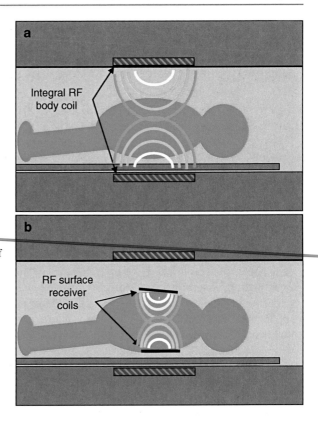

These are the key principles of surface coil imaging. In general, the smaller the coil, the better, although it is important that the coil is not too small that it cannot detect signal at depth.

RF Coils for Paediatric CMR

A good example the use of surface coils is in *paediatric CMR*. Whereas for adult imaging, the field of view used for most imaging protocols will not vary considerably, for paediatric subjects, the field of view will widely from teen-agers with almost the same field of view as adults, to neonates with a very small field of view. Not only does the field of view change but so does the demand for spatial resolution. The smaller structures within a neonatal heart will require significantly higher spatial resolution. As we saw from example 1 in Chap. 8, the need to increase spatial resolution over a small field of view, drastically reduces the SNR. The appropriate choice of surface coil is there-fore an essential step in designing paediatric imaging protocols in order to recover the SNR and to provide adequate image quality.

Array coils are now in common use (Fig. 9.2). They combine the advantages of a small coil, maximising SNR, while allowing imaging of a larger field of view. As the noise detected by each coil array element arises from a different region, the sum of the noise detected combines differently compared to a single large coil, giving an advantage of increased SNR. Array coils with elements distributed around the subject can also be used to provide information about the spatial distribution of the signal, allowing a reduced amount of phase encoding to be performed and therefore reducing the imaging time. This technique is known as *parallel imaging* (see section on this in Chap. 15). Most RF receiver coils used for adult imaging are *multi-element array coils*, both providing good SNR over the entire thorax and enabling parallel imaging to be employed.

Summary
- The choice of appropriate receiver coil is one of the most important factors in maximising image quality
- Dedicated receiver coils improve SNR by being closer to the region of interest while receiving less noise from outside the region of interest
- Appropriate coil selection is particularly important for paediatric applications
- Coil arrays with multiple receiver elements provide improved SNR over a large field of view
- Multi-element coils can also be used to provide information about the spatial distribution of the signal, reducing the number of phase encoding steps needed and therefore the image acquisition time (known as Parallel Imaging).

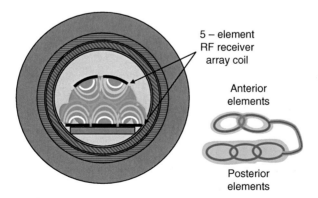

Fig. 9.2 Array coils consist of multiple receiver coil elements arranged in an array. Dedicated cardiac coils typically consist of 4–6 elements arranged as shown. The MR signal detected by each coil element can be directed through a separate receiver channel, providing high SNR imaging over a large field of view and enabling parallel imaging techniques to be employed

Further Reading

McRobbie DW, Moore EA, Graves MJ, Prince MR. Let's talk technical: MR equipment. In: MRI from picture to proton. 2nd ed. Cambridge: Cambridge University Press; 2007. p. 175–87.

Pulse Sequences and Image Contrast

10

John P. Ridgway

Abstract

Soft tissue contrast in MRI arises due to the differences between the tissues characteristic relaxation times. The type of pulse sequence and its parameters determines whether the image contrast is weighted by the T1, T2 or T2* relaxation processes. For Spin Echo (SE) pulse sequences, the TR controls the T1-weighting while the TE controls the T2* weighting. For Gradient echo (GE) pulse sequences, the TR and the flip angle control the T1-weighting while the TE controls the T2* weighting. A long TR and short TE produces proton density-weighted contrast, a short TR and short TE produces T1-weighted contrast and a long TR and a short TE produces T2- (or T2*) weighted contrast. Choosing a short TR and long TE combination for conventional pulse sequences generally produces an image with poor contrast and a low signal-to-noise ratio.

Keywords

Pixel intensity • Pulse sequence • Repetition time • TR • Echo time • TE • Proton density • Equilibrium • T1 relaxation time • T2 relaxation time • T2* relaxation time • Contrast • T1-weighted • T2-weighted • T2*-weighted • Proton density-weighted • Long TR • Long TE • Short TR • Short TE

J.P. Ridgway, PhD
Department of Medical Physics and Engineering, Leeds Teaching Hospitals NHS Trust, St James's University Hospital, 1st Floor, Bexley Wing, Leeds LS2 9TJ, UK
e-mail: j.p.ridgway@leeds.ac.uk

© Springer International Publishing 2015
S. Plein et al. (eds.), *Cardiovascular MR Manual*,
DOI 10.1007/978-3-319-20940-1_10

Dependence of the MR Signal on TR and TE

The MR signal intensity at a particular location is represented by the image *pixel intensity*. In Chaps. 8 and 9 it was shown that the strength of the MR signal relative to the background noise (SNR) depends on a number of instrumental factors including the magnetic field strength, the choice of receiver coil, and system electronics, as well as image acquisition parameters including the field of view, image acquisition matrix size and slice thickness (defining the voxel volume), the number of signal samples and the receiver bandwidth. It also depends on the sequence of RF pulses and gradient pulses used to generate the MR signal echo, commonly referred to as the *pulse sequence*. The two main types of pulse sequence are gradient echo and spin echo pulse sequences. The choice of pulse sequence and it's imaging parameters, including the timing parameters, *repetition time, TR* and *echo time, TE* determine the intrinsic strength of the MR signal from a particular tissue according to its *proton density* value and relaxation properties.

For a simple pulse sequence that uses a single RF excitation pulse (Fig. 10.1), the transverse magnetisation at the time of measurement depends on:

- The net longitudinal magnetisation at *equilibrium*, M_0. This is determined by the proton density of the tissue and the applied magnetic field strength.
- The value of the longitudinal (z) magnetisation, M_z, immediately before each RF excitation pulse is applied. This depends on the time allowed for recovery of the z magnetisation between pulses (usually the repetition time, TR), and the rate of recovery, determined by the *T1 relaxation time* of the particular tissue.
- The *flip angle* of the RF excitation pulse. This determines the proportion of that magnetisation that is transferred into the transverse (xy) plane by the RF pulse and therefore the initial value of the transverse magnetisation before it decays. In Fig. 10.1 the flip angle is 90° and all of the z-magnetisation is transferred into the xy plane.
- The rate of decay of the amplitude of the transverse magnetisation, determined by the *T2 relaxation time* of the particular tissue, together with the effect of magnetic field inhomogeneities (combined as the T2* relaxation time).
- The time after the excitation pulse at which the centre of the signal echo is generated and sampled (the echo time, TE).

In summary, the amplitude of the MR signal echo depends on the following:

- Decay of the transverse component of magnetisation (T2 and T2* relaxation), and the chosen echo time, TE.
- Recovery of the z-component of magnetisation (T1 relaxation), the chosen repetition time, TR, and the flip angle.
- Different tissues have different characteristic relaxation times. This gives rise to different signal amplitudes depending on the choice of the pulse sequence timing parameters TR and TE and the flip angle.

> *Both TR and flip angle control the differences due to T1 relaxation.*

> *TE controls the differences due to T2 and T2* relaxation.*

All of the above factors combine to determine the amplitude of the transverse magnetisation at the echo time for a particular tissue. This is translated into image pixel intensity according to the aforementioned instrumental factors (specific to each patient/receiver coil setup) and image acquisition parameters.

The above sequence describes a single repetition period, TR. After the excitation pulse, the longitudinal (z) component of magnetisation recovers back towards its equilibrium value at a rate determined by its longitudinal (T1) relaxation time (Fig. 10.1). The time at which the next excitation pulse is applied after the previous excitation pulse (the repetition time, TR), will determine the amount of recovery and therefore the value of the z-magnetisation before the next RF excitation pulse is applied. This then influences the signal amplitude in the following repetition period.

Image Contrast and Weighting

One of the most important advantages of MR imaging over other imaging modalities is the ability to generate contrast between different soft tissue types. This is because different types of soft tissue have different characteristic T1 and T2 relaxation times. The previous section showed that the dependence of the signal from a particular tissue on its T1 and T2 (or T2*) relaxation properties is controlled by the choice of the pulse sequence parameters, TR, TE and flip angle.

For spin echo pulse sequences the addition of a 180° refocusing pulse determines that the amplitude of the spin echo at the TE is influenced by T2 relaxation. As the excitation flip angle is fixed at 90°, the TR and TE are the only parameters used to control the image contrast. Typically, they are chosen to weight the image contrast so that it is either primarily dependent upon the differences in T1 relaxation times (*T1-weighted*), or primarily dependent on the differences in T2 relaxation times (*T2 weighted*).

For *gradient echo* pulse sequences the absence of a 180° refocusing pulse determines that the amplitude of the gradient echo at the TE, is influenced by T2* relaxation. Varying the flip angle of the excitation pulse, as well as the TR and TE, is used to control image contrast. Typically, these three parameters are chosen to weight the image contrast so that it is either primarily dependent upon the differences in T1 relaxation times (T1-weighted), or primarily dependent on the differences in T2* relaxation times (*T2*-weighted*).

For both Spin Echo and Gradient echo pulse sequences, if the parameters are chosen so that the image contrast is neither dependent on the differences in T1 or T2 (or T2*), the tissue signal is said to be primarily dependent on the proton density of the tissue and the image contrast is *'proton density' weighted.*

Sequence type	Parameters	Contrast weighting
Spin Echo	TR, TE	T1, T2 or Proton density
Gradient Echo	TR, TE, Flip angle	T1, T2* or Proton density

In the following examples, a simple pulse sequence with a fixed, 90° excitation pulse is used to demonstrate how the two parameters, TR and TE can be chosen to produce different contrast weightings. Whilst the pulse sequence is shown is gradient echo sequence without a 180° refocusing pulse, the trends for TR and TE are the

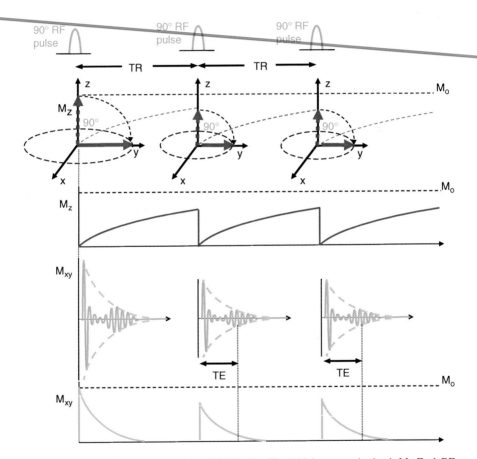

Fig. 10.1 Simple pulse sequence using a 90° RF pulse. The initial z-magnetisation is M_o. Each RF pulse fully transfers the z-magnetisation, M_z, into the xy plane. Recovery of the z-magnetisation with a time constant T1 during the repetition time, TR, determines its value prior to the next RF pulse. This in turn determines the magnetisation transferred into the xy plane after each RF pulse. The transverse magnetisation, M_{xy}, then decays with a time constant T2*. This and the choice of echo time, TE, at which the gradient echo is formed determines the MR signal echo amplitude

same for spin echo sequences, except that for the spin echo sequence, the amplitude of the signal echo at the TE, is governed by the T2 relaxation time rather than the T2* relaxation time. In these examples the terms 'long' and 'short' are used to describe the TR and TE as follows:

- *Long TR* means much longer than the T1 relaxation times of most of the tissues.
- *Short TR* means comparable to or shorter than the T1 relaxation times of most of the tissues.
- *Short TE* means much shorter than the T2* (or T2 for spin echo) values of all the tissues.
- *Long TE* means comparable to or longer than the T2* relaxation times of most of the tissues.

The possible combinations of TR and TE are as follows.

Long TR and Short TE (Fig. 10.2)

The choice of a long TR allows the *z*-magnetisation to recover close to the equilibrium values for most of the tissues. The 90° excitation pulse therefore transfers a similar amount of signal into the *xy* plane for all tissues. The choice of a short TE limits the amount of T2* decay for any tissue at the time of measurement. This results in a high signal from all tissues, with little difference between them. So the signal amplitude is not particularly affected by the T1 relaxation properties, or by

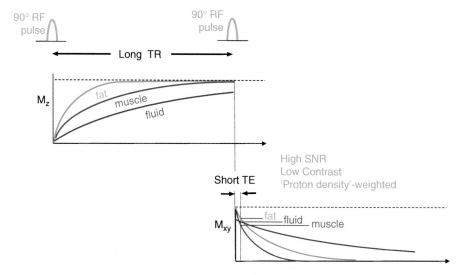

Fig. 10.2 Pulse sequence with a 'long TR' and 'short TE', produces 'proton density' weighted contrast

the T2* relaxation properties. The primary determinant of the signal amplitude is therefore the equilibrium magnetisation of the tissue and the image contrast is said to be *'proton density'* weighted. This type of weighting is useful where the depiction of anatomical structure is required, without the need to introduce soft tissue contrast.

Short TR, Short TE (Fig. 10.3)

The choice of a short TR determines that tissues with a short T1 (e.g., fat) will recover more than those with a long T1 (e.g., fluid). This determines the initial value of the transverse magnetisation, M_{xy}, when the next RF pulse is applied. Tissues that have recovered more quickly will have a greater longitudinal magnetisation before the next RF pulse, resulting in a greater transverse magnetisation after the RF pulse. The short TE limits the influence of the different T2* decay rates. The resultant contrast is therefore said to be *T1-weighted*. These images are typically characterised by bright fat signal and a low signal from fluid and are useful for anatomical imaging where high contrast is required between, fat, muscle and fluid.

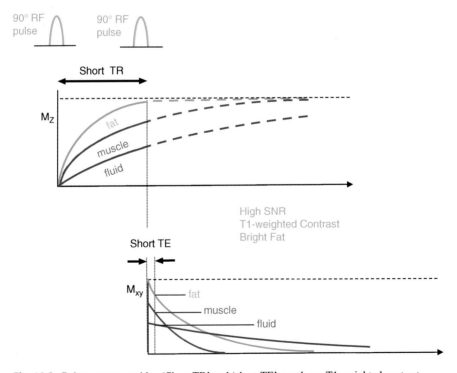

Fig. 10.3 Pulse sequence with a 'Short TR' and 'short TE', produces T1-weighted contrast

Long TR, Long TE (Fig. 10.4)

As with Fig. 10.2, the long TR allows recovery of the z-magnetisation for most tissues, therefore reducing the influence of differences in T1 relaxation time. The longer echo time however allows more decay of the xy component of the magnetisation. The differential rate of decay between a tissue with a short T2* (muscle) and a tissue with a long T2* (e.g., fluid) leads to a difference in signal that is said to be *T2* weighted* (For Spin Echo sequences this combination of TR and TE provides images that are T2-weighted). The short T2* leads to a reduced signal, while the long T2* leads to a high signal intensity. These images are characterised by bright fluid and are useful for the depiction of fluid collections and the characterisation of cardiac masses and oedema. For T2*weighted gradient echo, the image contrast is also strongly influenced by the presence of magnetic susceptibility effects and can be used to detect the presence of iron, for example where there is haemorrhage or iron loading of tissue.

Short TR, Long TE (Fig. 10.5)

This combination of timing parameter choices is generally not a good idea. The short TR reduces signal from tissue with long T1 relaxation times. The long TE reduces signal from tissues with short T2* values. Since the T1 and T2 (and T2*) relaxation times for most tissues follow similar trends, the result is a reduced signal from everything as well as poor contrast. i.e., a poor image.

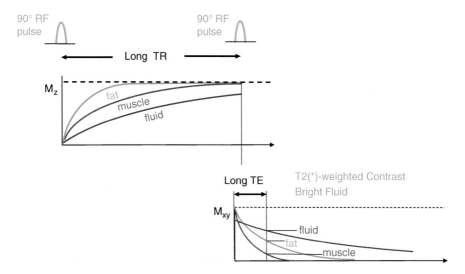

Fig. 10.4 Pulse sequence with a 'Long TR' and 'long TE', produces T2*-weighted contrast

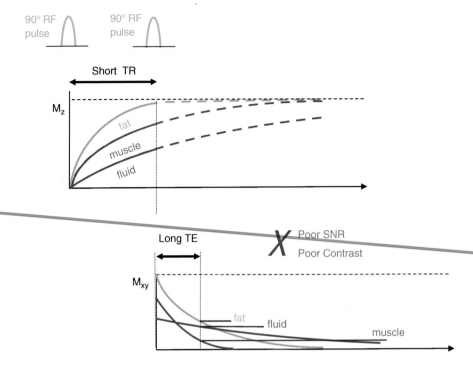

Fig. 10.5 Pulse sequence with a 'Short TR' and 'long TE', produces a poor contrast, low SNR image

Summary
- Soft tissue contrast in MRI arises due to the differences between the tissues' characteristic relaxation times.
- The type of pulse sequence and its parameters determines whether the image contrast is weighted by the T1, T2 or T2* relaxation processes.
- For Spin Echo (SE) pulse sequences, the TR controls the T1-weighting while the TE controls the T2* weighting.
- For Gradient echo (GE) pulse sequences, the TR and the flip angle control the T1-weighting while the TE controls the T2* weighting.
- Contrast weightings for TR and TE parameter choices with fixed flip angle:

	Short TE	Long TE
Long TR	*'Proton Density' weighted* Good SNR, No contrast	*T2*-weighted* *(T2-weighted for SE)* Bright Fluid
Short TR	*T1-weighted* Bright fat Low fluid signal	Poor SNR, Poor Contrast image

Further Reading

McRobbie DW, Moore EA, Graves MJ, Prince MR. Seeing is believing: introduction to image contrast. In: MRI from picture to proton. 2nd ed. Cambridge: Cambridge University Press; 2007. p. 30–40.

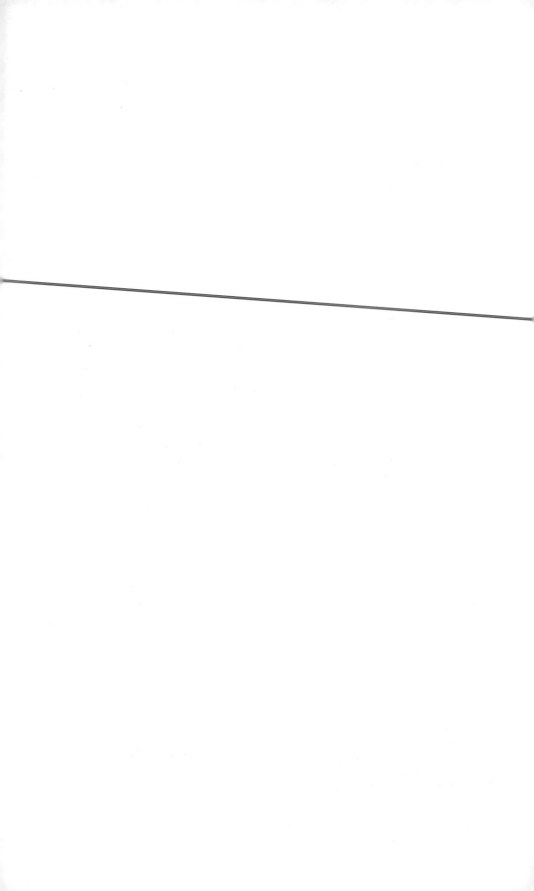

Gradient Echo Versus Spin Echo

11

John P. Ridgway

Abstract

Spin echo and gradient echo pulse sequences follow similar contrast behaviour but there are some key differences. The spin echo pulse sequence uses an excitation pulse that is normally 90°, and a 180° refocusing pulse that reverses the effect of field inhomogeneities. These two attributes make the spin echo technique ideally suited when the primary goal is to achieve good image quality, with a reduced sensitivity to artefacts caused by magnetic field distortions. The gradient echo pulse sequence uses an excitation pulse with a flip angle that is normally less than 90°. This causes only a proportion of the z-magnetisation is transferred into the xy plane, allowing faster recovery of the z -magnetisation towards the equilibrium shorter repetition times. This is known as low flip angle imaging and is the reason why gradient echo pulse sequences are suited to fast imaging. The absence of the 180° refocusing pulse in the gradient echo sequence leads to a greater influence of magnetic susceptibility effects, different appearances of the chemical shift artefact and flow blood in comparison with spin echo.

Keywords

Gradient echo • Spin echo • Pulse sequence • 180° refocusing pulse • Magnetic field inhomogeneities • Low flip angle • Fast gradient echo • Spoiled gradient echo • Magnetic susceptibility • Chemical shift • Flowing blood

J.P. Ridgway, PhD
Department of Medical Physics and Engineering, Leeds Teaching Hospitals NHS Trust,
St James's University Hospital, 1st Floor, Bexley Wing, Leeds LS2 9TJ, UK
e-mail: j.p.ridgway@leeds.ac.uk

© Springer International Publishing 2015
S. Plein et al. (eds.), *Cardiovascular MR Manual*,
DOI 10.1007/978-3-319-20940-1_11

91

Spin echo pulse sequences follow similar contrast behaviour to that described in the previous section however there are some key differences between gradient echo and spin echo pulse sequences (Fig. 11.1).

In the case of spin echo, a 180° refocusing pulse is applied at a time equal to half the echo time. This reverses the effect of the field inhomogeneities and the amplitude of the transverse magnetisation at the echo time is dependent on the pure T2 relaxation time of the tissue. As the T2 values for tissues are longer than the T2* values, the echo times chosen to achieve T2 weighting with spin echo pulse sequences are also longer than the echo times required to achieve T2* weighting with gradient echo pulse sequences.

The spin echo pulse sequence uses an excitation pulse that is normally 90°, so at each excitation pulse all of the z magnetisation is transferred into the transverse plane. This combined with the refocusing pulse gives the largest possible signal provided the magnetisation is allowed to recover sufficiently between repetitions.

These two attributes make the spin echo technique ideally suited when the primary goal is to achieve good image quality, with a reduced sensitivity to artefacts caused by magnetic field inhomogeneities.

The gradient echo pulse sequence uses an excitation pulse with a flip angle, α, that is normally less than 90° and typically 30° or less (Fig. 11.2). While this initially results in a smaller transverse magnetisation, as only a proportion of the z-magnetisation is transferred into the xy plane, the recovery of the z-magnetisation towards the equilibrium value is faster, allowing the repetition time to be reduced. In this case a much larger transverse magnetisation is achieved compared to that generated by a 90° pulse in combination with a very short TR. This is known as *low flip angle* imaging and is the basis for fast imaging with gradient echo pulse sequences. Much shorter repetition times can be used for gradient echo than for spin echo pulse sequences. *Fast gradient echo* pulse sequences are used where imaging speed is more important than SNR.

The contrast behaviour described in this section is only true for a gradient echo pulse sequence provided the TR is not too short (>100 ms). For fast imaging, very short TR values (<10 ms) are used and the contrast behaviour of the gradient echo sequence can change. The contrast behaviour described here is only applicable at very short TR values if particular type of gradient echo pulse sequence, *spoiled gradient echo* is used (See section on Spoiled gradient echo vs bSSFP in Chap. 13).

Further differences between spin echo and gradient echo pulse sequences arise due to the absence of the 180° refocusing pulse in the gradient echo sequence. This leads to signal loss in the presence of *magnetic susceptibility* effects (see section on this in Chap. 17), and at the boundaries between water and fat-based tissues (see section on Chemical shift artefact in Chap. 17). Flowing blood also appears differently between the two sequences. All of the above key differences are summarised in Table 11.1. Note that the description of TR as long or short is dependent on the choice of flip angle. A TR that may be described as short when a high flip angle is selected (e.g. TR=200 ms, flip angle 70°), becomes a long TR when a low flip angle is selected (e.g. TR=200 ms, flip angle 30°).

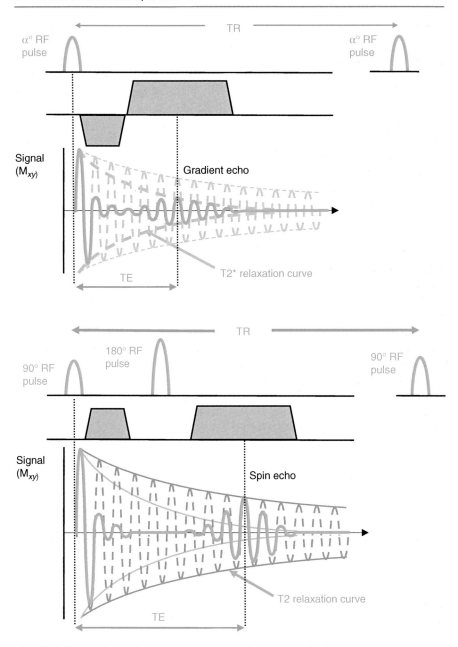

Fig. 11.1 Comparison between a gradient echo pulse sequence (*top*) and a spin echo sequence (*bottom*). The gradient echo sequence uses RF excitation pulses with low flip angles, α, that are typically much less than 90°. The gradient echo signal amplitude is determined by T2* decay and is therefore smaller. Echo times also tend to be shorter. The spin echo pulse sequence uses a 90° excitation pulse and a 180° RF pulse to reverse the effects of field inhomogeneities. The spin echo signal amplitude is determined primarily by T2 decay and is therefore larger

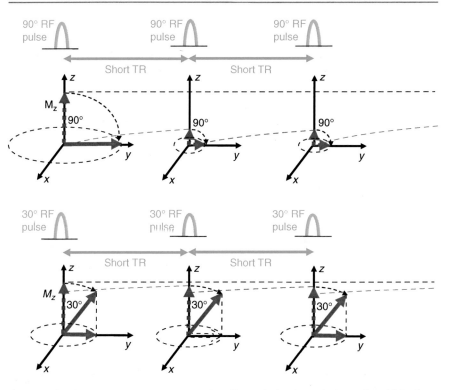

Fig. 11.2 Gradient echo sequences can use a low flip angle for the excitation pulse which allows much shorter TR values to be used without losing too much signal. When a 90° RF pulse is used (*top row*), the short TR allows very little recovery between RF pulses. The z-magnetisation quickly reduces, resulting in a low signal amplitude when it is transferred into the xy plane. The use of a low flip angle (in this case, 30°, *bottom row*), allows the z-magnetisation to remain much closer to its equilibrium value. This, when transferred into the xy plane, results in a much larger signal in comparison

Table 11.1 Summary of differences between conventional gradient echo and spin echo sequences

	Gradient echo (spoiled)	Spin echo
RF pulses	Variable excitation pulse	Excitation pulse and 180° refocusing pulse
Signal amplitude depends on decay of transverse magnetisation according to…	T2*	T2
Flip angle (excitation pulse)	5–70°	90°
Short echo time (minimise T2 or T2* weighting)	1–3 ms	6–25 ms
Long echo time (for T2 or T2* weighting)	7–15 ms	60–100 ms
Short Repetition time (T1 weighting)	3–400 ms (depends on flip angle)	400–800 ms
Long Repetition time (minimises T1 weighting)	400 ms – (depends on flip angle)	1500–2500 ms
Shortest practical TR	2–5 ms	200 ms
Intravoxel signal loss (susceptibility, iron)	Yes	No
Intravoxel signal loss (fat/water boundaries)	At out-of phase echo times	No
Signal from blood flowing through the slice	Bright (inflow enhancement)	Dark (spin washout)

Summary
- The contrast behaviour of conventional spin echo and gradient echo follow similar trends, but there are also key differences:
- Spin Echo (SE)
  - High quality T1- and T2-weighted imaging
  - Insensitive to magnetic susceptibility (T2*) effects including iron
  - Dark blood appearance (flowing blood)
  - Relatively long TR required – can't be used for fast imaging applications
- Gradient Echo (GE)
  - Relatively reduced signal
  - Short TR possible with variable low flip angle – suited to fast imaging applications
  - Bright blood appearance (flowing blood)
  - Increasing sensitivity to magnetic susceptibility (T2*) effects including iron as TE is increased.

Further Reading

Balaban RS, Peters DC. Basic principles of cardiovascular magnetic resonance. In: Manning WJ, Pennell DJ, editors. Cardiovascular magnetic resonance. 2nd ed. Philadelphia: Saunders; 2010. p. 3–18.
McRobbie DW, Moore EA, Graves MJ, Prince MR. MRI from picture to proton. 2nd ed. Cambridge: Cambridge University Press; 2007. p. 30–40. Chapter 3, Seeing is believing: introduction to image contrast.
Ridgway JP. Cardiac magnetic resonance physics for clinicians: part I. J Cardiovasc Magn Reson. 2010;12(1):71. doi:10.1186/1532-429X-12-71.

Black Blood Versus Bright Blood Imaging

12

John P. Ridgway

Abstract

Spin echo pulse sequences exhibit intrinsic black-blood contrast, caused by the movement of blood out of the image slice between the 90° and 180° pulses, known as spin washout. In the presence of slow blood flow, the intrinsic black blood contrast of spin echo pulse sequences becomes inconsistent. Black Blood Contrast can be improved by using a black blood preparation scheme, in combination with a spin echo pulse sequence. The black blood preparation scheme consists of two 180° inversion pulses, one non-selective and one slice selective, to invert the blood magnetisation outside the image slice. As the magnetisation recovers towards zero, the inverted blood moves into the slice. The spin echo pulse sequence is applied as the inverted blood magnetisation reaches zero leading to no signal from blood. Gradient Echo pulse sequences with short repetition times commonly exhibit an intrinsic bright blood appearance from flowing blood. The short TR causes saturation of the magnetisation and a reduction in signal of stationary tissue within the slice. Flowing blood entering the slice is fully magnetised and is able to yield a higher signal than the surrounding tissue, resulting in a bright blood appearance. This effect is known as inflow enhancement and it is the main contrast mechanism employed in time-of-flight TOF MR angiography, in addition to bright blood imaging of the heart.

Keywords

Spin echo • Black blood • Dark blood • Spin washout • Vessel patency • Black blood preparation • Double inversion preparation pulse • Time from inversion • TI • Signal voids • Gradient echo • Bright blood • Inflow enhancement • Time-of-flight • TOF • Angiography

J.P. Ridgway, PhD
Department of Medical Physics and Engineering, Leeds Teaching Hospitals NHS Trust,
St James's University Hospital, 1st Floor, Bexley Wing, Leeds LS2 9TJ, UK
e-mail: j.p.ridgway@leeds.ac.uk

© Springer International Publishing 2015
S. Plein et al. (eds.), *Cardiovascular MR Manual*,
DOI 10.1007/978-3-319-20940-1_12

Black Blood (Spin Echo Pulse Sequence)

The *spin echo* pulse sequence generates images that have intrinsic black blood contrast. This is because it uses two pulses, the 90° and 180° RF pulses, to produce the spin echo signal (Fig. 12.1). Both of these pulses are slice-selective but are separated by a time equal to half the echo time. The transverse magnetisation of blood flowing through the slice that moves out of the slice between the two pulses is not refocused by the 180° pulse and does not contribute to the generation of a spin echo. If the flow is sufficiently rapid for all the blood receiving the 90° pulse to move out of the slice, this results in a signal void, also known as a *'black blood'* or *'dark blood'* appearance. This effect is also known as the *spin washout* effect, referring to the 'washout' of proton spins form the image slice that would otherwise be refocused and contribute to the spin echo signal.

When there is significant blood flow *through* the slice, the black blood appearance provides high intrinsic contrast between the blood pool and the heart and blood vessel walls which is ideal for anatomical imaging (Fig. 12.2a).

Where blood is moving *slowly* however, or moves within the plane of the image slice, this effect is reduced and the dark blood contrast is lost (Fig. 12.2b).

> **Signal Voids and Vessel Patency**
> When a *signal void* is seen within the vessel lumen on spin echo images, it usually suggests that there is significant blood flow, confirming *vessel patency*. Conversely, if signal is seen within a vessel, this does not necessarily mean that it is occluded. It could either mean that there is thrombus or that the blood is moving slowly through, or remaining within in the image slice. This requires further imaging, such as velocity mapping, for confirmation.

Black Blood: Double Inversion Preparation Pulses

Reliance on the spin washout effect to produce dark blood contrast often leads to inconsistent results due to insufficient blood flow. In order to improve the effectiveness of black blood imaging it is common to use a black blood preparation pulse in combination with the spin echo pulse sequence. The preparation scheme consists of the addition of two 180° RF pulses followed by a delay, prior to the spin echo pulse sequence (Fig. 12.3). The effect of this preparation scheme is described as follows:

- The first 180° pulse inverts the magnetisation of all blood and tissues within range of the RF body transmitter coil.
- The second 180° pulse re-inverts the magnetisation only within a slice that encompasses the slice to be imaged.
- The net effect of these two pulses is to invert the magnetisation of blood and tissue outside the slice, while the magnetisation within the slice remains close to its equilibrium value.

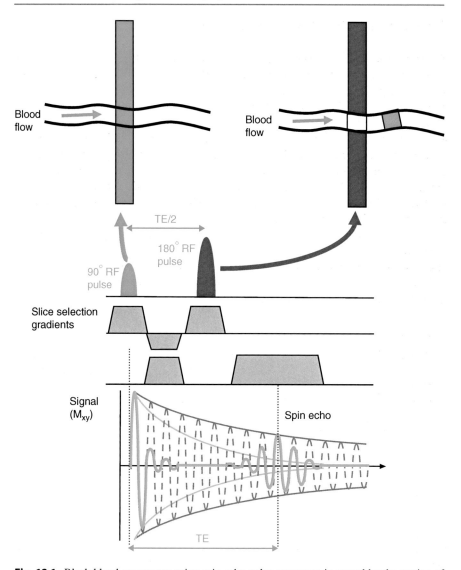

Fig. 12.1 Black blood appearance using spin echo pulse sequences is caused by the motion of blood through the image slice between the 90° and 180° RF pulses. The 90° pulse (*green*) causes resonance in all the tissue within the slice, however a spin echo signal is only produced when the same tissue and blood also receive the 180° refocusing pulse (*red*). Blood that moves out of the slice during the time between the 90° and 180° pulses does not produce a spin echo, resulting in a signal void

- There is then a time delay before the excitation pulse (*time from inversion, TI*). During this time, the inverted blood magnetisation recovers due to T1 relaxation from its initial negative value, towards its positive equilibrium value.
- The TI is calculated to be equal to the time it takes the inverted magnetisation of blood to pass through zero. At that time, the 90° excitation pulse of the spin echo pulse sequence is applied.

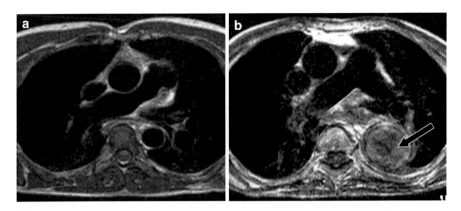

Fig. 12.2 The image in (a) is acquired using a Spin Echo pulse sequence. High blood flow velocities through the major vessels generate good contrast between the blood vessel walls and the blood due to the spin washout effect. Image (b) shows an image acquired in a patient with a dilated descending aorta. The slow blood flow reduces the spin washout effect and signal is seen from the blood within the descending aorta (*arrow*)

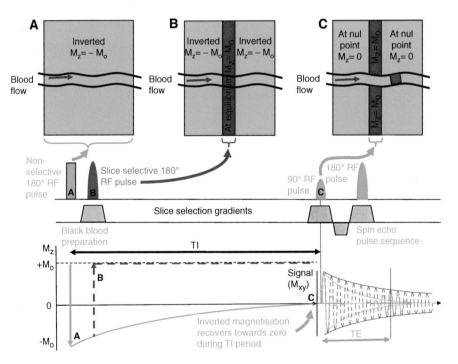

Fig. 12.3 Black-blood imaging commonly uses a double-inversion preparation pulse scheme to make the suppression of the blood signal more effective. The first inversion pulse, *A*, inverts the magnetisation of all the tissue within range of the RF transmitter coil. The second inversion pulse, *B*, restores the magnetisation of the tissue within the intended image slice. The net effect of pulses *A* and *B* is to invert the magnetisation of all the tissue outside the intended image slice (shown in *green*). After a prescribed recovery period, chosen as the time taken for the blood magnetisation to reach zero (*solid red line*), an excitation pulse, *C*, is applied to generate a signal dependent on the current value the z-magnetisation of tissue and blood within the slice. During that same period, blood from outside the slice that has been inverted (*green*) is likely to have replaced the non-inverted blood within the slice (*red*), resulting in a signal void within the vessel

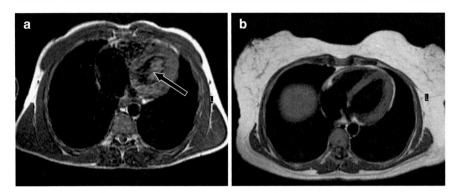

Fig. 12.4 Image (**a**) is acquired using a conventional spin echo pulse sequence. Note the imperfect suppression of the blood pool signal (*arrow*). This is because the spin washout effect is not always effective, either due to slower flow in diastole, or due to blood flowing more within the plane of the image slice. The image in (**b**) is acquired in diastole using a Black-Blood preparation pulse. Suppression of the blood pool signal is more consistent using this method

- At the same time, blood flow causes the blood with inverted magnetisation to move into the image slice, replacing the blood that has remained at equilibrium. As the excitation pulse of the spin echo pulse sequence is applied at the same time as the inverted blood magnetisation reaches zero, no signal is produced from the blood.

The double inversion pulse black blood preparation scheme provides much better signal suppression as the time delay used here is much greater than the half echo time period that gives rise to the intrinsic black blood contrast of the conventional spin echo pulse sequence (Fig. 12.4).

Bright Blood (Gradient Echo Pulse Sequence)

In contrast to the spin echo sequence, the gradient echo sequence only uses one rf pulse to generate the signal and so the spin washout effect does not apply and the signal from flowing blood is usually visible. Indeed, rather than suffering from a reduction in signal, flowing blood often appears with an apparently increased signal, compared to the surrounding tissues. The gradient echo pulse sequence is therefore commonly referred to as a *bright blood* imaging technique.

Gradient echo sequences are often used with a very short repetition time, (TR), for the purpose of fast imaging (e.g. TR <10 ms). This means that the magnetisation of tissue that remains in the image slice becomes saturated as rf pulses are rapidly applied to the same tissue, as there is little time for recovery of the z-magnetisation between pulses. This has the effect of reducing the signal from stationary tissue or blood that remains within the slice (Fig. 12.5). Blood moving into the slice, however, has not received any previous pulses and the spin population is therefore fully magnetised. The moving blood is therefore able to generate a much higher signal than the surrounding tissue, thus the blood signal appears enhanced or bright. This effect is known as *inflow enhancement*.

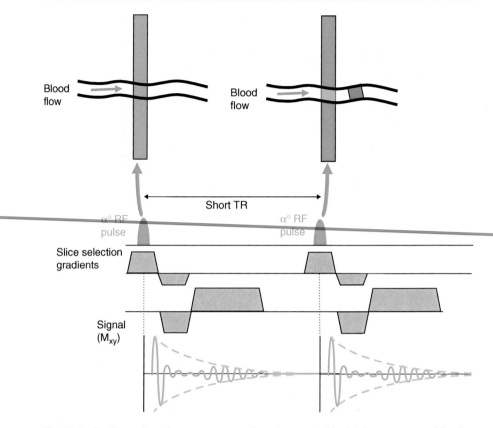

Fig. 12.5 Gradient echo pulse sequences are often characterised by bright appearance of flowing blood. This is because they often use very short repetition times. This results in limited recovery of the tissue magnetisation between pulses. Tissue that remains within the slice therefore has a reduced signal. Blood that flows through the image slice is constantly being replaced by fully magnetised blood which is able to generate a much higher signal when the excitation pulse is applied

When there is significant blood flow through the slice, the bright blood signal provides good intrinsic contrast between the blood pool and the heart and blood vessel walls (Fig. 12.6). The use of a much shorter repetition time (compared to spin echo for example) makes this technique useful for functional imaging of the heart and great vessels. The inflow enhancement effect is also used as the basis for *time-of-flight* MR *angiography* (TOF MRA). Where the blood flow is moving slowly through the slice or in a direction within the plane of the image slice, this effect is reduced and the bright blood contrast is reduced.

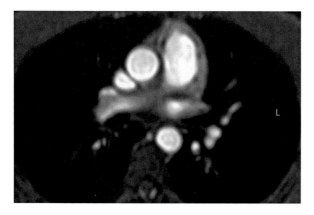

Fig. 12.6 A gradient echo pulse sequence showing 'bright blood' appearance within the major blood vessels, due to the inflow enhancement effect

Summary

- Spin echo pulse sequences exhibit intrinsic black-blood contrast, caused by the movement of blood out of the image slice between the 90° and 180° pulses.
- In the presence of slow blood flow, the intrinsic black blood contrast of spin echo pulse sequences becomes inconsistent.
- Black Blood Contrast can be improved by using a Black Blood preparation scheme, in combination with a spin echo pulse sequence.
- The black blood preparation scheme consists of two 180° inversion pulses, one non-selective and one slice selective, to invert the blood magnetisation outside the image slice.
- As the magnetisation recovers towards zero, the inverted blood moves into the slice. The spin echo pulse sequence is applied as the inverted blood magnetisation reaches zero leading to no signal from blood.
- Gradient Echo pulse sequences commonly exhibit an intrinsic 'bright blood' appearance from flowing blood.
- Gradient echo sequences use a short TR which causes saturation of the magnetisation and a reduction in signal of stationary tissue within the slice.
- Flowing blood entering the slice is fully magnetised and is able to yield a higher signal than the surrounding tissue, resulting in a bright blood appearance.

Further Reading

Balaban RS, Peters DC. Basic principles of cardiovascular magnetic resonance. In: Manning WJ, Pennell DJ, editors. Cardiovascular magnetic resonance. 2nd ed. Philadelphia: Saunders; 2010. p. 3–18.

McRobbie DW, Moore EA, Graves MJ, Prince MR. MRI from picture to proton. 2nd ed. Cambridge: Cambridge University Press; 2007a. p. 258–64. Chapter 13, Go with the flow: MR angiography.

McRobbie DW, Moore EA, Graves MJ, Prince MR. MRI from picture to proton. 2nd ed. Cambridge: Cambridge University Press; 2007b. p. 285–8. Chapter 14, A heart to heart discussion: cardiac MRI.

Ridgway JP. Cardiac magnetic resonance physics for clinicians: part I. J Cardiovasc Magn Reson. 2010;12(1):71. doi:10.1186/1532-429X-12-71.

Dealing with Cardiac Motion: How Do We Image the Beating Heart?

13

John P. Ridgway

Abstract

In order to acquire images of the beating heart, the MR pulse sequence and data acquisition must be synchronised with the patient's ECG signal. Still imaging uses the ECG signal to trigger the image data acquisition at a single chosen trigger delay after the R-wave. Still imaging is used to image cardiac anatomy, for tissue characterisation or to image the coronary arteries. Cine imaging acquires image data at multiple time points (cardiac phases) throughout the cardiac cycle to produce a sequence of images that can be viewed as a movie. Cine imaging that uses prospective ECG triggering does not image the last part of the cardiac cycle. Retrospective gating allows the pulse sequence to run continuously and the acquired data is assigned retrospectively to the cardiac phases, which enables the whole cardiac cycle to be imaged. Two main types of gradient echo sequence are used for cine imaging, Spoiled gradient echo and balanced Steady State Free Precession (bSSFP). For the spoiled gradient echo technique, the bright blood contrast is highly dependent on speed and direction of flow and flow jets are highly visible. For the bSSFP technique, the Bright Blood contrast depends more on the relaxation properties of blood and is more consistent, but flow jet are less visible. Cine gradient echo imaging is used to image cardiac function, ventricular wall motion and to qualitatively assess blood flow patterns.

Keywords

Fast imaging • Cardiac cycle • Cardiac synchronisation • ECG signal • Still imaging • Cine imaging • Triggering • ECG triggering • Trigger delay • Cardiac phase • Gating • ECG gating • r-wave • Prospective gating • Retrospective gating • Beat-to-beat variation • Arrhythmia rejection • Spoiled gradient echo • FLASH •

J.P. Ridgway, PhD
Department of Medical Physics and Engineering, Leeds Teaching Hospitals NHS Trust,
St James's University Hospital, 1st Floor, Bexley Wing, Leeds LS2 9TJ, UK
e-mail: j.p.ridgway@leeds.ac.uk

© Springer International Publishing 2015
S. Plein et al. (eds.), *Cardiovascular MR Manual*,
DOI 10.1007/978-3-319-20940-1_13

T1-FFE • SPGR • Spoiler gradient • Balanced steady state free precession • bSSFP • TrueFISP • bFFE • FIESTA

Imaging the beating heart is a challenge for MR imaging. To capture an image of the heart that is unaffected by motion would require an image to be acquired in just a few tens of milliseconds. In Chap. 8 it was shown that the minimum possible image acquisition time is limited by the repetition time and the need to acquire a sufficient number of phase encoding steps to achieve a particular image matrix size and therefore spatial resolution. To achieve an image acquisition in a few tens of milliseconds means both limiting the number of phase encoding steps (and thus the spatial resolution and SNR), and making the TR as short as possible. As Chap. 15 on *fast Imaging* will show, this can be done but only at the cost of accepting a significant reduction in image quality. One of the current main focuses of the development of MR technology is to devise imaging schemes that allow the fastest possible imaging whilst maintaining acceptable image quality.

For standard MR imaging, in order to achieve acceptable image quality, the image acquisition time is too long to 'freeze' heart motion. MR signals are therefore acquired over several heart beats, synchronising the pulse sequence and therefore the signal acquisition to a particular time point in the *cardiac cycle. Cardiac synchronisation* is achieved by using the patient's ECG signal, obtained by applying ECG pads and leads onto the patient's chest (Fig. 13.1)

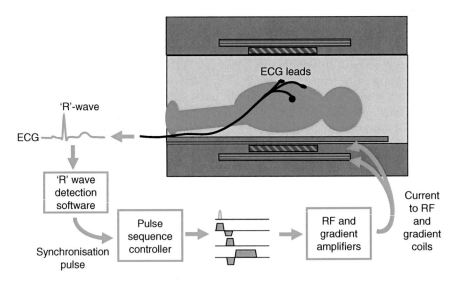

Fig. 13.1 Cardiac synchronisation is achieved by obtaining an ECG signal from the patient. A software algorithm is then used to detect the QRS complex and generate a synchronisation pulse. This can then be used as a trigger pulse to initiate the pulse sequence controller. This produces RF and gradient pulse waveforms that are amplified to drive the RF transmitter and gradient coils. This is then repeated, with each cardiac cycle triggering a new repetition of the pulse sequence

Software is used to detect the 'R' wave of the ECG and to generate a synchronisation pulse which is then used to synchronise the MR data acquisition. This enables images of the beating heart to be obtained either at a single time point (*still imaging*) or at multiple time points through the cardiac cycle (*cine imaging*).

Still Imaging

For still imaging the ECG synchronisation is known as *triggering*. The synchronisation pulse is used as a trigger to initiate the pulse sequence at a particular time point after the R-wave in each cardiac cycle. This time point is known as the *trigger delay* and is selectable by the system operator to determine the point in the cardiac cycle at which the heart is to be imaged (Fig. 13.2).

Examples of still imaging are given in Table 13.1. These techniques are used for anatomical imaging, tissue characterisation, myocardial viability assessment or coronary angiography and are discussed in more detail in Chaps. 16 and 21.

In order to improve the efficiency of still imaging, MR signal data can be acquired from multiple slice locations within each cardiac cycle (Fig. 13.3). At the end of the acquisition, the multiple slices are reconstructed with each slice acquired at a different time point in the cardiac cycle.

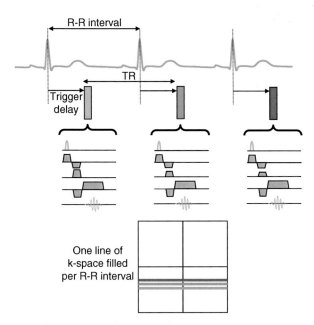

Fig. 13.2 Still imaging is achieved by acquiring data at a single time point in the cardiac cycle after the cardiac synchronisation pulse, determined by an operator-selected trigger delay. One line of k-space is filled with each heartbeat. Once k-space has been filled, a single image is reconstructed, corresponding to that time point

Table 13.1 Still imaging techniques and their common applications

'Still' imaging technique	Pulse sequence	Information
T1w or T2w Black Blood SE	Double Inversion 2D T1w SE	Anatomy and Tissue Characterisation
Black Blood STIR	Triple Inversion 2D T2w SE	Tissue Characterisation/Oedema
Late Enhancement	Inversion recovery 2D Gradient echo	Tissue Characterisation/Myocardial scar
Coronary MRA	3D Gradient echo	Coronary Vessel lumen

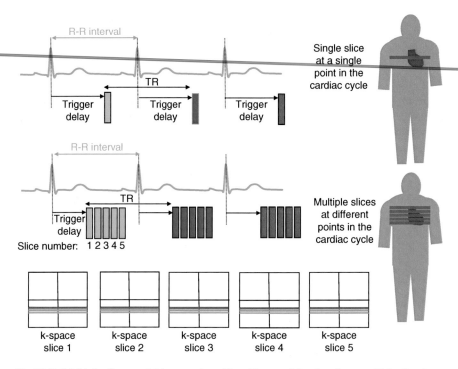

Fig. 13.3 Multiple slice acquisitions can be achieved by acquiring data from multiple slice locations at different time points within the cardiac cycle. The total imaging time is the same as for a single slice acquisition

Cine Imaging

Cine imaging involves the acquisition of data at multiple time points, known as a *cardiac phases*, throughout the cardiac cycle (Fig. 13.4). The trigger delay for the first time point is set to the shortest possible time after the R wave to enable images to be acquired from the beginning of the cardiac cycle. Data acquired within each cardiac phase fills a separate k-space, resulting in the reconstruction of a separate image corresponding to each cardiac phase. The images for all the cardiac phases

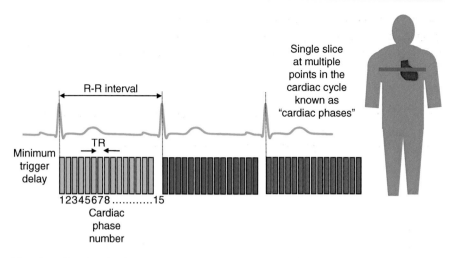

Fig. 13.4 Cine imaging is achieved by acquiring data for a single slice location at multiple time points throughout the cardiac cycle. Multiple images are then reconstructed at the corresponding time points, known as cardiac phases. These images may then be viewed as a movie to allow the visualisation of cardiac motion and blood flow patterns

are then viewed as a movie sequence or cine, allowing functional assessment of the heart, its wall motion and a visual, qualitative assessment of blood flow.

Triggering Versus Gating for Cine Imaging

For cine imaging, cardiac synchronisation can be performed in either of two ways: ECG triggering or ECG *gating.*

ECG triggering can be used to commence data acquisition immediately after the QRS complex (Fig. 13.5a). Data is then acquired for multiple consecutive cardiac phases until nearly at the end of the cardiac cycle. Data acquisition is then stopped until the synchronisation pulse from the next 'R'-wave is received. This method requires the system to estimate an average R-R interval for the patient being imaged (This can be either entered by the operator or captured from the ECG trace by the MR system). This is then used to determine the average length of the cardiac cycle over which data can be acquired and therefore how many cardiac phases can be acquired. A consequence of this approach is that there is a 'blind spot' where no data is acquired at the end of the cardiac cycle while the system waits for the next trigger pulse. This is a disadvantage if imaging of diastolic function or mitral and tricuspid valve function is important.

An alternative is to use *ECG gating* (Fig. 13.5b). Here the pulse sequence runs continuously with a short TR. The synchronisation pulse is used to mark when a repetition of the pulse sequence is coincident with the 'R'-wave. The signals from this and subsequent repetitions are then related to the corresponding time points in the cardiac cycle. This can be done either prospectively or retrospectively.

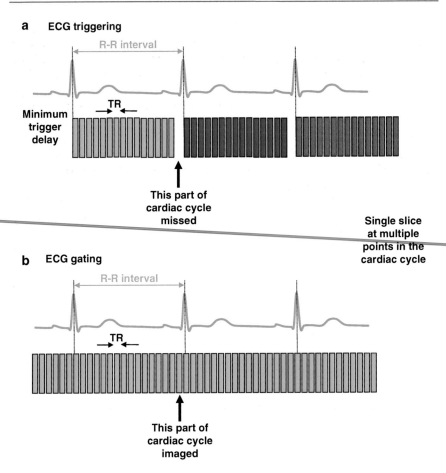

Fig. 13.5 (**a**) ECG triggering initiates the data acquisition immediately after the QRS complex and must stop before the next QRS complex. This results in the last part of the cardiac cycle not being imaged. (**b**) For ECG gating data acquisition is continuous. If the data is sorted retrospectively, data can be assigned accurately to the end of the cardiac cycle, ensuring the whole of the cardiac cycle is imaged

Prospective Versus Retrospective ECG Gating

Prospective gating allocates the MR signal data to points in the cardiac cycle as it is acquired. As with triggering, the number of imaged time points is pre-selected. This selection allows for an estimate of the shortest heart beat that is likely to occur during the acquisition. This will always lead to the last few time points in most heart beats being excluded, resulting in a 'blind spot' at the end of the cardiac cycle.

Retrospective gating allocates the MR signal data at the end of the entire k-space acquisition. This approach provides more flexibility when imaging patients with beat-to-beat variations in heart rates (most patients!) The method acquires data from the whole of each heartbeat, so that heart beats of different lengths will have different numbers of data points recorded. At the end of the data acquisition, an average heart beat interval is calculated from the whole acquisition. Data points acquired from short heart beats are stretched and data from long heart beats are compressed to fit the average heart beat interval, ensuring that all points in the cardiac cycle are imaged. This is particularly important for functional imaging where diastolic ventricular function, mitral or tricuspid valve function, diastolic flow measurement or atrial contraction are of interest.

Retrospective gating works well for normal beat-to-beat variations in the R-R interval. There is also usually an option for data points acquired from excessively long or short heart beats to be rejected and reacquired. This is known as *arrhythmia rejection*. In cases where there are many arrhythmias however, rejection of data is not practical and the only option is to use a 'real-time' image data acquisition for which ECG synchronisation is not required (see section on cine gradient echo in Chap. 16).

Spoiled Gradient Echo Versus bSSFP

In general, cine imaging requires very short repetition times to be used and therefore can only be achieved using gradient echo-based pulse sequences.

There are two main types of gradient echo pulse sequence used for cine imaging. These have the generic names, *spoiled gradient echo* and *balanced steady state free precession (bSSFP)*. MR manufacturers also have their own names for these pulse sequences and these are also given in the following sections.

Spoiled Gradient Echo

Siemens:	FLASH	Fast Low Angle Shot
Philips:	T1 FFE	T1-weighted Fast Field Echo
GE:	SPGR	Spoiled GRASS (Gradient Recalled Acquisition in the Steady State)

The need for very short TR values means that the transverse magnetisation generated by one RF excitation pulse still exists when the next RF pulse is applied. This can potentially contribute to, or interfere with, the signal during the following TR. In spoiled gradient echo, this signal is de-phased (or spoiled) using a *spoiler gradient* at the end of each TR period, so that its contribution to subsequent TR periods is removed (Fig. 13.6a). The resultant sequence, with a short TR and TE, essentially behaves as a T1-weighted pulse sequence. As a very short TR is used, tissue or blood that remains in the slice becomes saturated (Fig. 13.7). This sequence thus relies on the flow of blood to generate contrast as described in Chap. 12.

Fig. 13.6 (a) Spoiled gradient echo pulse sequence. The spoiler gradients (shown in *red*) destroy any residual transverse magnetisation prior to the next RF pulse. The contrast is therefore essentially T1 weighted. (b) SSFP Pulse sequence. Additional gradient pulses (shown in *blue*, *red* and *green*) are added to ensure that the all transverse magnetisation is in phase when the next RF pulse is applied. This modifies the contrast behaviour so that it is related to the T2/T1 ratio

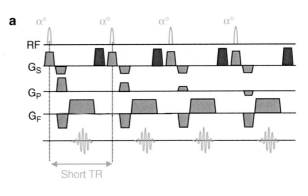

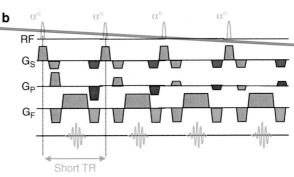

Balanced Steady State Free Precession (bSSFP)

Siemens:	True FISP	True Fast Imaging with Steady Precession
Philips:	bFFE	Balanced Fast Field Echo
GE:	FIESTA	Fast Imaging Employing Steady sTate Acquisition

Balanced SSFP gradient echo sequences are designed to ensure that the transverse magnetisation is not spoiled but fully re-phased at the end of each TR period (Fig. 13.6b) when the next RF pulse is applied. This then carries over into the next repetition and is superimposed onto the to the transverse magnetisation generated by that RF pulse. After a number of repetitions this gives rise to a steady state condition where the transverse magnetisation from two or three successive repetition periods combine to give a much greater signal.

The contrast behaviour of bSSFP sequences is very different to the spoiled gradient echo sequences (Fig. 13.7). SSFP contrast is related to the T2/T1 ratio, with fluid and fat in particular appearing as brighter than other tissues. Because the transverse magnetisation originating from several TR's are combined, the SNR for bSSFP is much greater compared to spoiled gradient echo. The increased SNR

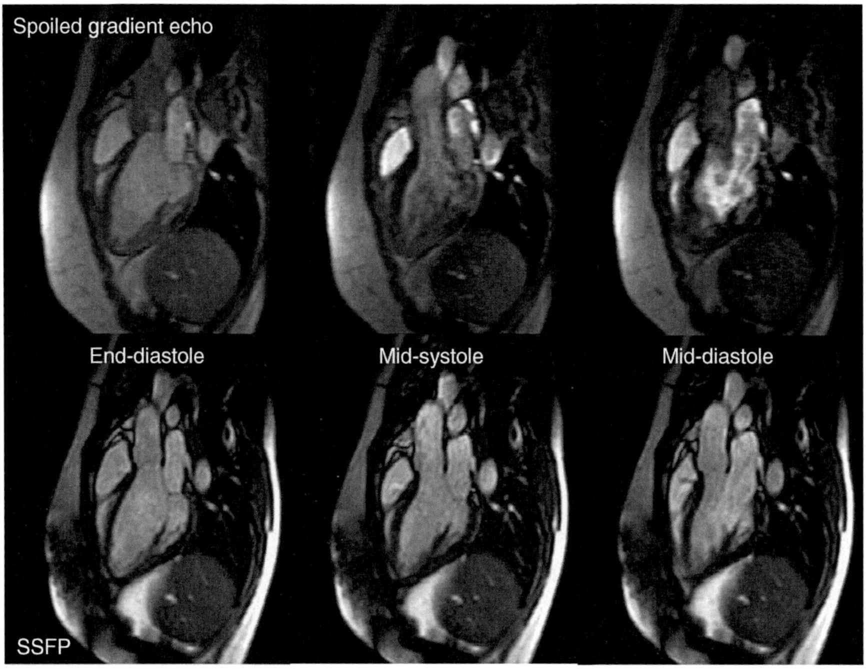

Fig. 13.7 Images taken from a cine gradient echo series using (*top row*) spoiled gradient echo pulse sequence and (*bottom row*) a balanced SSFP pulse sequence. The images shown correspond to the end diastolic, mid-systolic and mid-diastolic time points within the cardiac cycle. Note how the blood signal intensity varies through the cardiac cycle when using the spoiled gradient echo pulse sequence due to the speed and direction of flow, enabling the qualitative assessment of blood flow patterns. The blood signal intensity is more consistent through the cardiac cycle bSSFP, providing better definition of the endo-cardial boundary and the valve leaflets

allows a higher bandwidth to be used, resulting in a shorter TE, TR and therefore improved imaging efficiency. However, if the magnetic field is not uniform, the transverse magnetisation from different TRs can destructively cancel rather than add together in areas of magnetic field inhomogeneity, making the SSFP technique prone to dark banding artefacts across the image (known as off-resonance artefacts). Patient-specific dynamic shimming (see Chap. 1) is therefore very important to achieve images that are free of banding artefacts over the region of interest. Keeping the TR as short as possible also helps to minimise the banding artefacts observed in bSSFP imaging.

Cine imaging is generally used to image cardiac function and blood flow patterns. The choice of whether to use a spoiled gradient echo or bSSFP pulse sequence depends on the information required. Table 13.2 describes the most common applications of cine imaging techniques and choice of pulse sequence in each case. These are discussed in more detail in Chaps. 16 and 21.

Table 13.2 Cine imaging techniques and their common applications

Cine imaging technique	Pulse sequence	Information
Cine gradient echo	Spoiled Gradient echo	Function, qualitative flow assessment, flow jets, regurgitation
Cine SSFP imaging	Balanced SSFP	Function, volumetric measurements
Velocity Mapping	Spoiled Gradient echo	Flow velocity, flow rate
Myocardial Tagging	Gradient echo or bSSFP	Intra-myocardial motion/contraction

Summary

- In order to acquire images of the beating heart, the MR pulse sequence and data acquisition must be synchronised with the patient's ECG signal.
- Still imaging uses the ECG signal to 'trigger' the image data acquisition at a single chosen time point (trigger delay) after the R-wave.
- Still imaging is used to image cardiac anatomy, for tissue characterisation or to image the coronary arteries.
- Cine imaging acquires image data at multiple time points (cardiac phases) throughout the cardiac cycle to produce a sequence of images that can be viewed as a movie.
- Cine imaging that uses ECG triggering does not image the last part of the cardiac cycle.
- Retrospective gating allows the pulse sequence to run continuously and the acquired data is assigned retrospectively to the cardiac phases. This ensures that the whole cardiac cycle is imaged.
- Cine gradient echo imaging is used to image cardiac function, ventricular wall motion and to qualitatively assess blood flow patterns.
- Two main types of gradient echo sequence are used for cine imaging, Spoiled Gradient echo and balanced Steady State Free Precession (bSSFP).
- For the spoiled gradient echo technique, the bright blood contrast is highly dependent on speed and direction of flow and flow jets are highly visible
- For the bSSFP technique, the Bright Blood contrast depends more on the relaxation properties of blood and is more consistent, but flow jet are less visible.

Further Reading

McRobbie DW, Moore EA, Graves MJ, Prince MR. MRI from picture to proton. 2nd ed. Cambridge: Cambridge University Press; 2007. p. 282–97. Chapter 14, A heart to heart discussion: cardiac MRI.

Rehwald WG, Wagner A, Albert TSE, Sievers B, Dyke CK, Elliott MD, Grizzard JD, Kim RJ, Judd RM. Clinical cardiovascular magnetic resonance imaging techniques. In: Manning WJ, Pennell DJ, editors. Cardiovascular magnetic resonance. 2nd ed. Philadelphia: Saunders; 2010. p. 19–38.

Ridgway JP. Cardiac magnetic resonance physics for clinicians: part I. J Cardiovasc Magn Reson. 2010;12(1):71. doi:10.1186/1532-429X-12-71.

Dealing with Respiratory Motion

14

John P. Ridgway

Abstract

MR images acquired using conventional spin echo or gradient echo methods over several minutes are degraded by respiratory motion artefacts. The effects of respiratory motion can be limited by respiratory compensation or respiratory gating. Respiratory gating only accepts image data that is acquired at one phase of the respiratory cycle (usually end expiration). The respiratory position is monitored either by a pneumatic bellows device, or by the acquisition of navigator echoes. The navigator echo is produced during each cardiac cycle immediately prior to data acquisition. An RF pulse scheme excites a column of tissue that cuts through the patient's diaphragm, producing an echo which can be used to produce a trace showing the diaphragm position. This allows more accurate monitoring of the diaphragm, position for high resolution applications such as coronary artery imaging.

Keywords

Respiratory motion • Ghosting artefacts • Respiratory compensation • Respiratory curve • Respiratory gating • Navigator pulse • Navigator echo • Gating threshold • Gating window

For conventional imaging methods, the phase encoding gradient is incremented with each successive heartbeat, acquiring a single line of k-space each heart beat and resulting in imaging times of several minutes. This means that images using

J.P. Ridgway, PhD
Department of Medical Physics and Engineering,
Leeds Teaching Hospitals NHS Trust, St James's University Hospital,
1st Floor, Bexley Wing, Leeds LS2 9TJ, UK
e-mail: j.p.ridgway@leeds.ac.uk

© Springer International Publishing 2015
S. Plein et al. (eds.), *Cardiovascular MR Manual*,
DOI 10.1007/978-3-319-20940-1_14

115

these techniques are degraded by *respiratory motion* (see section on Ghosting artefacts in Chap. 17).

Image degradation caused by respiratory motion can be reduced by using one of three possible approaches:

- *Respiratory Compensation* methods (*respiratory gating*)
- Fast imaging techniques with patient breath-holding
- Ultra-fast (single-shot) imaging techniques (real-time imaging)

In practice, most cardiac imaging is performed with patient breath-holding combined with fast imaging techniques and these are described in Chap. 15. Respiratory compensation methods are described in this section.

Respiratory Compensation (Respiratory Gating)

These require the patient's respiratory cycle to be monitored. The simplest way to do this is to use a pneumatic bellows system attached to the abdomen by a Velcro band (Fig. 14.1). The data acquisition is then controlled or gated (Fig. 14.2), such that data is acquired predominantly from one part of the respiratory cycle (Usually end expiration as it is assumed that most patients spend longer periods there). Typically a gating threshold is set automatically and data from each cardiac cycle is either accepted or rejected depending on whether it is acquired either above or below the respiratory gating threshold. More sophisticated methods acquired data throughout a greater part or the whole of the respiratory cycle, but restrict the acquisition of the central lines of k-space to within the gating threshold. In this case, the phase encoding steps can be re-ordered on the fly, according to the respiratory cycle.

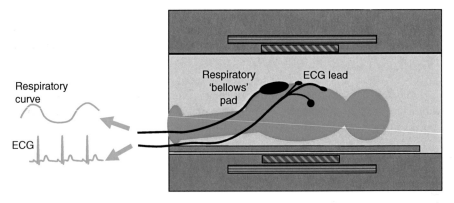

Fig. 14.1 The patient respiratory cycle is monitored by placing a pneumatic bellows device on the patient's abdomen held in place using a Velcro band. The change in pressure caused by movement of the abdomen generates a waveform that is related to the respiratory cycle

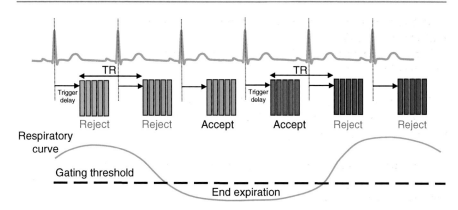

Fig. 14.2 A respiratory gating threshold is set automatically such that data is accepted as stored in k-space if the data acquisition occurs when the respiratory curve is below the threshold (assumed to correspond to end-expiration). When the respiratory curve lies above the threshold the acquired data is rejected and the same line of k-space is re-acquired until data acquisition again falls within the end-expiratory period

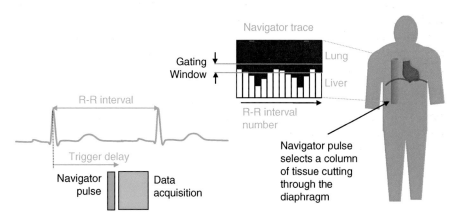

Fig. 14.3 Respiratory gating using navigator echoes uses a specially designed RF pulse (or pulses) to excite a column of tissue through the diaphragm, generating an echo immediately before each image data acquisition. A line of signal is reconstructed from each navigator echo and displayed as a trace. The boundary between the low signal intensity in the lung and the relatively high signal intensity in the liver creates an edge that can easily be detected and used as a gating signal which accurately reflects the diaphragm position and is used to determine whether the data is accepted or rejected. The accuracy of this method allows a narrow gating window to be set (typically 5 mm) for high resolution applications such as coronary artery imaging

Respiratory Gating Using Navigator Echoes

A more accurate method is to use real-time monitoring of the diaphragm position by the use of a *navigator echo* (Fig. 14.3). This method is commonly used to image the coronary arteries (see Chap. 16).

Summary

- MR images acquired using conventional spin echo or gradient echo methods over several minutes are degraded by respiratory motion artefacts.
- The effects of respiratory motion can be limited by:
  - respiratory compensation or gating
  - patient breath-holding combined with fast image acquisition
  - ultra-fast (real-time) image acquisition.
- Respiratory gating only accepts image data that is acquired at one phase of the respiratory cycle (usually end expiration).
- The respiratory position is monitored either by a pneumatic bellows device, or by the acquisition of navigator echoes.
- The navigator echo is produced immediately prior to data acquisition by an RF pulse scheme that excites a column of tissue that cuts through the patient's diaphragm.
- This allows more accurate monitoring of the diaphragm, position for high resolution applications such as coronary artery imaging.

Further Reading

Biglands JD, Radjenovic A, Ridgway JP. Cardiac magnetic resonance physics for clinicians: part II. J Cardiovasc Magn Reson. 2012;14:66. doi:10.1186/1532-429X-14-66.

Firmin D, Keegan J. Use of navigator echoes in cardiovascular magnetic resonance and factors affecting their implementation. In: Manning WJ, Pennell DJ, editors. Cardiovascular magnetic resonance. 2nd ed. Philadelphia: Saunders; 2010. p. 129–39.

Fast Imaging: How Do We Speed Up the Image Acquisition?

15

John P. Ridgway

Abstract

The key method of faster image acquisition techniques is to acquire more than one line of k-space within each heartbeat. This fills up k-space more rapidly, leading to shorter image acquisition times.

Fast (or turbo) spin echo fills multiple lines of k-space by generating a train of spin echoes with multiple 180° refocusing pulses. Fast (or turbo) gradient echo fills multiple lines of k-space within the same heart beat by the rapid repetition of several TR periods, known as a shot. The number of lines of k-space acquired in each determines the acceleration factor. Image acquisition time can also be shortened by reducing the number of phase encoding steps acquired. This can be done by reducing the image acquisition matrix or the field of view in the phase encoding direction. The symmetry property of k-space also allows image acquisition time to be reduced by sampling only just over one half of k-space, either by omitting phase encoding steps, or by not sampling first part of the echo. Parallel imaging makes use of multi-element array coils to reduce the amount of phase encoding required, resulting in faster image acquisition times.

Keywords

Fast imaging • *k*-space • Turbo spin echo • TSE • Fast spin echo • FSE • Echo train length • ETL • Turbofactor • Effective echo time • Turbo gradient echo • Fast gradient echo • Shot • Multiple shot imaging • Segmented *k*-space • Number of segments • Views per segment • Echo planar imaging • EPI • Segmented EPI • Rectangular field of view • Half Fourier • 0.5 Nex • Partial echo • Asymmetric echo • Parallel imaging • Coil sensitivity map • Reference scan

J.P. Ridgway, PhD
Department of Medical Physics and Engineering, Leeds Teaching Hospitals NHS Trust,
St James's University Hospital, 1st Floor, Bexley Wing, Leeds LS2 9TJ, UK
e-mail: j.p.ridgway@leeds.ac.uk

© Springer International Publishing 2015
S. Plein et al. (eds.), *Cardiovascular MR Manual*,
DOI 10.1007/978-3-319-20940-1_15

Conventional imaging techniques acquire only one phase encoding step (one line of k-space) per heartbeat. It therefore invariably takes several minutes to acquire an anatomical image dataset with conventional spin echo (SE) or a cine image dataset with conventional gradient echo sequences (FLASH, SPGR, FFE).

In order to overcome this limitation to achieve shorter image acquisition times, *fast imaging* techniques acquire more than one line of k-space in each heartbeat. This fills up *k-space* more rapidly, leading to shorter image acquisition times. Pulse sequences that use this principle are known as *fast* or *turbo* pulse sequences. It can be applied to both Spin Echo and Gradient echo pulse sequences.

Turbo (or Fast) Spin Echo

Philips, Siemens	TSE	Turbo Spin Echo
GE	FSE	Fast Spin Echo

The spin echo (SE) pulse sequence generates a spin echo signal by the use of an excitation pulse followed by a 180° RF refocusing pulse. Further echoes can be generated from the same transverse magnetisation by applying additional 180° refocusing pulses. Each time the echo is de-phased due to the presence of magnetic field inhomogeneities, the de-phasing can be reversed by the application of a further 180° pulse. The turbo/fast spin echo pulse sequence generates multiple echoes by applying multiple 180° pulses after the initial 90° pulse (Fig. 15.1). After each 180° pulse there is a corresponding spin echo. Each echo is used to fill a new line of k-space by applying a different amount of phase encoding to each one, prior to data sampling.

The number of echoes acquired for each excitation pulse is known as the *echo train length (ETL)* or *turbofactor* and this defines the acceleration factor for the pulse sequence. Typically echo train lengths of 15 or 16 are used in order to reduce the imaging time to within a breath-hold period. Each successive echo in the echo train has a different echo time. The amplitude of each echo diminishes as its echo time increases according to T2 decay. The echo which is acquired closest to the centre of k-space (with the smallest phase encoding gradient) defines the *effective echo time* for the sequence, as this is the echo time that has the greatest influence on the image contrast.

For cardiac imaging, fast (or turbo) spin echo pulse sequences are commonly used in combination with a double inversion black-blood magnetisation preparation scheme (see Chap. 12) to acquire anatomical images of the heart and major vessels. One or two slices are typically acquired within each breath hold period.

Turbo (or Fast) Gradient Echo

Acceleration of cine gradient echo imaging is achieved by simply repeating the gradient echo pulse sequence a number of times rapidly acquiring a number of lines of k-space within each cardiac phase (Fig. 15.2). Each group of k-space lines acquired is known as a *shot*. This is repeated for each cardiac phase and then for each heartbeat, each time acquiring a different group of lines in each successive

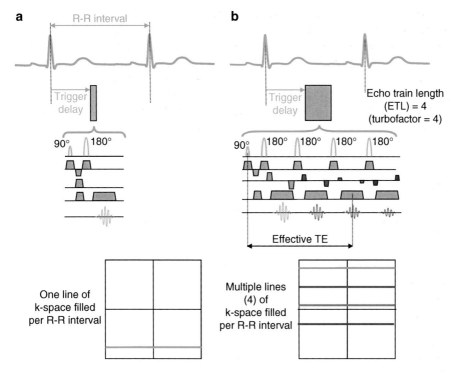

Fig. 15.1 The conventional spin echo pulse sequence (**a**) applies a single 180° pulse following the 90° pulse to generate a single spin echo. One line of k-space is filled each R-R interval. The Fast/turbo spin echo pulse sequence (**b**) applies multiple 180° pulses following the 90° pulse to generate multiple spin echoes. Multiple lines of k-space are filled within each R-R interval by applying a different amplitude of the phase encoding gradient to each echo. In this diagram each phase encoding gradient is colour coded corresponding to the line of k-space filled. The phase encoding applied to each echo is removed by applying an equal and opposite phase encoding gradient after each echo is sampled. In this example, four 180° pulses are applied to generate four spin echoes (so in this case the turbofactor = 4). This provides a fourfold reduction in scan time

heart beat until the whole of k-space is filled. This is known as *multiple shot imaging*, and is also known as *segmented k-space* gradient echo imaging, as k-space is segmented into a series of groups of lines.

The parameter that defines the number of lines of k-space acquired in each shot is dependent upon the manufacturer as follows:

Philips	Turbofactor
Siemens	No of segments
GE	Views per segment

This determines the acceleration factor for a particular pulse sequence. For functional imaging it also determines the length of the acquisition window corresponding to each phase of the cardiac cycle. Increasing the 'turbofactor' decreases the scan time (shortens the length of breath-hold) but increases the acquisition window for each cardiac phase, thus limiting the number of cardiac phases that can be imaged (the cine frame rate or temporal resolution). In order to maximise the

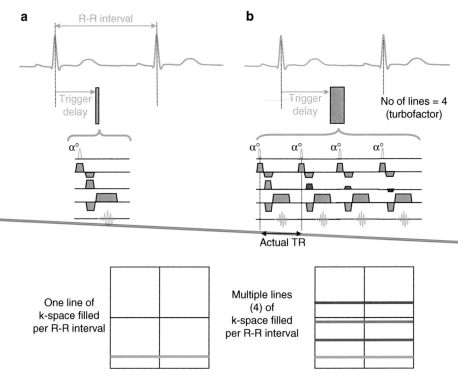

Fig. 15.2 The conventional gradient echo pulse sequence (**a**) applies a single low flip angle RF pulse to generate a single gradient echo. One line of k-space is filled each R-R interval for each cardiac phase. The Fast/turbo gradient echo pulse sequence (**b**) rapidly repeats the low flip angle RF pulse to generate multiple gradient echoes. Multiple lines of k-space are filled within each R-R interval by applying a different amplitude of phase encoding gradient to each echo. In this diagram each phase encoding gradient is colour coded corresponding to the line of k-space filled. In this example, four RF pulses are applied to generate four gradient echoes, so that the turbofactor=4 (Philips), no of segments=4 (Siemens), or no of views per segment=4 (GE). This provides a four-fold reduction in scan time

number of cardiac phases and minimise the breath-hold period, a very short TR must be used.

For breath hold cine gradient echo imaging, this method of accelerated image acquisition can be applied to both the commonly used types of gradient echo pulse sequence described in section Prospective versus retrospective ECG gating of Chap. 13. The vendor-specific names for the 'turbo' or 'fast' versions of these sequences are given below:

Fast Spoiled Gradient Echo

Siemens	TFL	TurboFLASH
Philips	T1-TFE	T1-weighted Turbo Field Echo
GE	FSPGR	Fast SPoiled GRASS

Steady State Free Precession (SSFP)

Siemens		SegmentedTrue FISP
Philips	BTFE	Balanced Turbo Field Echo
GE	FIESTA	Fast Imaging Employing Steady sTate Acquisition

When the whole of k-space is filled in a *single shot*, the cine sequence can be acquired within a single heart beat and cardiac synchronisation is no longer necessary. This is known as '*real-time*' imaging.

Echo Planar Imaging (EPI)

One of the fastest techniques available is known as *echo planar imaging (EPI)*. This is a gradient echo technique that generates multiple gradient echoes following a single RF pulse (Fig. 15.3). The first echo is generated as usual by applying a de-phasing gradient followed by a frequency encoding gradient applied in the opposite direction. Once the first echo has been sampled and de-phased, the frequency encoding gradient is then successively reapplied with alternating sign, each time re-phasing and de-phasing the transverse magnetisation to form a new gradient echo. The amplitude of each successive echo rapidly diminishes according to T2* decay so it is necessary to switch the gradient rapidly and acquire the echoes before the signal decays into the background noise level. To ensure that each echo fills a different line in k-space, a small phase encoding gradient is applied as the frequency encoding gradient is switched in order to increment the amount of phase encoding applied to each echo. In order to sample each echo as quickly as possible, a high bandwidth is used. The use of a high bandwidth, together with the low signal level caused by T2* decay, results in a low SNR for this technique. EPI is only therefore used for applications where reduced image quality is acceptable in return for greater

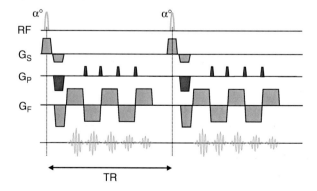

Fig. 15.3 The Echo Planar Imaging (EPI) pulse sequence is a gradient echo pulse sequence that rapidly alternates the direction of the frequency encoding gradient. Each time the gradient is switched a gradient echo is formed. Multiple lines of k-space are filled within each R-R interval by applying a small phase encoding gradient (shown in *red*) prior to sampling each echo. In this example, the frequency encoding gradient is switched five times after the initial de-phasing gradient to generate five gradient echoes. This provides a five-fold reduction in scan time

imaging speed. For cardiac imaging, a hybrid approach is often employed that combines the segmented gradient echo approach and an EPI readout with a short echo train length (known as *segmented EPI*). Such an approach has been used for perfusion imaging.

Reducing the Total Number of Phase Encoding Steps Acquired for Each Image

Another common approach to achieve faster imaging is to reduce the number of phase encoding steps required to complete the data acquisition (*scan percentage, phase percentage*). This can be done by reducing the image acquisition matrix or by reducing the field of view in the phase encoding direction (*rectangular field of view*). Both these approaches have drawbacks as illustrated by the examples in Chap. 8.

The number of phase encoding steps can also be reduced by exploiting the symmetry properties of k-space by using *half Fourier* imaging (also known as *half Nex, 0.5 Nex or half scan*). In this case the acquisition is completed when just over half the lines of k-space are acquired (Fig. 15.4). The missing information from the lines not acquired can be predicted by using the symmetry properties of k-space. Typically 65 % of the lines are acquired, giving a corresponding reduction in scan time. As fewer lines are acquired, the SNR is reduced due to the reduction in the number of signal samples (see Chap. 8).

A alternative approach is sometimes used in gradient echo imaging where less de-phasing is applied prior to echo sampling and the echo is re-phased early by the readout gradient. Because the centre of the echo occurs earlier than with full echo sampling, this results in a shorter minimum TE and shorter minimum TR, allowing faster imaging (Fig. 15.5). This is known as *partial echo* or *asymmetric echo*

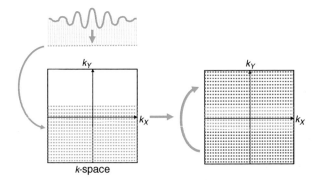

Fig. 15.4 Half Fourier image acquisition fills only about 65 % of the lines of k-space. The symmetry of k-space allows the missing information to be synthesised. The acquired lines of k-space shown in *blue* are used to synthesise the missing lines in *red*

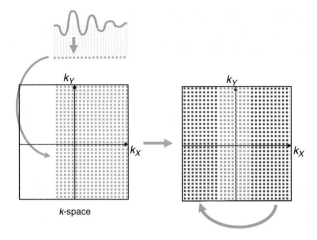

Fig. 15.5 Partial echo or asymmetric echo is achieved by applying less de-phasing to the FID so that when the readout gradient is applied the centre of the echo is attained earlier. This essentially truncates the front of the signal echo, resulting in a shorter TE and therefore a shorter minimum TR and a faster imaging acquisition. As with Half Fourier imaging, the symmetry of k-space is exploited with the acquired lines in *blue* used to synthesise the information for the missing lines in *red*

imaging. As with half Fourier imaging a reduced number of points in k-space is sampled, resulting in a reduced image SNR.

Parallel Imaging

Parallel imaging is an additional method that can be used to achieve shorter imaging acquisition times by exploiting the spatial distribution of coil elements in an array coil (Fig. 15.6). Here, the number of phase encoding steps required to reconstruct the image is reduced by a certain factor, known as the *reduction factor.* MR signal data covering the full extent of k-space is acquired, but lines of k-space spaced further apart (k-space is under-sampled). This would normally result in aliasing of information in the image. For example, for a reduction factor of 2, alternate lines of k-space are skipped. This is equivalent to acquiring a rectangular field of view of 50 %. In order to reconstruct a full field of view and avoid image aliasing, parallel imaging relies on the distribution of at least two elements of an RF coil array, along the phase encoding direction, to provide the information missed by under-sampling k-space. The reconstruction process requires knowledge of the coil sensitivity profile (a 3D plot of how the detected signal varies with distance from each coil element). By comparing the signal from each coil element, together with the coil sensitivity profile, this allows reconstruction of an image without aliasing. This reconstruction step can either be performed in the image space (SENSE) or in k-space (SMASH). A knowledge of the *coil sensitivity map* or signal intensity

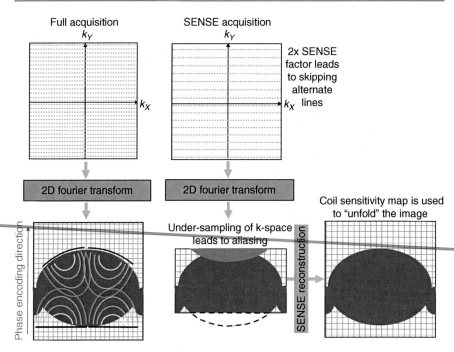

Fig. 15.6 Parallel imaging uses the spatial distribution of coil array elements and their characteristic sensitivity maps to provide spatial information. This allows under-sampling of k-space (skipping of phase encoding steps) during the acquisition, shortening the image acquisition time. In this example, a SENSE factor of 2 leads to skipping of alternate lines of k-space. Without the SENSE reconstruction this would lead to an effective reduction of the field of view and image aliasing or 'foldover'. The coil element sensitivity maps acquired from the reference data are used during the image reconstruction to 'unfold' the image to a full field of view

Table 15.1 Parallel imaging techniques offered by the different vendors

	Image based reconstruction (SENSE)		k-SPACE-based reconstruction
Sensitivity map (reference scan)	Separate acquisition	Concurrent	Concurrent
Philips	SENSE		
Siemens		mSENSE	GRAPPA
GE	ASSET		ARC

SENSE SENSitivity Encoding, *mSENSE* modified SENSE, *GRAPPA* GeneRalised, Autocalibrating Partially Parallel Acquisition, *ASSET* Array Spatial Sensitivity Encoding Technique, *ARC* Autocalibrating Reconstruction for Cartesian Sampling

distribution for each patient, coil array element and image slice geometry is essential for this technique to work. Sensitivity maps are formed from the central lines of k-space and can either be acquired as a separate *reference scan* with SENSE, or concurrently as part of the acquisition (mSENSE, GRAPPA). The most common parallel imaging techniques and their acronyms currently supplied by MR equipment vendors is summarised in Table 15.1.

Summary
- The key principle of fast imaging techniques is to acquire more than one line of k-space within each heartbeat.
- This fills up k-space more rapidly, leading to shorter image acquisition times.
- Fast (or turbo) spin echo fills multiple lines of k-space by generating multiple spin echoes with multiple 180° refocusing pulses.
- Fast (or turbo) Gradient echo fills multiple lines of k-space within the same heart beat by rapid repetition of several TR periods (a shot).
- The number of lines of k-space acquired in each determines the acceleration factor:
  - turbofactor (Philips)
  - no of segments (Siemens)
  - no of views per segment (GE)
- The symmetry property of k-space also allows image acquisition time to be reduced by sampling only just over one half of k-space, either by omitting phase encoding steps (Half Fourier, Half Scan, Half NEX) or by not sampling first part of the echo (Partial Echo, asymmetric echo).
- Parallel imaging exploits the spatial distribution of elements of array coils to reduce the amount of phase encoding required, resulting in faster image acquisition times.

Further Reading

Balaban RS, Peters DC. Basic principles of cardiovascular magnetic resonance. In: Manning WJ, Pennell DJ, editors. Cardiovascular magnetic resonance. 2nd ed. Philadelphia: Saunders; 2010. p. 3–18.

Glockner JF, Hu HH, Stanley DW, Angelos L, King K. Parallel MR imaging: a user's guide. Radiographics. 2005;25:1279–97. doi:10.1148/rg.255045202.

McRobbie DW, Moore EA, Graves MJ, Prince MR. MRI from picture to proton. 2nd ed. Cambridge: Cambridge University Press; 2007. p. 346–73. Chapter 17, The parallel universe: parallel imaging and novel image acquisition.

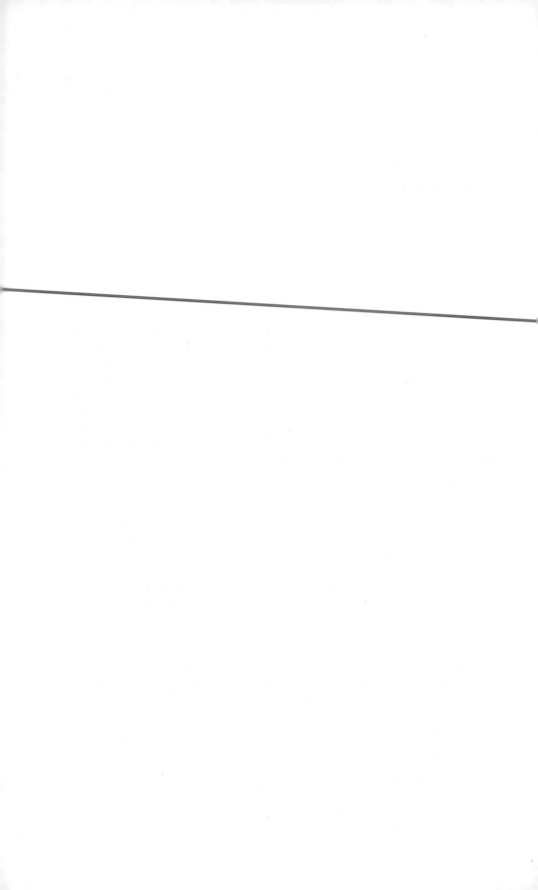

Special Pulse Sequences for Cardiac Imaging

16

John P. Ridgway

Abstract

Fast/turbo spin echo pulse sequences and fast/turbo gradient echo pulse sequences, in combination with magnetisation preparation schemes used to modify contrast or suppress signal from specific tissues or regions, form the basis for all advanced cardiac MR imaging techniques: Spatially selective tissue saturation and frequency-selective fat suppression are used to suppress unwanted tissue signal. Black blood preparation schemes are combined with T1- and T2-weighted fast/turbo spin echo for anatomical imaging. Black blood preparation is also combined with turboSTIR technique to provide fat suppression and high fluid signal weighting for imaging of myocardial oedema. Inversion recovery fast/turbo gradient echo is used with a contrast medium for imaging of myocardial infarction (late gadolinium enhancement imaging). Coronary artery imaging uses a combination of 3D fast/turbo gradient echo with respiratory navigator gating. Retrospectively-gated cine gradient echo imaging is used for functional imaging, while velocity-encoded cine gradient echo imaging is used for flow quantification. The assessment of intra-myocardial contraction is possible using myocardial tagging pulses combined with cine gradient echo imaging and myocardial perfusion assessment uses of a saturation-recovery preparation scheme combined with a single-shot, fast gradient echo pulse sequence to image dynamic contrast enhancement within the myocardium.

Keywords

Fast spin echo • Turbo spin echo • Fast gradient echo • Turbo gradient echo • Preparation pulses • Magnetisation preparation • Tissue saturation • Frequency-selective fat suppression • Fat suppression • Spoiler gradient • Inversion recovery

J.P. Ridgway, PhD
Department of Medical Physics and Engineering, Leeds Teaching Hospitals NHS Trust,
St James's University Hospital, 1st Floor, Leeds LS2 9TJ, UK
e-mail: j.p.ridgway@leeds.ac.uk

© Springer International Publishing 2015
S. Plein et al. (eds.), *Cardiovascular MR Manual*,
DOI 10.1007/978-3-319-20940-1_16

• IR • Time from inversion • TI • Short TI inversion recovery • STIR • TurboSTIR • Black blood TSE • Black blood FSE • Black blood turboSTIR • Triple inversion recovery • Myocardial oedema • Contrast agent • Gadolinium • Paramagnetic • Late gadolinium enhancement • LGE • Delayed enhancement • Viability imaging • TI scout • Coronary artery imaging • Three-dimensional gradient echo • Navigator echo • T2 preparation • Cardiac function • Bright blood cine gradient echo • Retrospective gating • Balanced SSFP • Spoiled gradient echo • Blood flow • Velocity mapping • Bipolar gradient • Phase map • Velocity map • Velocity range • VENC • Tagging • Myocardial tagging • Binomial pulse

Spin echo and gradient echo pulse sequences form the basis for all the advanced pulse sequences that are used in cardiac applications. For most cardiac synchronised applications, the 'Fast' or 'turbo' variant of the pulse sequence is used, i.e. *fast* or *turbo spin echo* and *fast* or *turbo gradient echo* (see Chap. 15). Depending on the application, further pulses may be added as *preparation pulses* in order to modify the contrast or to suppress the signal from particular tissue types or regions. The addition of preparation pulses is known as m*agnetisation preparation*. The following sections describe the most common preparation scheme and pulse sequence combinations that are in use for cardiac imaging. Where possible, the common generic and vendor-specific names are given for each technique.

Selective Tissue Saturation

Common Names: Sat Bands

REST Slabs

Spatially selective tissue saturation is a magnetisation preparation scheme that is used to suppress the signal from a prescribed region of tissue. It may be a region that is outside the field of view in the phase encoding direction, where the signal is suppressed in order to prevent aliasing (see Chap. 17), or a region that is subject to physiological motion (respiratory, peristaltic or swallowing) in order to prevent motion artefacts (see Chap. 17). Saturation regions may also be used to suppress the signal from blood flowing into the image slice to remove artefacts caused by pulsatile blood flow (see Chap. 17). In this case they are positioned at an upstream location parallel to the image slice. The saturation region is selected as a slab (thick slice) of tissue, by using a selective 90° RF pulse in combination with one or more selection gradients (Fig. 16.1). The combination of gradients determines the orientation of the slab. The RF pulse saturates the magnetisation within the slab and the transverse magnetisation is de-phased using a Spoiler gradient. The pulse sequence used for image data acquisition is then applied immediately afterwards. As the magnetisation of the tissue within the slab is saturated, it does not contribute any signal

Fig. 16.1 Selective tissue saturation is achieved by applying a 90° saturation pulse in combination with selection gradients immediately prior to the imaging pulse sequence (in this case, spin echo). This causes saturation of the magnetisation within a slab of tissue. The spoiler gradient de-phases any signal contribution from the saturation region

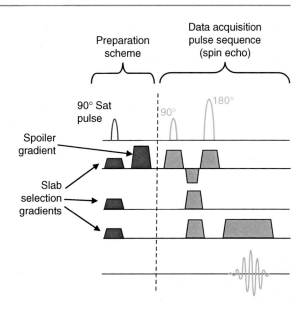

and the region appears on the image as a signal void. Saturation regions can be placed by the operator manually using the graphical user interface and for some applications they may be placed automatically.

Application	Placement of saturation region
To prevent aliasing	Slab at right angles to image slice, over the tissue outside the field of view in the phase encoding direction
To prevent motion artefact (respiratory, peristaltic, swallowing)	Slab at right angles to image slice, over the tissue that is moving and in line with the region of interest in the phase encoding direction
To prevent suppress signal from flowing blood.	Slab parallel and adjacent to the image slice, upstream relative to the direction of flow.

Frequency Selective Fat Suppression

Common Names:	CHESS (CHEmical Shift Selective) pulse
(GE, Siemens)	Fat Sat
(Philips)	SPIR (Spectral Inversion Recovery)
	(SPIR is not really inversion recovery; it uses a 120° RF pulse, producing a partial inversion)

The suppression of signal from fat is often desirable as the high intensity fat signal can mask other lower intensity features. One method of achieving this is to exploit the difference in Larmor frequency between the hydrogen nuclei in lipid molecules

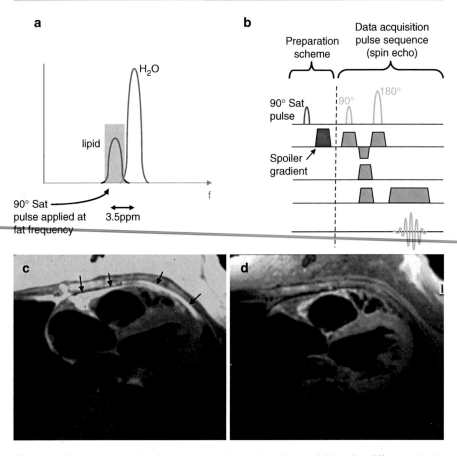

Fig. 16.2 Frequency selective fat suppression is achieved by exploiting the difference in the Larmor frequency between lipid and water (**a**). The fat suppression preparation scheme applies a 90° saturation pulse at the Larmor frequency of fat immediately prior to the imaging pulse sequence (**b**). The transverse magnetisation produced by this pulse is suppressed by a spoiler gradient. As the magnetisation of fat is saturated (reduced to zero), it does not contribute to the signal generated by the spin echo pulse sequence. The image in (**c**) is acquired using a T1-weighted spin echo pulse sequence and an anterior surface receiver coil. Bright signal from pericardial fat is seen anterior to the heart. The image in (**d**) is acquired using the same pulse sequence, but with a frequency selective fat suppression pulse. Note that the signal from fat is now suppressed, providing better assessment of the myocardial thickness around the right ventricular outflow tract

and water molecules (see also section on "Chemical shift artefact" in Chap. 17). There is a difference of 3.5 parts per million in the frequency between them (Fig. 16.2a). At 1.5 T this is a difference of approximately 220 Hz. The signal from the lipid molecules is suppressed by applying a 90° RF pulse at the Larmor frequency of fat (Fig. 16.2b). As no magnetic field gradient is applied, this pulse will saturate (reduce to zero) the z-magnetisation of fat within the entire imaging volume, provided that the Larmor frequency is constant (i.e. the magnetic field is uniform throughout the volume). The transverse magnetisation produced by the RF pulse is de-phased using a *spoiler gradient* and the pulse sequence used for image data acquisition is then applied immediately afterwards. As the fat magnetisation is already saturated, it does not contribute any signal and appears on the image as a signal void (Fig. 16.2c, d). For fat suppression to be effective using this method the magnetic field must be particularly uniform and dynamic shimming over the field of view is mandatory.

Pros and Cons of Frequency-Selective Fat Suppression (cf. STIR)

Pros	Cons
Can be applied to any pulse sequence (gradient echo, spin echo)	Requires dynamic shimming to ensure a highly uniform magnetic field across the region of interest.
Can be applied to T1- or T2-weighted pulse sequences without altering the intrinsic contrast	Does not work well in the presence of metal due to local magnetic field inhomogeneities
Does not introduce a significantly increase the time duration of the pulse sequence	Does not work well at low field strengths <1.0 T, where the Larmor frequency difference becomes too small

STIR and Turbo STIR

Another method of suppressing the signal from fat exploits the differences in T1 relaxation time between fat and other tissues. It uses a preparation scheme with a 180° inversion RF pulse, followed by a delay prior to the imaging pulse sequence (Fig. 16.3). This is known as an *inversion recovery* (*IR*) pulse sequence and the delay is known as the *time from inversion, TI*. The inversion pulse is usually slice selective and inverts the magnetisation of all the tissue within the image slice. During the subsequent TI period, the magnetisation of each tissue recovers according to its characteristic T1 relaxation time. As fat has the shortest T1 of all the tissues, its magnetisation is the fastest to recover back towards its equilibrium value. The TI is chosen so that the imaging pulse sequence is applied at the time when the magnetisation value of fat is zero (typically 160 ms at 1.5 T). It therefore contributes no signal to the acquired image. This particular instance of inversion recovery sequence with a short TI value is known as a *short TI inversion recovery* or *STIR* pulse sequence. It is normally combined with spin echo pulse sequences. When combined with Fast or Turbo Spin Echo it may be referred to as *turboSTIR*. In addition to the suppressed fat signal, a useful characteristic of this pulse sequence is the high signal from fluid. The high fluid signal weighting can be further increased by increasing the TE to introduce T2 weighting in addition to the intrinsic T1 weighting. This pulse sequence is therefore particularly suited for the detection of inflammatory processes and oedema. For CMR applications, it is usually combined with a black-blood preparation scheme for myocardial oedema imaging (see later section in this chapter on "Black blood turboSTIR").

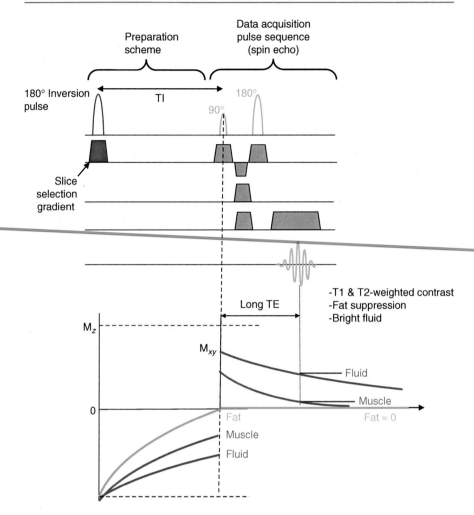

Fig. 16.3 The STIR pulse sequence consists of a slice-selective 180° inversion pulse followed by a time delay, TI, prior to the imaging pulse sequence (in this case spin echo). The inversion pulse inverts the magnetisation of all tissues. The magnetisation recovers according to the T1 relaxation time if each tissue. The TI is chosen so that the imaging pulse sequence is applied when the fat magnetisation is zero. In the resultant image, the fat signal is suppressed while fluid signal is bright

Pros and Cons of STIR (cf. Frequency-Selective Fat Suppression)

Pros	Cons
Does not require a highly uniform magnetic field & fat suppression works well in the presence of distortion of the magnetic field by metallic implants.	Single type of pulse sequence and a limited range of contrast weighting.
Combined T1 and T2 weighting gives High fluid signal, useful for oedema, inflammation.	IR pulse and TI delay significantly increases the time duration of the pulse sequence

Pros	Cons
Works well at low field strengths <1.0 T.	Cannot be used with contrast agent as this reduces the T1 of the other tissues

Black Blood FSE/TSE

The most commonly-used advanced pulse sequence for anatomical imaging combines the *black-blood preparation* scheme described in Chap. 12 with the *fast (or turbo) spin echo* pulse sequence described in Chap. 15 (Fig. 16.4a). The black blood preparation scheme provides consistently high contrast between the heart and vessel walls and the blood pool. The use of the fast (or turbo) spin echo pulse sequence with an echo train length (turbofactor) of between 15 and 20, shortens the image acquisition time so that it falls within a typical breath-hold period. One or two slices are typically acquired within each breath-hold period. Adjustment of the k-space order within the echo train controls the effective echo time and therefore the T2-weighting of the contrast. For T1 weighting (Fig. 16.4b), a short effective echo time is chosen and the pulse sequence is triggered every heart beat to keep the repetition time short. For T2 weighting (Fig. 16.4c), a long effective echo time is used

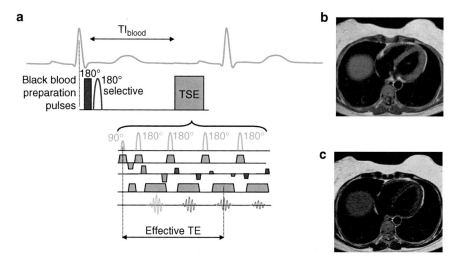

Fig. 16.4 The black blood fast (turbo) spin echo pulse sequence used for anatomical imaging (**a**). The black blood preparation scheme is applied at the beginning of the cardiac cycle with the image acquisition in diastole. The exact duration of the black blood inversion time, TI_{Blood} is calculated to provide the best blood suppression and depends on the heart rate and the number of heart beats between each trigger pulse (typically $TI_{Blood} = 400–600$ ms). The image in (**b**) is acquired with short effective echo time every heart beat to generate T1-weighted contrast. The image in (**c**) is acquired with a long effective echo time every two heart beats to generate T2-weighted contrast. Note the lower signal from the myocardium compared to that in image (**b**), due to the short T2 relaxation time of myocardial muscle

and the pulse sequence is triggered only every two or three heart beats to make a long repetition time. Frequency selective fat suppression may also be applied to suppress the signal from fat if required.

The time delay after the black blood preparation scheme is automatically calculated by the MR system software to provide the best suppression of signal from blood. This depends on the TR of the pulse sequence which is determined by the patient's heart rate and the number of heart beats between each trigger pulse.

A common problem with this pulse sequence is loss of signal from the myocardium due motion of the re-inverted myocardial tissue out if the image slice between the time of the black-blood preparation scheme and the time of the fast (turbo) spin echo data acquisition. This effect can be reduced by increasing the thickness of the slice of tissue that is re-inverted by the second 180° pulse of the black-blood preparation scheme. While the image slice thickness may be typically 6–8 mm, a typical value for the black blood inversion preparation pulse is 20 mm. The exact choice depends on how much displacement of the myocardium there is through the slice and requires some adjustment depending on the trigger delay, slice orientation and location within the heart.

Black Blood TurboSTIR (Triple Inversion Recovery)

The black blood preparation scheme can also be combined with the turboSTIR pulse sequence described earlier (Fig. 16.5). This provides a pulse sequence that has strong fluid weighting but with no signal from blood within the cardiac chambers and it is particularly useful for the assessment of *myocardial oedema*. This pulse sequence consists of the two 180° pulses for the black blood preparation, followed by a third 180° pulse to provide the STIR contrast. It is therefore sometimes known as a triple inversion recovery pulse sequence. The sequence has two inversion times, TI_{Blood} and TI_{fat}. TI_{fat} has the same value for fat suppression as in the STIR sequence (approx. 160 ms). Calculation of the value for TI_{Blood} is more complicated and depends on the heart rate, the number of heart beats between trigger pulses and whether the third inversion pulse is slice selective or not. The setting of other imaging parameter values is similar to the Black Blood FSE/TSE pulse sequence in the previous section.

Inversion Recovery Fast/Turbo Gradient Echo

Common names:	Late gadolinium enhancement (LGE)
	Delayed enhancement
	Viability imaging

Inversion recovery preparation schemes can also be combined with fast (or turbo) gradient echo pulse sequences. The most common application for this combination is for the imaging of the myocardium after intravenous administration of an MR

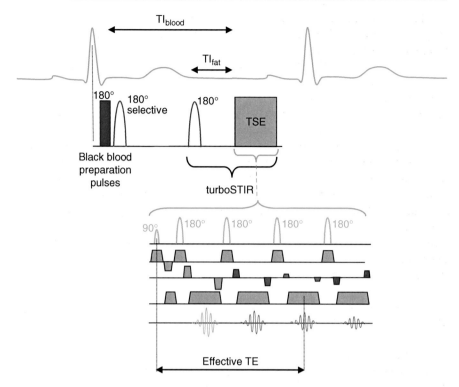

Fig. 16.5 The black-blood turboSTIR (triple inversion) pulse sequence used to achieve image contrast with a high signal from fluid. The black blood preparation scheme is applied at the beginning of the cardiac cycle with a further 180° inversion pulse approx. 150 ms prior to image acquisition in diastole. The exact duration of the black blood inversion, TI_{Blood} is calculated to provide the best blood suppression

contrast medium to differentiate viable myocardial tissue from non-viable, infarcted myocardial tissue. The *contrast agent* is based on the element *Gadolinium*. Gadolinium is a highly is a *paramagnetic* substance that mediates the T1 relaxation time of water molecules when it is in close proximity to them. The T1 relaxation time is therefore reduced, demonstrated by an increase in signal intensity when using T1-weighted imaging methods. The contrast agent is carried within the blood pool into the myocardial muscle where it enters extra-cellular space. Wash-in and wash-out of the contrast is relatively fast for normal myocardium, whereas wash-in and wash-out is delayed for infarcted muscle. Delayed imaging after contrast agent injection using a T1-weighted pulse sequence is therefore able demonstrate areas of infarction as areas with increased signal where there is a greater concentration of contrast agent. The inversion recovery technique provides T1-weighting and enhances the signal difference between normal and infarcted myocardium by suppressing the signal from normal myocardium (Fig. 16.6). The use of the fast or turbo gradient echo pulse sequence allows image acquisition to be kept within a breath-hold period. The delay required following administration of the contrast agent and

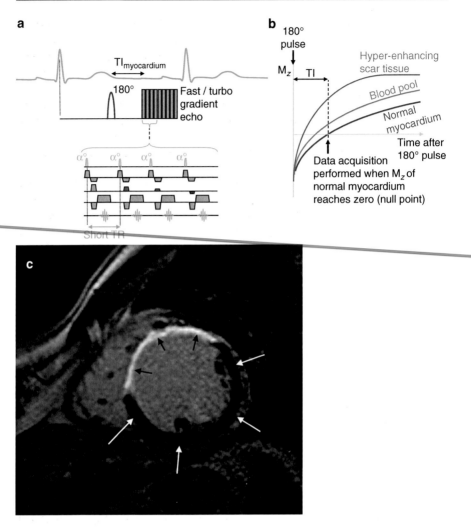

Fig. 16.6 Late Enhancement imaging is performed using an inversion recovery fast (or turbo) gradient echo pulse sequence (**a**). The fast (or turbo) gradient echo pulse sequence allows the image acquisition to be completed within a few heart beats. Image acquisition is normally performed in diastole to minimise the effects of heart motion. The 180° inversion pulse is followed by a delay, TI$_{myocardium}$, selected to suppress the signal from normal myocardium. The graph in (**b**) shows the relaxation curves for normal myocardium, the blood pool and scar tissue. The higher concentration of contrast agent within scar tissue results in a faster T1 relaxation rate and therefore an increased signal compared to the blood pool and normal myocardium. Nulling the signal from normal myocardium maximises the scar tissue contrast. The image in (**c**) shows the enhanced signal from scar tissue (*small black arrows*), and the nulled signal within the normal, viable myocardium (*white arrows*)

the enhanced signal from infracted tissue gives this technique the name *late gadolinium enhancement,* abbreviated *LGE* (previously *delayed enhancement*). As this technique is able to differentiate normal (viable) myocardial tissue from infracted (non-viable) myocardial tissue, it is also sometimes referred to as *viability imaging.*

The quality of LGE imaging depends on the effective suppression of the signal from normal myocardium. This requires very precise selection of the appropriate inversion time, $TI_{myocardium}$, which depends on many factors, including the dose of contrast, the delay after administration and the rate of renal excretion. The TI is therefore chosen by performing a number of fast, low-resolution test image acquisitions at different TIs, typically within the range from 200–250 ms in steps of 25–50 ms. The TI from the test image that demonstrates the best suppression of normal myocardium is then used to perform imaging at full resolution. This can also be achieved by performing a so-called *TI-scout,* which acquires images at multiple time delays after a single inversion pulse within the same acquisition.

Navigator-Gated 3D Fast/Turbo Gradient Echo (Coronary Artery Imaging)

Coronary artery imaging is one of the most challenging applications of cardiac MR imaging due to their small size and their motion with the cardiac and respiratory cycles. The most common pulse sequence used to image the coronary vessel lumen is a *three dimensional (3D) gradient echo* pulse sequence, combined with a series of preparation pulses to optimise the vessel contrast (Fig. 16.7). The use of a gradient echo pulse sequence for data acquisition provides a relatively enhanced signal from flowing blood. The 3D data acquisition allows thin slices to be acquired to achieve a high resolution data set (see Chap. 8). The acquisition of a high resolution 3D data set requires a long acquisition time, even when using a fast/turbo sequence. This acquisition method cannot therefore be combined with breath-holding and the acquisition must therefore be both cardiac triggered and respiratory gated.

The preparation scheme includes a RF pulse that is used to produce a *navigator echo* that is used to gate the MR acquisition with respect to the respiratory cycle (see Chap. 14). *Frequency-selective fat suppression* is used to suppress the fat signal surrounding the coronary arteries. The image data acquisition is also preceded by a *T2-preparation* scheme. This scheme uses the same series of pulses as a fast spin echo train (90°-180°-180°-180°-180°) which produces a transverse magnetisation that is T2-weighted. The final pulse in this scheme is a 90° that restores this magnetisation along the z-axis. This pulse scheme helps to suppress the signal from the myocardium (short T2) relative to the blood signal (long T2).

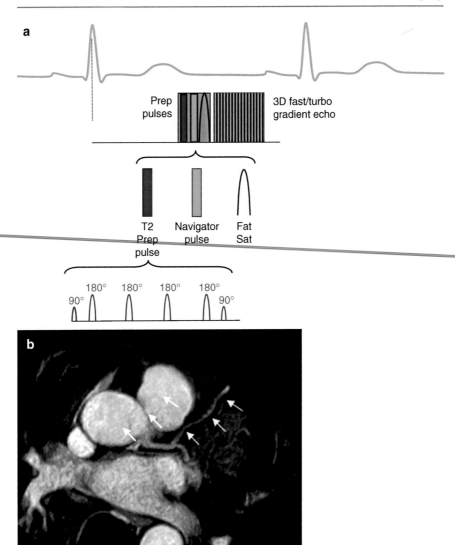

Fig. 16.7 Navigator-gated three dimensional (3D) fast gradient echo pulse sequence for coronary artery imaging (**a**). The preparation scheme consists of a T2-preparation pulse, a navigator RF pulse and a frequency selective fat suppression pulse. The data acquisition window is positioned in mid-diastole to minimise the effect of cardiac motion. The coronary artery image in (**b**) is generated from a 3D data set acquired using the pulse sequence in (**a**). This produced by post-processing the 3D data set on a workstation to produce a curved reformat that follows the course of the left anterior descending artery (*arrows*)

Key Features of a Navigator-Gated 3D Coronary Artery Imaging Sequence

Fast/turbo Gradient echo Pulse sequence	Enhanced signal from flowing blood and fast image data acquisition window (short TR)
3D data acquisition	Thin slices, high isotropic resolution
Cardiac triggered with data acquisition window in mid diastole	Minimise cardiac motion
Respiratory Navigator	Minimise effects of Cardiac motion
T2 preparation pulse scheme	Enhance contrast between coronary artery and muscle
Frequency selective fat suppression	Suppress fat bright signal surrounding arteries

Cine Gradient Echo

Imaging of *cardiac function*, including the assessment of wall motion and volumetric assessment is done using a *'bright-blood' cine gradient echo* technique that acquires images at multiple heart phases which are displayed as a movie. The most common approach to cine imaging is to combine *retrospective gating* (see Chap. 13) with a fast or turbo gradient echo method (see Chap. 15). This allows imaging of the entire cardiac within a single breath-hold period (Fig. 16.8). The choice of gradient echo pulse sequence depends on the field strength and the specific application. At 1.5 T the *balanced SSFP* gradient echo sequence is used for most functional imaging applications volumetric assessments due to its high contrast between blood and myocardium throughout the cardiac cycle. The *spoiled gradient echo* pulse sequence is often used for assessment of valvular disease and flow jets, due to its greater flow sensitivity.

A key parameter for this pulse sequence is the number of lines of k-space acquired within each heart phase (turbofactor, no of segments or number of views per segment). Increasing the value of this parameter shortens the acquisition time (Chap. 15), but also increases the time between cardiac phases. This reduces the number of cardiac phases within the cardiac cycle and therefore the cine frame rate or 'temporal resolution' of the image acquisition (the ability to resolve faster motion). *'Real-Time' imaging* is achieved by selecting a very high turbofactor, such that the whole image acquisition is completed in a single cardiac phase in a single heart beat (a single-shot acquisition). Since all the phase encoding steps are acquired in a single heartbeat, cardiac synchronisation is not required for real time imaging.

Velocity Encoded Cine Gradient Echo (*Velocity Mapping*)

Qualitative assessment of blood flow patterns can be performed using cine gradient echo pulse sequences. Spoiled gradient echo (non-SSPF) pulse sequences are particularly useful for the visualisation of flow jets associated with regurgitant and

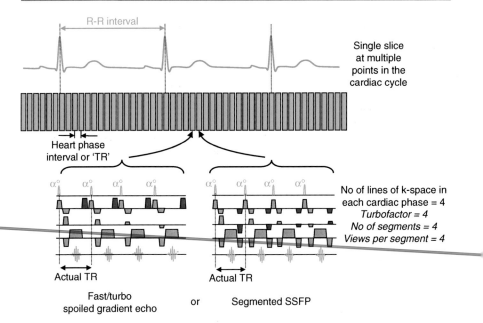

Fig. 16.8 A retrospectively-gated cine gradient echo pulse sequence used for 'bright-blood' functional imaging. Either Spoiled Gradient Echo or balanced SSFP Pulse sequences may be used for this application. The number of lines of k-space acquired in each cardiac phase (in this example=4) determines the acquisition time for this sequence (typically within a single breath-hold period). Increasing the number of lines (the turbofactor, no of segments or no of views per segment) shortens the acquisition time but increases the time between heart phases (the heart phase interval or 'TR'), resulting in poorer temporal resolution

stenotic valves, stenotic vessels and septal defects, due to their inherent sensitivity to the presence of these flow jets (see Chap. 17). This sensitivity arises due to the motion of spins within the flowing blood along the magnetic field gradients that are applied as part of the gradient echo pulse sequence. The formation of the gradient echo requires that any de-phasing of the magnetisation caused by either the slice selection or frequency encoding gradients to be reversed at the echo time (TE). This is achieved by applying two gradients along the same direction but with opposite signs. This combination is known as a *bipolar gradient* pulse pair. The second gradient reverses (re-phases) the de-phasing caused by the first gradient. For stationary tissue this is generally true, but for spins within flowing blood that change their position along the gradient during the interval between the de-phasing and re-phasing gradients, the complete reversal of the phase changes that cause de-phasing is not achieved (Fig. 16.9). As a result, the phase of the transverse magnetisation within flowing blood is different from the phase of transverse magnetisation within stationary tissue and the difference is proportional to the velocity of the blood in the direction of the applied gradient. For a certain velocity, the size of this phase difference depends on the flow sensitivity of the pulse sequence. This depends on the amplitude (or slope) of the bipolar gradients, their duration and the time interval between the two gradient pulses.

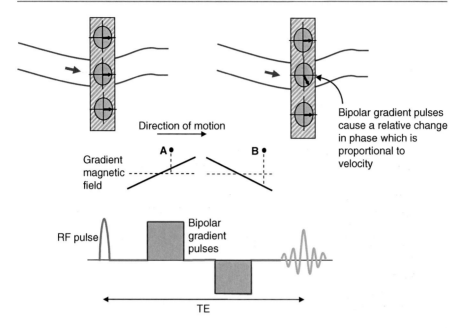

Fig. 16.9 All imaging pulse sequences use magnetic gradients for purposes such as slice selection and frequency encoding. These usually consist of two gradients applied in the same direction but with opposite sign (known as a bipolar gradient pulse pair). The second 're-phasing' gradient pulse reverses the de-phasing caused by the first gradient to ensure the transverse magnetisation is fully re-phased at the echo time, TE. Whilst this is achievable for stationary tissue, proton magnetic moments (spins) within flowing blood that move along the gradient during the time interval between the two gradient pulses do not experience the same change in magnetic field when the second gradient magnetic field is applied. The transverse magnetisation within the flowing blood therefore acquires a different phase relative to the transverse magnetisation within the stationary tissue. This difference in phase is proportional to the blood flow velocity along the direction of the gradient

This inherent flow sensitivity is exploited to enable the quantification of blood flow velocity by generating images, known as *phase maps*, which depend upon the phase of the transverse magnetisation, rather than its magnitude. There are however a number potential of causes of relative change in phase of the transverse magnetisation. These include:

- Phase changes due to motion along more than one gradient direction (multiple velocity components)
- Phase changes due to magnetic field inhomogeneities

The phase changes due to the above causes must be accounted for in order to isolate the change that is due to motion along the desired gradient direction. This is achieved by performing two consecutive acquisitions for each phase encoding step. The two acquisitions are identical other than that they have different flow sensitivities in the chosen direction of flow measurement, known as the velocity encoding

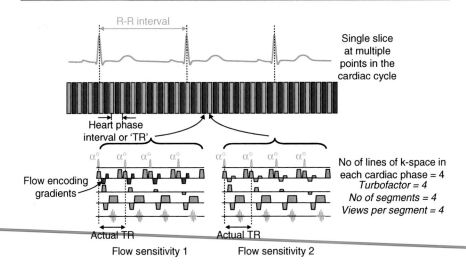

Fig. 16.10 Velocity mapping uses a fast or turbo cine gradient echo pulse sequence combined with retrospective gating. Two acquisitions are performed for each encoding step with different flow sensitivities. This is achieved by changing the amplitude of the bipolar flow encoding gradients between the two acquisitions. In this example the 4 k-space lines for each cardiac phase are played out twice; once for each flow sensitivity. Alternatively, the change in flow sensitivity may be interleaved with the change in phase encoding step. In either case the use of two acquisitions for velocity encoding doubles the time between the cardiac phases (heart phase interval or 'TR'), leading to poorer temporal resolution compared with an equivalent cine gradient echo pulse sequence without velocity encoding

direction (Fig. 16.10). The flow sensitivity and is determined by the amplitude, duration and time separation of the bipolar flow-encoding gradients in that direction. Once the image data acquisition is complete, phase maps from the two acquisitions are calculated and subtracted to produce a *velocity map*. The subtracted velocity map contains only phase shifts that are related to velocity components in the velocity-encoding direction. Phase changes due to other causes, including velocity components in other directions and magnetic field inhomogeneities are removed by the subtraction.

Velocity maps are generally displayed using a grey scale with stationary tissue being displayed as mid-grey, with velocities in forward (positive) and reverse (negative) directions being represented as higher (towards white) and lower (towards black) intensities (Fig. 16.11).

The maximum measurable *velocity range*, sometimes known as the *VENC*, is defined by the MR operator. It is determined by the difference in the flow sensitivities of the two acquisitions. The imaging of blood flow with velocities that are higher than the chosen VENC results in aliasing of the velocity value, with positive velocities being displayed as negative velocities and vice versa (Fig. 16.12). Selecting a VENC that is too low is a common pitfall of velocity-encoded cine MR imaging. The presence of flow jets or turbulence presents a further pitfall when attempting to quantify blood flow velocities as they can cause signal loss (see Chap.

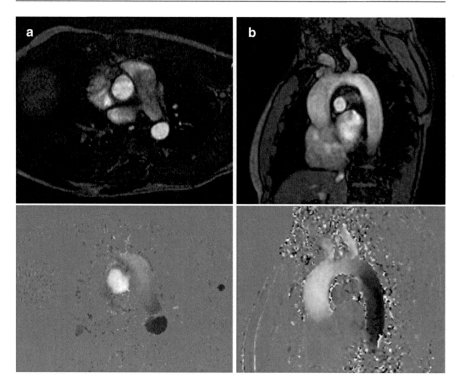

Fig. 16.11 Examples of velocity-encoded cine gradient echo imaging. The images in (**a**) show the signal 'magnitude' (*top*) and velocity map (*bottom*) of an axial slice acquired through the level of the great arteries. Velocity encoding is for through-plane flow (inferior-superior direction) with flow towards the head displayed as higher intensity grey levels (*towards white*) while flow towards the feet is displayed as lower grey levels. Stationary tissue (zero velocity) is displayed as mid-grey. The images in (**b**) show an oblique sagittal image slice through the aortic arch. In this case the velocity encoding direction is selected to be along the image plane in the superior-inferior direction. In both examples, the images shown correspond to mid-systole, and therefore show significant forward blood flow through the aorta

17). At low signal magnitudes, calculation of the signal phase becomes unreliable, resulting in spurious velocity measurements. This pitfall can be avoided by selecting a short echo time for the cine velocity mapping gradient echo pulse sequence (Fig. 16.13).

Myocardial Tagging (Binomial Preparation Pulses)

Imaging of heart wall motion is routinely performed using cine gradient echo pulse sequences. In addition, it is possible to assess intra-myocardial motion by '*tagging*' the myocardium at end diastole with a line or grid pattern, which then deforms as the heart wall contracts. *Myocardial tagging* is done using a specialised preparation scheme consisting of series of non-selective RF pulses, (together known as a

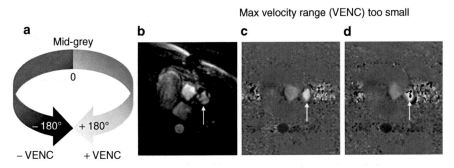

Fig. 16.12 The selection of the velocity encoding sensitivity (VENC) determines the maximum velocity that can be measured with a velocity-encoded cine pulse sequence, corresponding to a velocity-related phase shift of ±180° in the flow encoding direction (**a**). Blood flow velocities above that selected range are aliased, appearing as velocities in the opposite direction. The image in (**b**) shows a magnitude image taken from a cine series at the level of the pulmonary valve (*arrow*). (**c**) shows the corresponding velocity map during early systole, showing high forward blood flow velocity through the pulmonary value (*arrow*). The image in (**d**) shows a velocity map further into systole, where the velocity at the centre of the pulmonary outflow tract has increased to a value greater than the VENC. Velocity aliasing is seen as a few black pixels at the centre of the vessel. This acquisition would normally be repeated with a higher VENC in order to remove the aliasing

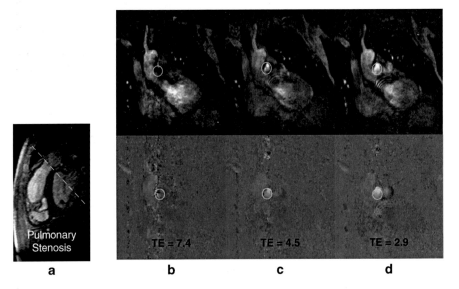

Fig. 16.13 The dotted line in (**a**) shows the image orientation used to acquire velocity encoded measurements at the level of the pulmonary valve in a patient with pulmonary valve stenosis. The subsequent images show the magnitude image (*top*) and corresponding velocity map acquired through the valve during mid-systole. A circle indicates the location of the pulmonary artery cross section. In (**b**) an echo time of 7.4 ms is used, resulting in complete loss of signal in the magnitude image and an unreliable velocity calculation. In (**c**) a shorter echo time of 4.5 ms is used, resulting in reduced signal loss, although the velocity map is still unreliable and underestimates the velocity within the pulmonary artery. In (**d**) an echo time of 2.9 ms is used, minimising the signal loss and providing a more reliable estimate of velocity

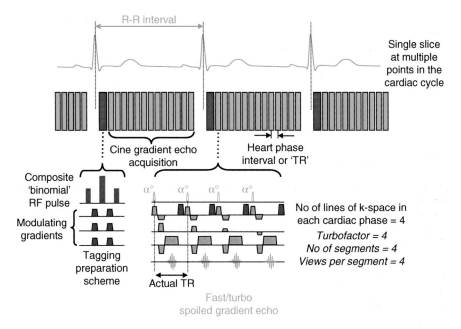

Fig. 16.14 Myocardial tagging pulse sequence with a tagging preparation scheme applied immediately after the R-wave followed by a fast cine gradient echo acquisition. The tagging preparation scheme consists of a composite 'binomial' RF pulse (in this example consisting of three non-selective RF pulses) combined with modulating gradient pulses. The modulating gradients (two gradient pulses in this example) are applied in between the RF pulses along a direction parallel to the image slice. This generates a magnetisation pattern across the image consisting of parallel lines of saturated tissue

composite or binomial pulse) combined with a series of gradient pulses, known as modulating gradients (Fig. 16.14). The effective flip angle of the composite RF pulse is around 90°. The modulating gradients are applied in between the RF pulses and along a direction that is parallel to the image slice. The tagging preparation scheme is applied immediately after the R-wave (at end diastole) and superimposes a 'magnetisation' pattern across the image slice consisting of lines of tissue that are alternately saturated or at equilibrium. A cine image data acquisition is then performed using a gradient echo pulse sequence.

On the first image of the cine series (immediately after the tagging pulse), the magnetisation pattern appears as a series of low-signal-intensity parallel lines across the image. As the heart contracts through systole the magnetisation pattern deforms as it follows the contraction of the myocardial muscle (Fig. 16.15). As the pattern is generated though saturation of the tissue magnetisation, the pattern fades during the cardiac cycle as T1-relaxation causes the magnetisation to return towards its equilibrium value. Typically two line patterns are generated at right angles to form a grid pattern. This can be done by using two tagging preparation pulses within the same acquisition (known as grid tagging), or by performing two separate acquisitions with line tagging at right angles, and subsequently combining the two data sets as a post-processing step.

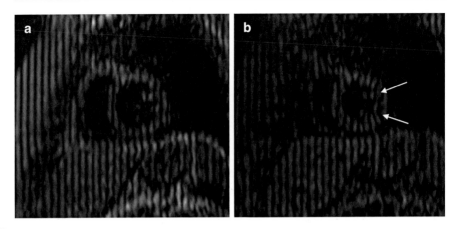

Fig. 16.15 Example images from a myocardial tagging cine pulse sequence. Image (**a**) is taken from the cine series immediately after the tagging preparation scheme has superimposed a magnetisation pattern of vertical lines across the image slice. Image (**b**) is taken from the same cine series at end-systole when the left ventricle has fully contracted. Note the deformation of the line pattern due to contraction of the myocardial muscle, especially in the left ventricular free wall (*arrows*). Analysis of the tagged line displacement can provide a quantitative assessment of myocardial strain

Saturation Recovery, Single-Shot Fast Gradient Echo for Dynamic, Contrast-Enhanced Myocardial Perfusion Imaging

Assessment of myocardial perfusion is achieved by imaging the heart during the first-pass of an MR contrast agent through the coronary circulation and the myocardial tissue. This requires a technique that is rapid enough to acquire an entire image at several slice locations within a single heartbeat. A single-shot gradient echo based technique is used for data acquisition (Fig. 16.16). Fast gradient echo, balanced SSFP and segmented EPI pulse sequences have all been used and each has advantages and disadvantages. T1 contrast is generated by using a saturation recovery (90°) preparation pulse as the effect of this pulse is independent of heart rate variations. Methods to further accelerate the data acquisition such as half Fourier imaging and parallel imaging are also commonly used in order to improve the spatial resolution of the technique.

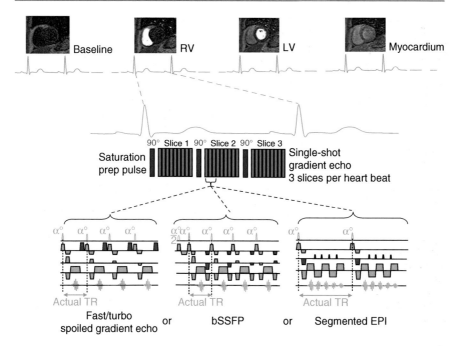

Fig. 16.16 A schematic diagram showing the key features of a myocardial perfusion imaging sequence. Imaging is performed as a dynamic series, during which a short bolus of MR contrast agent is injected intravenously. The image acquisition is performed using single-shot gradient echo-based acquisition with a 90° saturation-recovery preparation pulse. The single shot acquisition must be sufficiently rapid to enable the acquisition of a complete image at several slice locations (in this example, 3 slices) within a single heartbeat. The pulse sequence may be a fast (or turbo) gradient echo, balanced SSFP or segmented EPI pulse sequence. The saturation recovery preparation generates T1-weighted contrast so that contrast agent appears bright in areas of high concentration. Typical appearances of the images during the first pass of contrast agent through the heart are shown including a baseline image (before contrast medium arrives in the heart), as the contrast arrives in the right ventricle, the left ventricle and then as it perfuses the myocardium

Summary
- Fast (or turbo) spin echo pulse sequences and fast (or turbo) gradient echo pulse sequences form the basis for all advanced cardiac MR imaging techniques.
- Magnetisation preparation schemes are used to modify contrast or suppress signal from specific tissues or regions.
- Different combinations of the above provide the following special pulse sequences for cardiac imaging:
  - Selective (regional) tissue saturation
  - Frequency selective fat suppression
  - Use of short TI inversion recovery for fat suppression and high fluid signal weighting (STIR, turboSTIR)
  - Use of black blood preparation for T1- and T2-weighted fast(turbo) spin echo for anatomical imaging
  - Combination of black blood preparation with turboSTIR technique for imaging of myocardial oedema.
  - Inversion recovery fast (turbo) gradient echo in combination with contrast medium for imaging of myocardial infarction (Late gadolinium enhancement imaging, LGE).
  - Combination of 3D fast(turbo) gradient echo with respiratory navigator gating for coronary artery imaging
  - Retrospectively-gated cine gradient echo imaging for imaging cardiac function
  - Velocity-encoded cine gradient echo imaging for flow quantification
  - Myocardial tagging pulse combined with cine gradient echo Imaging for the assessment of intra-myocardial contraction
  - Use of a saturation recovery preparation combined with single-shot, fast gradient echo for dynamic, contrast enhanced myocardial perfusion imaging.

Further Reading

Biglands JD, Radjenovic A, Ridgway JP. Cardiac magnetic resonance physics for clinicians: part II. J Cardiovasc Magn Reson. 2012;14:66. doi:10.1186/1532-429X-14-66.

Gerber BL, Raman SV, Nayak K, Epstein FH, Ferreira P, Axel L, Kraitchman DL. Myocardial first-pass perfusion cardiovascular magnetic resonance: history, theory, and current state of the art. J Cardiovasc Magn Reson. 2008;18(10):1–18.

Ibrahim EH. Myocardial tagging by cardiovascular magnetic resonance: evolution of techniques, pulse sequences, analysis algorithms and applications. J Cardiovasc Magn Reson. 2012;13:36.

Kellman P, Arai AE. Imaging sequences for first pass perfusion – a review. J Cardiovasc Magn Reson. 2007;9(3):525–37.

Lotz J, Meier C, Leppert A, Galanski M. Cardiovascular flow measurement with phase-contrast MR imaging: basic facts and implementation. Radiographics. 2022;22:651–71. doi:10.1186/1532-429X-14-66.

Rehwald WG, Wagner A, Albert TSE, Sievers B, Dyke CK, Elliott MD, Grizzard JD, Kim RJ, Judd RM. Clinical cardiovascular magnetic resonance imaging techniques. In: Manning WJ, Pennell DJ, editors. Cardiovascular magnetic resonance. 2nd ed. Philadelphia: Saunders; 2010. p. 19–38.

Common Artefacts

17

John P. Ridgway

Abstract

The causes and remedies of a number of common image artefacts are discussed, including image examples of each. They include those that are a result of the image encoding and reconstruction process image aliasing in the phase encoding direction and image aliasing (or residual fold-over) that occurs with parallel imaging; Motion artefacts including image ghosting due to respiratory motion, image ghosting caused by pulsatile blood flow and flow-related signal loss in the presence of flow jets or turbulence with high velocity gradients; Artefacts related to differences in the resonant frequency of fat and water, including chemical shift artefact in spin echo imaging and in gradient echo imaging; Artefacts that relate to signal de-phasing caused by magnetic susceptibility differences in tissue and metallic artefacts; Artefacts that are caused by both continuous radiofrequency interference and noise spikes. The technique of flow compensation can be used to reduce motion artefacts from flowing blood. In-phase and out-of-phase gradient echo imaging exploits the chemical shift effect in gradient echo imaging.

Keywords

Artefacts • Aliasing • Fold-over • Wrap-around • Over-sampling • Parallel imaging • Residual fold-over • Ghosting • Motion artefacts • Respiratory motion • Pulsatile flow • Flow compensation • Flow-related signal void • Velocity gradient • Chemical shift • In-phase • Out-of-phase • Magnetic susceptibility • Paramagnetic • Diamagnetic • Metallic artefact • Deoxyhaemoglobin • Venous blood • Radiofrequency interference • Noise spike

J.P. Ridgway, PhD
Department of Medical Physics and Engineering,
Leeds Teaching Hospitals NHS Trust, St James's University Hospital,
1st Floor, Bexley Wing, Leeds LS2 9TJ, UK
e-mail: j.p.ridgway@leeds.ac.uk

© Springer International Publishing 2015
S. Plein et al. (eds.), *Cardiovascular MR Manual*,
DOI 10.1007/978-3-319-20940-1_17

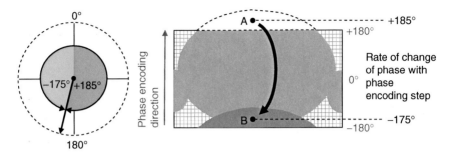

Fig. 17.1 Diagram demonstrating the cause of image aliasing or fold-over. The phase encoding process is designed to encode locations in the phase-encoding direction only within the pre-defined field of view. As the phase encoding gradient is incremented, the phase of the transverse magnetisation at locations within the field view, changes with steps in the range of from +180° to −180°, enabling reconstruction at the correct location The location at A, outside the field of view, has a phase that changes in steps of +185°. This is indistinguishable from the phase change of −175° at point B, inside the field of view. Signal from point A therefore appears at point B

Image Aliasing

Common Names:	*Aliasing*
	Fold-over
	Back-folding
	Wrap-around

Image *aliasing* occurs when the imaged subject is larger than the field of view in the phase encoding direction. Aliasing is a consequence of the phase encoding process: Whilst the number of phase encoding steps used to complete the image acquisition is sufficient to uniquely encode all the locations within the field of view, locations outside the field of view are not uniquely encoded (Fig. 17.1). At the edge of the field of view, the phase increments in steps of 180° with each phase encoding step (see Chap. 6). A little further beyond the edge of the field of view (point A) phase changes in steps of 185° are indistinguishable from phase changes in steps of -175° corresponding to locations just inside the opposite edge of the field of view. Signal originating at point A is therefore reconstructed to appear at point B and aliasing occurs (Fig. 17.2a).

A number of common solutions that can be used to reduce or remove image aliasing are listed in Table 17.1.

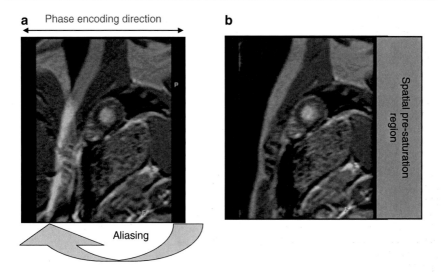

Fig. 17.2 Short-axis image of the heart (**a**) showing aliasing of signal from the posterior chest wall from outside the field of view onto the anterior chest wall. The use of a Selective Tissue Saturation Region placed outside the field of view posteriorly (**b**) suppresses the signal from the posterior chest wall and removes the aliased signal

Table 17.1 Common solutions to remove/reduce image aliasing

Solution	Disadvantage/comment
Increase field of view	Reduced spatial resolution
Acquire additional phase encoding steps (phase-oversampling, fold-over suppression, no phase wrap)	Increases image acquisition time
Swap phase and frequency direction	May introduce aliasing in the other direction
Use selective tissue saturation (Sat bands). See Fig. 17.2b.	Slight increase in image acquisition time
Use a surface coil or switch off unwanted elements of array coil	May reduce SNR over part of region of interest

Why Doesn't Aliasing Occur in the Frequency Encoding Direction?
In theory aliasing could also occur in the frequency encoding direction but this is easily avoided by data *over-sampling*. Over-sampling doubles the rate at which the MR signal echo is digitally sampled to acquire double the number of data samples. This doubles the frequency range (bandwidth) that can be

accurately detected, effectively doubling the field of view in the frequency encoding direction. Once the image has been reconstructed, image data outside the prescribed field of view is discarded. As over-sampling when frequency encoding is achieved by doubling the sampling rate, the sampling time of the MR signal echo is unchanged and there is no penalty of increased imaging time (unlike phase-oversampling). Frequencies originating from outside the prescribed field of view can also be easily removed prior to image reconstruction by electronic or digital filtering with high-pass filters as the signal is digitally sampled and stored. Both of these methods are commonly used in practice.

Aliasing Artefacts with Parallel Imaging

| Common Name: | *Residual fold-over* |

Image aliasing can be a particular problem when using parallel imaging techniques such as SENSE. These techniques achieve a reduction in image acquisition time by reducing the number of acquired phase encoding steps, and under-sampling k-space. This has the same effect as reducing the field of view in the phase encoding direction, which causes image aliasing. The subsequent SENSE reconstruction, making use of coil sensitivity information, removes any aliasing due to this under-sampling process and reconstructs a full field of view image. If the field of view in the phase encoding direction after SENSE reconstruction is still too small to encompass the subject, this will cause aliasing that cannot be removed by the SENSE reconstruction. Furthermore, it appears at the centre of the image rather than the edge (Fig. 17.3).

The approaches to remove SENSE aliasing artefacts are the same as the approaches listed in Table 17.1 for standard aliasing. An additional option here is to fractionally reduce the SENSE factor at the expense of a slightly longer acquisition time.

Ghosting Artefacts from Motion (Respiratory)

Patient motion during the image acquisition typically results in smearing or ghosting of signal across the image in the phase encoding direction. This is because the phase encoding process is the method by which signal is correctly assigned to a location in the phase encoding direction. If tissue is changing position between each TR (or phase encoding step) this leads to misplacement of the signal in the image. Motion that is random or asynchronous with the TR typically results in smearing of signal in the phase encoding direction. A typical example of such an artefact is that caused by *respiratory motion* (Fig. 17.4).

Motion artefacts are more prominent when the motion occurs when the data acquisition is close to the centre of k-space (usually the middle of the image acquisition). Motion that is more periodic (cardiac or respiratory will result in discrete,

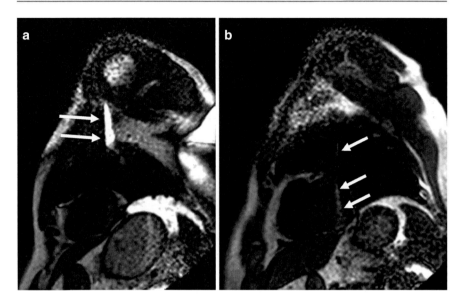

Fig. 17.3 (**a, b**) Short axis images taken from a dynamic series of saturation recovery-prepared gradient echo perfusion imaging sequence acquired with parallel imaging (SENSE factor 2). Note the SENSE aliasing artefact at the centre of the field of view (*straight arrows*). In these examples the artefact could be removed by repeating the acquisition after re-centring the field of view to the right, ensuring that the posterior chest wall is included in the field of view

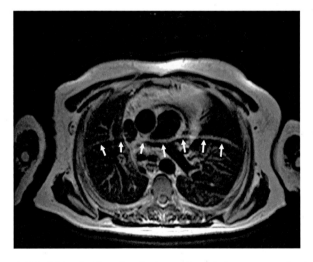

Fig. 17.4 An axial black-blood turbo spin echo image through the great vessels where the patient has been unable to completely suspend respiration. A respiratory ghost artefact is clearly seen (*arrows*). Note that the shape of the artefact is the same as the anterior chest wall, suggesting that this is the main source of the artefact

repeated ghosts in the phase encoding direction. Motion that has a periodicity that is close to a multiple or the pulse sequence TR results in particularly strong ghosting common solutions to remove or reduce respiratory ghosting are given in (Table 17.2).

Table 17.2 Common solutions to remove/reduce respiratory ghosting

Solution	Comment
Patient breath-holding combined with Fast Imaging techniques	Limits acquisition time and therefore spatial resolution
Respiratory gating using bellows or Navigator echoes	Increases image acquisition time (due to rejection of data.
Swap phase and frequency direction	May introduce ghosting in the other direction
Use selective tissue saturation (sat bands) to suppress the signal from anterior abdominal wall	Slight increase in image acquisition time

Ghosting Artefacts from Motion (Pulsatile Flow)

Another type of *ghosting* caused by motion is that seen from blood vessels carrying *pulsatile blood flow*. Even if the vessel itself is not moving during the cardiac cycle, ghosts are often still visible. This is particularly common with arterial vessels that carry highly pulsatile blood flow, or with pulsatile cerebrospinal fluid (CSF) motion in the spinal column. The ghosting in this case is due to motion of proton magnetic moments (spins) in the blood (or CSF) along the gradient magnetic fields used for imaging. Motion along magnetic field gradients results in the transverse magnetisation of flowing blood having a different phase relative to that of stationary tissue (see section on "Velocity-encoded cine imaging" in Fig. 16.9). This relative phase difference is proportional to the velocity of motion. If the blood flow velocity is constant, the relative phase difference is always the same and is ignored by the image reconstruction process. For pulsatile flow, unless the pulse sequence is synchronised with the cardiac cycle, the velocity, and therefore, the relative phase difference, will be different for each repetition of the pulse sequence. The varying phase change with each repetition is misinterpreted by the image reconstruction process as being a result of the phase encoding process. This results in a series of ghost images of the vessel appearing in line with the true vessel in the phase encoding direction (Fig. 17.5). Common solutions for removal of ghosting related to pulsatile flow are given in Table 17.3

What Is Flow Compensation?
Flow compensation applies a modification to the gradient pulses to reduce the flow sensitivity of a pulse sequence. It is normally achieved by adding one or more gradient pulses to the pulse sequence where there is already a bipolar gradient pulse. The purpose of the additional gradient pulse(s) is to reduce or nullify the velocity-dependent phase shift caused by motion along the gradient. This reduces flow de-phasing and ghosting artefacts from pulsatile flow.

Common Names:	Flow compensation
	Gradient moment nulling
	Gradient motion re-phasing

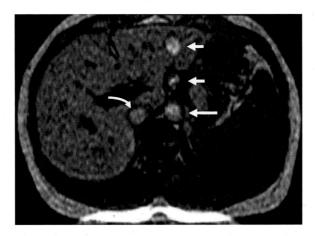

Fig. 17.5 An axial spoiled gradient echo image through the abdomen showing the abdominal aorta (*large arrow*) and ghosting due to pulsatile blood flow (*small arrows*). Note that absence of ghosting from the much less pulsatile inferior vena cava (*curved arrow*). The phase encoding direction is anterior-posterior. Note also aliasing from the anterior abdominal wall onto the posterior abdominal wall

Table 17.3 Common solutions to remove/reduce ghosting from pulsatile flow

Solution	Comment
Use cardiac synchronisation (ECG triggering or gating) (Chap. 13)	Limits acquisition time and therefore spatial resolution
Use flow compensation (see box)	Increases image acquisition time (increases minimum TE)
Use selective tissue saturation parallel to the image slice positioned 'upstream' (parallel sat bands) to suppress the blood signal flowing into the slice. (See section on this in Chap. 16).	Slight increase in image acquisition time
Swap phase and frequency direction	May introduce ghosting in the other direction

Flow Related Signal Loss & Flow Jets

Gradient echo-based pulse sequences normally produce images with a 'bright-blood' appearance. In the presence of flow jets however, a signal void is often seen at the location of the jet (Fig. 17.6). This effect is commonly observed when imaging regurgitant valves, stenotic vessels or flow through septal defects. The signal void is caused by a de-phasing of the magnetisation in the presence of the jet. This is another consequence of the velocity-related phase shift caused by motion along the magnetic field gradients (section on "Velocity-encoded cine imaging" in Fig. 16.9). The flow jet contains a large range of velocities (sometimes referred to as a *velocity gradient*). This causes a large range of phase shifts, causing de-phasing of the transverse magnetisation and therefore resulting in signal loss. The *flow-related signal void* is often qualitatively related to the size and severity of the flow jet and is

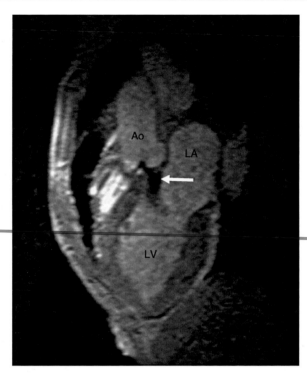

Fig. 17.6 An image taken from a cine gradient echo series, corresponding to diastole. The image is a left ventricular outflow tract (LVOT) view, showing the Aorta (*Ao*), Left Ventricle (*LV*) and Left Atrium (*LA*). The aortic valve is closed while the mitral valve is open. Note the signal void due to the regurgitant flow jet through the aortic valve (*arrow*)

Table 17.4 Common solutions to remove/reduce flow-related signal loss

Solution	Comment
Reduce echo time.	A TE of less than 3.5 ms significantly reduces signal loss (Kilner et al. 1991) but may require use of a high receiver bandwidth, and or partial (asymmetric) echo sampling, reducing SNR
Use flow compensation (see box)	Increases image acquisition time (increases minimum TE)
Use a balanced SSFP pulse sequence	Balanced SSFP pulse sequences are less flow sensitive than spoiled gradient echo pulse sequences

sometimes used to grade regurgitation for example. Qualitative assessment of this kind must be done with caution, as the size of the signal void also depends on the pulse sequence type, the echo time and a number of other parameters that affect the imaging gradients strength and duration. For example, increasing the echo time increases the apparent size of the flow jet. Additionally, the same flow jet visualised using a balanced SSFP pulse sequence is smaller than when visualised using a spoiled gradient echo pulse sequence with equivalent imaging parameters. Common approaches used to reduce flow-related signal loss are summarised in Table 17.4.

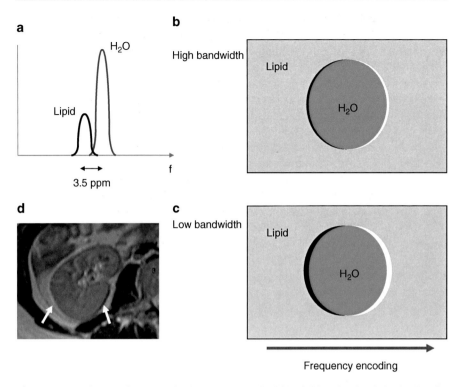

Fig. 17.7 The Larmor frequency for hydrogen nuclei within lipid molecules is lower that the Larmor frequency for those within water molecules (**a**). This results in a relative shift in the true position of lipid-based tissue and water-based tissue in the frequency encoding direction (**b**). This shift is increased when selecting a lower bandwidth (**c**). This results in bright (signal overlap) or dark (signal gap) artefacts at the interfaces between water and lipid-based tissues, such as the kidneys surrounded by fat (*arrows* in **d**)

Chemical Shift Artefact

Chemical shift artefact occurs due to the difference in resonant frequency between fat and water-based tissue. The Larmor frequency for hydrogen nuclei within lipid molecules is lower than that within water molecules by approximately 3.5 parts-per-million (Fig. 17.7a). This shift in frequency, due to the difference in the molecular structure of these two molecules is known as the *chemical shift*. The way in which chemical shift artefacts appear depends on the pulse sequence and its imaging parameters.

When using Spin Echo-based pulse sequences, the chemical shift artefact is most commonly seen when a low imaging bandwidth is selected (e.g. on T2-weighted imaging). As frequency is used to encode position, (in the frequency encoding direction), the signals from fat and water based tissues become misregistered relative to one another in the frequency encoding direction (Fig. 17.7). This effect is particularly marked when using a low imaging bandwidth as the bandwidth corresponding to each pixel becomes comparable to, or smaller than the chemical shift between fat and water. The amount of mis-registration may be several pixels, resulting in overlapping of signal at some interfaces and a gap in signal at others.

When using gradient echo pulse sequences, a second chemical shift artefact effect is seen as a signal void in pixels that contain both fat and water-based tissue. This is again the result of the signals from the lipid and water at the same location having different frequencies. Immediately after the RF excitation pulse the two signals are in phase but gradually move out of phase as the signals evolve until they cancel (Fig. 17.8). At a later time, they move back into phase, their signals combining. As the two signals continue to evolve, they alternately move out of phase and back into phase. The time at which the gradient echo is sampled (the TE) will determine whether the signals cancel or combine. If the TE for the pulse sequence is chosen to coincide with the point when the signals cancel, all pixels containing fat and water appear as a signal void (out-of-phase image, Fig. 17.9a). If the echo time is chosen at the point where the signals are in phase and combine then the same pixels will have a high signal (in-phase image, Fig. 17.9b). As this effect depends on the difference in Larmor frequency between fat and water, the chosen echo times will depend on field strength (see Table 17.5).

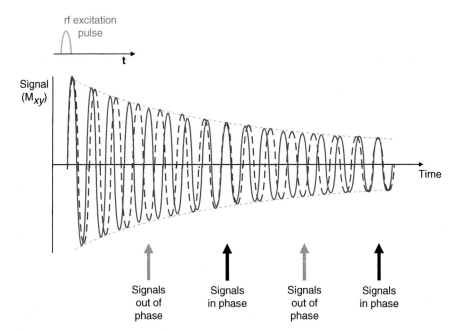

Fig. 17.8 Diagram showing FID signals from water- (*blue*) and lipid- (*red*) based tissue. Immediately after the RF excitation pulse, the two signals are in phase. As the FID signals evolve they alternately move out-of-phase (peaks and troughs oppose each other) and back into phase (peaks and troughs coincide)

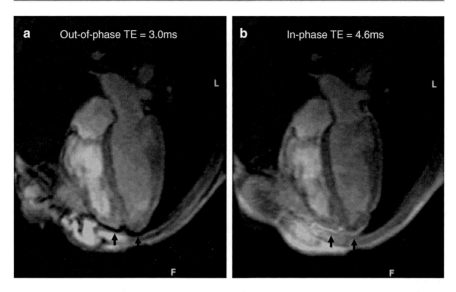

Fig. 17.9 Images from two cine gradient echo series with different echo times showing a four-chamber view of the heart acquired at 1.5 T. The echo time in (**a**) is 3.0 ms which is close to the out-of-phase echo time at 1.5 T (2.3 ms). There is a signal void at the interface between the pericardial fat layer and the surrounding water based tissue (*arrows*). Image (**b**) is acquired with an in-phase echo time (4.6 ms) and shows the pericardial fat layer as a bright signal (*arrows*)

Table 17.5 Echo times for in-phase and out-of-phase gradient echo imaging

Field strength (T)	Out of phase (ms)	In phase (ms)	Out of phase (ms)	In phase (ms)
1.0	3.4	6.8	10.2	13.6
1.5	2.3	4.6	6.9	9.2
3.0	1.2	2.3	3.4	4.6

Magnetic Susceptibility Artefacts

Magnetic susceptibility artefact arises from variations in the local magnetic field caused by the presence of materials with differing magnetic susceptibility. This is a property of any material that, when placed in a magnetic field, it causes the value of the field to either increase (*paramagnetic*) or decrease (*diamagnetic*). Most soft tissues are diamagnetic, but there significant differences between soft tissue and air, bone and venous blood (*deoxyhaemoglobin*). Artefacts related to magnetic susceptibility appear when there two or more tissues or substances that cause a localised change in the magnetic field, effectively creating a small local magnetic field gradient, thus contributing to T2* relaxation. This causes local de-phasing of the transverse magnetisation. For spin echo sequences, the de-phasing is reversed by the 180° refocusing pulse so it has a negligible effect on the image. For gradient echo pulse sequence, however, the de-phasing causes local signal loss. This signal loss is commonly seen at the boundary between two tissues with different magnetic

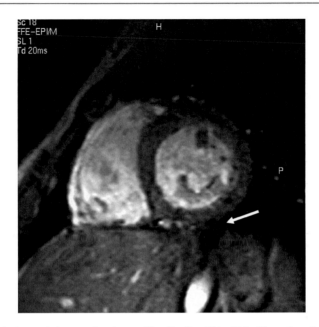

Fig. 17.10 A short-axis image taken from a Cine Gradient Echo-Echo Planar Imaging (EPI) pulse sequence. Note the signal loss around the great vein (*arrow*) caused by the susceptibility effect of deoxygenated blood

susceptibilities, or within tissues such as trabecular bone which contains many interfaces within a single voxel.

The signal loss caused by magnetic susceptibility effects increases with increasing echo time as it is a T2* relaxation effect. The effect is particularly marked at tissue-air interfaces around the lungs or bowel and around venous blood in the great veins around the heart. T2*- weighted gradient echo techniques such as echo planar imaging are particularly affected by this (Fig. 17.10).

Metallic Artefact

The presence of metal, such as clips used in surgery, sternal wires and heart valves with metallic components, create what is effectively an extreme case of magnetic susceptibility artefact, commonly referred to as *metallic artefact*. The local field distortion caused by metal causes de-phasing of the transverse magnetisation over a volume that is typically much greater than the size of the implant (Fig. 17.11). The artefact appears as a large signal void on images acquired using gradient echo based techniques. Images acquired using spin echo based methods will have smaller voids with bright 'arc shaped' artefacts where the magnetisation has been partially refocused in the distorted field by the 180° refocusing pulse. In both cases, the size of artefact can be minimised by selecting the shortest possible echo time. In severe cases, the magnetic field distortion also causes significant localised geometric distortion of the image.

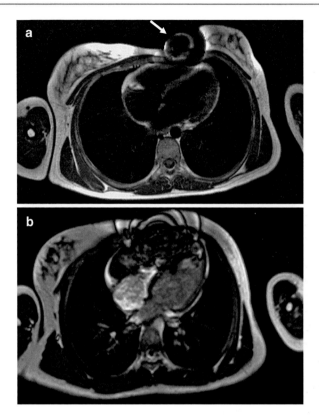

Fig. 17.11 Two axial images acquired from a patient with a Reveal device implanted in the chest wall. The black-blood turbo spin echo image (**a**) shows an area of signal loss within the anterior chest wall, containing a bright 'ring' artefact where the 180° pulses have refocused some of the signal within the distorted magnetic field. The balanced SSFP image (**b**) shows an area of signal loss that extends into the anterior heart. Note the dark fringes within the subcutaneous fat of the anterior chest wall. This is a characteristic appearance of balanced SSFP pulse sequences in the presence of an inhomogeneous magnetic field. The fringe pattern is indicative of the shape of the magnetic field distortion

Radiofrequency Interference Artefacts

Radiofrequency interference can originate from outside the MR environment if the RF shield is damaged or the RF room door is left open (see Chap. 2). It can also originate from inside the MR examination room if a piece of electronic equipment that is not MR compatible is taken inside the RF shield, or if the MR equipment itself is faulty.

There are two main kinds of interference: Continuous interference may appear as a line or band of noise across the image in the phase encoding direction (Fig. 17.12a). This is usually caused by bringing non-MR compatible electrical equipment into the exam room, but may also be caused by MR system faults.

An electrical spike (*noise spike*) generates interference that appears on the image as parallel stripes at any angle across the whole image (Fig. 17.12b). The angle and

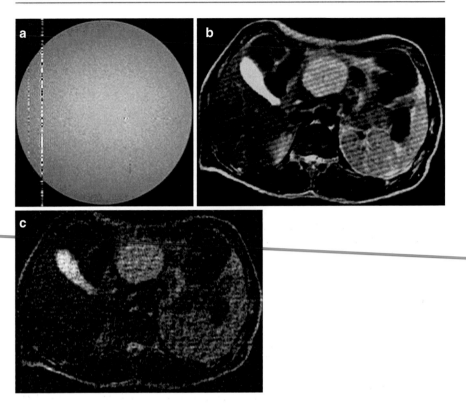

Fig. 17.12 Examples of artefacts caused by RF interference. (**a**) An image of a test object showing continuous interference at two frequencies, (one weak, one strong). (**b**) An abdominal image showing interference from a single interference spike and (**c**) multiple noise spikes

spacing of the stripes depends on where the spike occurs in k-space (see Chap. 7). Several spikes will add multiple stripe patterns, giving a herringbone appearance Fig. 17.12c). These may be caused by faulty MR equipment, very low humidity in the exam room, faulty light bulbs or even by nylon clothing worn by the patient, producing discharges of static electricity.

Summary
- Discusses the causes of the following common image artefacts:
  - Image aliasing in the phase encoding direction
  - Image aliasing with parallel imaging
  - Ghosting due to respiratory motion
  - Ghosting due to pulsatile blood flow
  - Flow-related signal loss (flow jets)
  - Chemical shift artefact (spin echo)

  - Chemical shift artefact (gradient echo) and in-phase and out-of-phase imaging
  - Magnetic susceptibility effects
  - Metal artefacts
  - Radiofrequency interference (continuous and noise spikes)
- Remedies and examples are given where appropriate.
- The technique of flow compensation is explained

Reference

Kilner PJ, Firmin DN, Rees RS, Martinez J, Pennell DJ, Mohiaddin RH, Underwood SR, Longmore DB. Valve and great vessel stenosis: assessment with MR jet velocity mapping. Radiology. 1991;178(1):229–35.

Further Reading

Ferreira PF, Gatehouse PD, Mohiaddin RH, Firmin DN. Cardiovascular magnetic resonance artefacts. J Cardiovasc Magn Reson. 2013;15:41. doi:10.1186/1532-429X-15-41.

Morelli JN, Runge VN, Ai F, Attenberger U, Vu L, Schmeets SH, Nitz WR, Kirsch JE. An Image-based approach to understanding the physics of MR artifacts. Radiographics. 2011;31:849–66. doi:10.1148/rg.313105115.

Scott AD, Keegan J, Firmin DN. Motion in cardiovascular MR imaging. Radiology. 2009;250(2):331–51.

Stadler A, Schima W, Ba-Ssalamah A, Kettenbach J, Eisenhuber E. Artifacts in body MR imaging: their appearance and how to eliminate them. Eur Radiol. 2007;17:1242–55. doi:10.1007/s00330-006-0470-4.

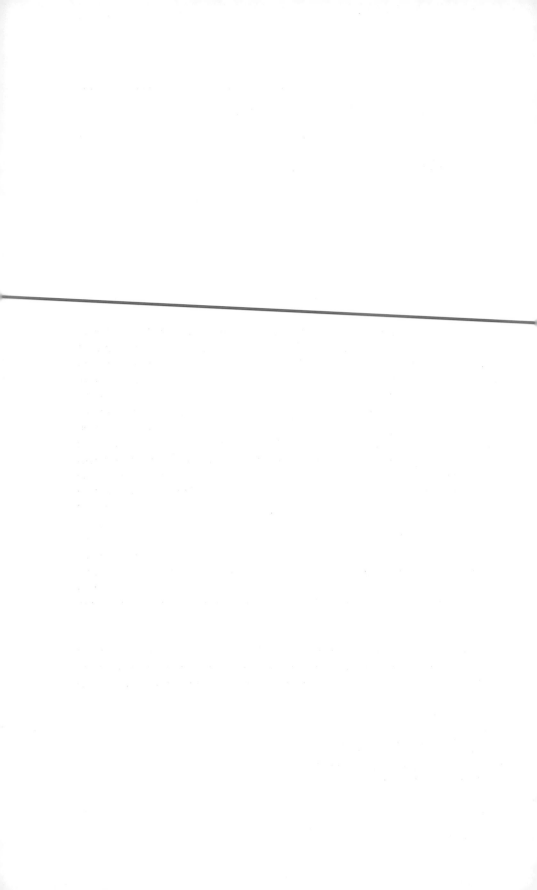

Influence of Field Strength on CMR

18

John P. Ridgway

Abstract

The twofold increase in the equilibrium net magnetisation at 3.0 T theoretically leads to a doubling in signal-to-noise ratio (SNR) in comparison to that at 1.5 T. In general, this can be traded for an increase in spatial resolution or in combination with parallel imaging it can be used to allow a reduction in image acquisition time or to improve the temporal resolution of functional imaging techniques. T1 relaxation times are significantly increased at 3.0 T, which leads to improved tag persistence for myocardial tagging techniques, improved background tissue suppression for MRA, and improved contrast for late gadolinium enhancement (LGE) and myocardial perfusion imaging. Drawbacks of imaging at 3.0 T include increased ECG artefacts, increased magnetic susceptibility artefacts, (most notably off-resonance banding artefacts on bSSFP pulse sequences), higher specific absorption rates (SAR) leading to increased tissue heating, RF field inhomogeneity, and greater safety restrictions relating to implanted devices. These drawbacks have presented a technical challenge to MR manufacturers, leading to the development of a number of solutions, including vector-cardiogram (VCG) triggering, resonant frequency scouts, high order shimming, and multi-channel RF body transmitter coils. All the CMR techniques used at 1.5 T can be applied at 3.0 T, each with some advantages and disadvantages.

Keywords

Field strength • 3.0 T • Signal-to noise ratio • SNR • Contrast-to-noise ratio • CNR • Parallel imaging • Resonant frequency • Larmor frequency • Relaxation times • ECG artefact • Magneto-hydrodynamic effect • Vector-cardiogram • VCG

J.P. Ridgway, PhD
Department of Medical Physics and Engineering,
Leeds Teaching Hospitals NHS Trust, St James's University Hospital,
1st Floor, Bexley Wing, Leeds LS2 9TJ, UK
e-mail: j.p.ridgway@leeds.ac.uk

© Springer International Publishing 2015   167
S. Plein et al. (eds.), *Cardiovascular MR Manual*,
DOI 10.1007/978-3-319-20940-1_18

• Magnetic susceptibility artefact • Spoiled gradient echo • bSSFP • Off-resonance artefacts • High-order shimming • Frequency scout • Specific absorption rate • SAR • Tissue heating • Permittivity • Conductivity • B_1 non-uniformity • Multi-transmit • Safety • Implanted devices • Implant heating • Black-blood • Functional cine imaging • Velocity-encoded imaging • Myocardial tagging • Late gadolinium enhancement • LGE • Myocardial perfusion imaging • MRA • Coronary MRA

The predominant field strength currently in use for CMR is 1.5 T however the use of 3.0 T MR systems for CMR is increasing. The increased field strength at 3.0 T has some clear benefits but there are also some significant drawbacks which have presented technical challenges to the adoption of 3.0 T for all CMR applications.

Potential Benefits of Increasing Field Strength from 1.5 to 3.0 T

The net magnetisation at equilibrium increases with field strength (see Chap. 1), so in theory the increase in field strength from 1.5 to 3.0 T doubles the net magnetisation and therefore the available signal. This is the major benefit of increasing field strength to 3.0 T as it should theoretically lead to a doubling of *signal-to-noise ratio (SNR)*, although this is not fully achieved in practice due to some of the drawbacks which are discussed later in this chapter. The increase in SNR at 3.0 T can be used simply to improve image quality for techniques which are limited by poor SNR at 1.5 T, or it can be traded for an increase in spatial resolution or in combination with *parallel imaging* (see Chap. 15) it can be used to allow a reduction in image acquisition time or to improve temporal resolution of functional imaging techniques. The overall increase in SNR for all tissues, together with careful optimisation of pulse sequence parameters (see below) can lead to improvements in *contrast-to-noise ratio (CNR)* for specific tissues of interest.

Doubling of the field strength from 1.5 to 3.0 T also results in a doubling of the *resonant (Larmor) frequency* from 63 to 126 MHz. The first benefit of this is that the chemical shift between the Larmor frequency of fat and water is doubled from about 220 Hz at 1.5 T to 440 Hz at 3.0 T. This increased separation in water and fat has the potential to make frequency-selective fat suppression techniques more effective and it makes the clinical application of proton MR spectroscopy more feasible at 3.0 T.

The dependence of tissue *relaxation times* on field strength also brings some potential benefits. T1 relaxation times are significantly *increased* at 3.0 T by up to 40 % for myocardial and blood T1 values. This means that pulse sequence parameters may need adjustment for some imaging protocols derived at 1.5 T in order to optimise image contrast at 3.0 T. The increase in myocardial T1 means that myocardial tagging techniques benefit from prolonged persistence of the tagging pattern further into the cardiac cycle. There are also advantages for techniques that use gadolinium-based contrast agents, such as contrast-enhanced magnetic resonance angiography (CE-MRA), late gadolinium enhancement (LGE) and first-pass contrast-enhanced perfusion imaging. Whilst the native T1 of tissue is increased at 3.0 T, the T1 of the contrast-enhanced tissue is relatively unchanged, leading to greater contrast between the enhanced and unenhanced tissue. This leads to improved background tissue suppression for CE-MRA, increased CNR for LGE imaging, and improved contrast between normal and ischaemic tissue in perfusion imaging.

T2 relaxation times are on the whole relatively *unchanged* or slightly *decreased* at 3.0 T, but T2* relaxation times are significantly *decreased* at 3.0 T. Magnetic field inhomogeneity caused by magnetic susceptibility differences increases with increasing field strength. This is both a drawback for some imaging techniques at 3.0 T, causing greater magnetic susceptibility-related artefacts and signal loss, and a benefit for other techniques which rely on T2*-weighted contrast, such as for the evaluation of iron loading. At 3.0 T it also becomes potentially feasible to exploit techniques such as blood-oxygenation-level-dependent (BOLD) imaging, widely used for fMRI imaging of the brain, as an alternative method for evaluation of myocardial perfusion.

The potential benefits of performing CMR at 3.0T compared to 1.5 T are summarised in Table 18.1.

Drawbacks and Technical Challenges of Imaging at 3.0 T

The drawbacks and technical challenges associated with CMR at 3.0 T are discussed in the following sections and summarised in Table 18.2.

Increased ECG Artefact

The first drawback of CMR at 3.0 T is the increased artefact superimposed onto the T-wave of the subject's ECG. This artefact which is the result of blood flow within

Table 18.1 Summary of potential benefits of 3.0 T compared to 1.5 T

Change in parameter	Benefit
Field strength is doubled, leading to two-fold increase in net magnetisation at equilibrium.	Potential for significant increases in SNR and CNR which can be traded for improvements in spatial resolution, temporal resolution or shorter acquisition times
Larmor frequency is doubled.	Increased separation of fat and water frequencies (chemical shift) leading to more robust frequency-selective fat suppression and improved feasibility for CMR spectroscopy
Increase in T1 relaxation times	Prolonged persistence of myocardial tagging patterns and improvements in CNR for techniques using contrast agents including CE-MRA, LGE and first-pass perfusion imaging
T2* relaxation times decreased	Greater sensitivity for iron loading and opens possibility of using the BOLD effect to assess perfusion

Table 18.2 Summary of main drawbacks of 3.0 T compared to 1.5 T

Drawback	Technical challenge/solution
Increased T-wave artefact on the patient's ECG	Improved R-wave detection software algorithms, based on techniques such as vector-cardiogram
Increased magnetic field inhomogeneity related to magnetic susceptibility effects leading to banding on bSSFP sequences	High order shimming, frequency scout for bSSFP pulse sequences
Increased Specific Absorption Rate (SAR)	Reduce refocusing pulse flip angles for fast/turbo SE pulse sequences. Reduce flip angle or increase TR for bSSFP.
RF field inhomogeneity, leading to RF pulse flip angle non-uniformity	Multi-channel transmit coils, improved RF pulse design
Increased T1 relaxation times	Optimisation of pulse sequence parameters necessary: Increase TI values for black-blood and late gadolinium enhanced sequences
Additional safety restrictions for implanted devices	Further testing of implanted devices at 3.0 T needed. Manufacture of devices that MR safe or conditional at 3.0 T.

the aorta is present at 1.5 T but greatly increased at 3.0 T. As blood is an electrical conductor, fast motion of blood within the aorta during systole through the magnetic field generates a voltage that is superimposed onto the ECG. This is known as the *magneto-hydrodynamic effect*. As the magnetic field strength is increased, so also is the voltage generated leading to increased T-wave artefacts. The augmented T-wave can be misinterpreted as an R-wave by the detection software (see Chap. 13), causing incorrect synchronisation of the MR acquisition with the cardiac cycle. Improvements in R-wave detection algorithms and ECG lead positions, including the use of the *vector-cardiogram (VCG)* principle (Fischer et al. 1999), have now largely overcome this drawback.

Increased Magnetic Susceptibility Artefacts

Inhomogeneity of the B_0 magnetic field is caused by differences in magnetic susceptibility of different tissues, leading to increased T2* decay (Chap. 5) and the presence of magnetic susceptibility artefacts (Chap. 17). This effect increases with field strength, so that there are greater field inhomogeneities at 3.0 T compared to 1.5 T in areas where there are tissues of significantly different magnetic susceptibilities. This is a particular problem for cardiac imaging, due to the adjacent lungs, (air/tissue interfaces) and the presence of large veins such as the coronary sinus which contain deoxygenated blood which has a very different magnetic susceptibility and shorter T2* value compared to that of oxygenated blood and cardiac tissue. This is mostly a problem for gradient echo based techniques which are T2* dependent. *Spoiled gradient echo* and *EPI* pulse sequences suffer from localised signal loss, in addition to overall reduction in signal-to-noise ratio (SNR) due to reduced tissue T2* values. Signal loss increases when using longer echo times and longer EPI echo trains and so can be minimised by keeping TE as short as possible and minimising EPI echo train lengths. *Balanced SSFP* pulse sequences suffer from dark banding artefacts where the magnetic field inhomogeneities cause the actual resonant (Larmor) frequency in some parts of the image to deviate from the resonant frequency set for the RF pulses. These are often referred to as *'off-resonance' artefacts* and these become more prominent for as the TR of the bSSFP sequence increases. Off-resonance banding artefacts can be reduced by keeping the TR as short as possible. Local shimming of the magnetic field is mandatory for bSSFP sequences in order to make the magnetic field as uniform as possible and to adjust the resonant frequency. At 3.0 T this becomes even more important. Normally, the gradient magnetic fields are used to provide a linear correction of the magnetic field inhomogeneities across the region of interest, but it has been shown that at 3.0 T, additional *'high order shimming'* coils can provide additional benefit by correcting for non-linear variations in the magnetic field (Schar et al. 2004). At 3.0 T and to a lesser extent at 1.5 T, it is also beneficial to perform a 'frequency scout' which is an additional preparation step that allows the operator to visually determine the most optimum resonant RF pulse frequency for the region of interest in order to minimise off-resonance artefacts on bSSFP pulse sequences.

Increased Specific Absorption Rate (SAR)

The increase in resonant (Larmor) frequency with increasing field strength leads to an increase in heat deposition in the patient's tissues. The energy deposited by each RF pulse is related to the square of the resonant frequency and the square of the flip angle. This means that 180° pulses deposit four times the energy of 90° pulses and that these energies are also four times greater at 3.0 T compared to 1.5 T. The tissue heating effect (measured by SAR) also increases with the rate at which the RF pulses are applied. Techniques that rapidly apply pulses with higher flip angles such as fast/turbo spin echo with long echo trains, or those that apply medium flip angles rapidly and continuously, such as retrospectively-gated bSSFP techniques or velocity-encoded pulse sequences have high SAR values and are more likely to cause tissue heating. Pulse sequences that are within safe SAR limits at 1.5 T may therefore exceed those limits at 3.0 T. This is a particular problem for patients with implanted devices, neonates and infants or in pregnancy where the SAR limits are restricted. It is therefore often a requirement to modify these sequences to reduce energy deposition. Fast/turbo spin echo pulses often have echo train refocusing pulses which are less than 180° which can reduce SNR. The SAR for retrospectively-gated bSSFP pulse sequences can be reduced by reducing the flip angle, which reduces SNR and contrast, or by increasing TR which causes an increase is susceptibility related banding artefacts (see previous section). These measures either increase the image acquisition time or lead to poorer spatial or temporal resolution for cine imaging. Parallel imaging therefore has a significant role to play at 3.0 T, as it can offset some of the loss in image acquisition speed, spatial and temporal resolution imposed by SAR restrictions.

Increased Inhomogeneity of the RF (B₁) Field

The electrical properties of patient's tissue, *permittivity* and *conductivity*, have an effect on the uniformity of the RF field which is negligible at 1.5 T but becomes significant at 3.0 T. This is a consequence of the higher frequency of the RF field and it leads to a variation in the effective RF pulse flip angle across the patient and a loss of image uniformity. At this higher frequency, the wavelength of the RF field becomes comparable to the body size and typical field of view used for cardiac imaging, which causes standing wave effects, seen as a variation in signal intensity across the field of view. In addition RF eddy currents induced by the B_1 field can cause signal loss in areas of high tissue conductivity or brightening of signal in regions of high permittivity. This variation in flip angle across the field of view also causes the SAR to vary across the patient, making it difficult to predict the maximum local tissue heating effect. These effects have been a major challenge to MR manufacturers for body imaging at 3.0 T. Solutions have included the design of new body transmitter coils with two of more elements (*multi-transmit*) to allow greater spatial control of the RF field, the design of RF pulses which are less dependent on *B1 non-uniformity* effects and the use of dielectric pads to counter the heterogeneity of the patient's tissue.

Changes to Relaxation Times

Whilst the increase in the T1 relaxation time of tissues at 3.0 T has some advantages, it requires the modification of parameters such as repetition times (TR) and inversion Times (TI) used for protocols which are successful at 1.5 T to be adjusted for use at 3.0 T. In particular, inversion times used in black-blood imaging pulse sequences must be increased which may cause difficulties at faster heart rates as it may not be possible to complete the data acquisition for each shot within the same cardiac cycle. For gradient echo techniques, the doubling of the Larmor frequency at 3.0 T also leads to halving of the echo times at which phase cancellation between fat and water occurs. This may lead to the appearance of dark boundaries (sometimes referred to as the India ink effect) at fat/water interfaces which are not visible at 1.5 T when using a gradient echo pulse sequence with the same echo time.

Safety of Implanted Devices at 3.0 T

A further drawback relates to the *safety* of patients with *implanted devices*. Whilst displacement or torque (twisting) forces acting on weakly ferromagnetic implants tested at 1.5 T may be negligible, they may become significant at 3.0 T. Increased risk of implant heating at 3.0 T is also a consideration, both due to the four-fold increase in SAR compared to 1.5 T, and also due to the associated decrease in wavelength of the transmitted RF field. Implants of dimensions close to this shorter wavelength have a significantly increased risk of heating compared to the risk at 1.5 T for the same SAR value, as these implants will act as antennae if oriented predominantly along the direction of the B_1 field. In general, when assessing the safety of implants for 3.0 T, it must not be assumed that implants which are 'MR safe' (or more correctly, MR conditional) at 1.5 T are MR safe at 3.0 T. There are many implants which are MR safe or MR conditional which can undergo CMR at 1.5 T but not at 3.0 T. This may because the conditions exclude imaging at 3.0 T, or it may be that those particular implants have not yet been tested at 3.0 T. MR conditional pacemakers are an example of a device that has been tested and can undergo CMR examination subject to conditions at 1.5 T, but not at 3.0 T. Further development and testing of devices such as these may lead to them being able to undergo CMR examination at 3.0 T under specified conditions in the future. Conversely, more rigorous testing by the manufacturers may lead to some devices previously considered 'MR safe', becoming MR conditional at either field strength. The most current guidelines provided by the implant manufacturers should therefore always be checked and local screening procedures updated accordingly on a regular basis.

Clinical CMR Techniques at 3.0 T

The advantages and disadvantages of using different CMR techniques at 3.0 T compared to 1.5 T are discussed in the following sections and are summarised in Table 18.3.

Black-Blood Fast/Turbo Spin Echo

Anatomical imaging at 3.0 T using dark-blood fast/turbo spin echo pulses should benefit from increased SNR. This can be traded for higher spatial resolution or for the use of parallel imaging to reduce the echo train length or to reduce breath-hold periods. The increase in SAR at 3.0 T can be mitigated by the use of reduced refocusing pulse flip angles and by shortening the echo train length in combination with parallel imaging. Longer TI values to null the signal from blood will be required but these may be difficult to apply at higher heart rates.

Functional Cine Imaging

At 3.0 T bSSFP pulse sequences benefit from increased SNR, but suffer from dark-banding artefacts caused by off-resonance effects in regions of poor magnetic field homogeneity. Banding artefacts can be reduced by performing a frequency scout,

Table 18.3 Summary of CMR techniques at 3.0 T compared to 1.5 T

CMR technique	Advantage	Disadvantage
Black-blood fast/turbo spin echo	Increased SNR, improved fat suppression, Parallel imaging to shorten echo train/breath-hold	Higher SAR, Longer TIs to achieve blood suppression.
Functional cine imaging – bSSFP	Increased SNR. Parallel imaging can be used to improve performance of segmented cine acquisition.	Dark banding off-resonance artefacts, High SAR values.
Functional cine imaging – spoiled gradient echo	Suffers less from artefacts at 3.0 T compared to bSSFP. Parallel imaging can be used to improve performance of segmented cine acquisition.	Lower SNR than bSSFP sequences; Increased flow artefacts at 3.0 T
Velocity-encoded cine imaging	Parallel imaging can be used to improve performance of segmented cine acquisition and 4D flow becomes clinically feasible	None specific to this technique.
Myocardial tagging	Higher SNR and improved persistence of the tagging pattern throughout the cardiac cycle.	Use of bSSFP for image acquisition suffers from artefacts, so spoiled gradient echo must be used
Late gadolinium enhanced imaging (LGE)	Increased contrast-to-noise ratio (CNR) between the infarcted region and the normal myocardium; possibility to reduce contrast dose.	Inhomogeneity of the 180° inversion pulse flip angle can lead to non-uniform suppression of the normal myocardium
Myocardial perfusion imaging	Increased SNR allows use of increased parallel imaging factors and other acceleration methods. Improved CNR for areas of ischaemia	Use of bSSFP for image acquisition suffers from artefacts; spoiled gradient echo preferred with lower SNR
Contrast-enhanced MRA	Increased SNR at 3.0 T allows increased use of parallel imaging. Increase in tissue T1 relaxation times leads to better suppression of background tissues	None specific to this technique.
Non-breath-hold coronary MRA	Increased SNR leads to gain in image quality or in combination with parallel imaging leads to higher spatial resolution or reduced image acquisition times	Increased magnetic field inhomogeneity may require modification of navigator RF pulse design. Use of bSSFP for image acquisition suffers from artefacts.

and high order shimming may also be beneficial (Schar et al. 2004). SAR values are high due to the very short TR, but can be reduced by reducing the flip angle at the expense of SNR, or increasing TR which may increase banding artefacts. The increase in SNR allows parallel imaging to be used to improve the temporal resolution of the segmented bSSFP cine acquisition, or to reduce breath-hold periods. *Spoiled gradient echo* pulse sequences do not suffer from off-resonance banding artefacts and so are often used in preference to bSSFP pulse sequences for functional cine imaging at 3.0 T, but they still suffer from signal loss in regions where there are large susceptibility differences (e.g. adjacent to the coronary sinus). There is however an increased dependence of signal intensity on flow at 3.0 T including flow voids.

Velocity-Encoded Cine Imaging

Velocity encoded imaging at 3.0 T has been shown to have similar precision and accuracy to 1.5 T (Lotz et al. 2005), however the gain in SNR at 3.0 T enables the use of acceleration techniques such as parallel imaging or kt-BLAST to improve the temporal resolution or to reduce the image acquisition time. This potentially enables the acquisition of 4D flow velocity data sets within a clinically acceptable imaging time (Carlsson et al. 2011).

Myocardial Tagging

Myocardial tagging techniques benefit from higher SNR at 3.0 T and in addition the longer T1 relaxation time of the myocardium leads to better persistence of the tagging pattern throughout the cardiac cycle. At 1.5 T the tagging grid or line pattern fades becoming indistinguishable beyond the systolic period, whereas at 3.0 T the tagging pattern is more clearly visible well into the diastolic period. The cine image acquisition is normally performed using a spoiled gradient echo pulse sequences. Use of a bSSFP sequence will suffer from the same drawbacks as those related to functional cine imaging.

Late Gadolinium Enhancement (LGE) Imaging

LGE imaging at 3.0 T is similarly effective as at 1.5 T although the general increase in SNR leads to an increased contrast-to-noise ratio (CNR) between the infarcted region and the normal myocardium and blood pool. This gain in CNR may allow the dose of contrast agent to be reduced. Inhomogeneity of the 180° inversion pulse flip angle is a potential drawback of 3.0 T for LGE imaging, as if this is significant it can lead to spatially varying incomplete suppression of the normal myocardium and variation of the blood pool signal. A key practical difference at 3.0 T is that the TI values determined by the TI scout to null the signal from normal myocardium will be increased in comparison to 1.5 T, due to the relative increase in T1 relaxation times at 3.0 T.

Myocardial Perfusion Imaging

MR Perfusion imaging benefits from both increased SNR and CNR at 3.0 T. The increase in SNR allows parallel imaging or other acceleration methods to be used, which in turn which can be translated into improvements in spatial resolution or reduced image data acquisition periods. This potentially allows an increase in the number of slices that can be imaged each heartbeat, particularly at higher heart rates during stress imaging. The increase in T1 relaxation time of the myocardium at 3.0 T leads to greater differences between enhanced and non-enhanced tissue, providing improved CNR. As for functional cine imaging, spoiled gradient echo pulse sequence are a more robust choice for data acquisition as bSSFP pulse sequences, which although they provide greater SNR, can suffer from off-resonance artefacts.

Magnetic Resonance Angiography (MRA)

Contrast-enhanced MRA particularly benefits from the increased SNR at 3.0 T and suppression of background tissues is improved due to the relative increase in T1 relaxation times which leads to greater saturation of background tissue signal. The improvements in SNR enables increased use of parallel imaging, leading to higher spatial resolution, greater coverage (no of slices) or shorter scan times.

3D Navigator-Gated Coronary MRA

Relative improvements in SNR can either lead to gains in image quality or, in combination with parallel imaging, allow imaging at higher spatial resolution or with reduced image acquisition times. The special two-dimensional selective RF pulses used in some approaches to generate the navigator echo require modification at 3.0 T to minimise effects of increased magnetic field inhomogeneity and T2* effects. The use of bSSFP pulse sequences for image acquisition can suffer from off-resonance artefacts, so a spoiled gradient echo or spiral k-space acquisition may be preferred.

Summary

The benefits of imaging at 3.0 T are:

- Increase SNR and CNR, leading to improvements in spatial resolution, temporal resolution or reduce image acquisition times
- Increased chemical shift, leading to improved fat suppression and MR spectroscopy
- Increased T1 relaxation times, leading to improved myocardial tagging and improved CNR of contrast enhanced techniques

The drawbacks of imaging at 3.0 T are:

- Increased ECG artefacts
- Increased magnetic susceptibility artefacts (off-resonance dark banding on bSSFP pulse sequences)
- Increased specific absorption rate, (SAR) increased tissue heating
- Significant inhomogeneity of the RF field, causing image artefacts
- Increased T1 relaxation times, requiring modification to pulse sequence parameters
- Additional safety restrictions for implanted devices

Many of these drawbacks have technical solutions which are developed or are under development

These technical developments allow all of the CMR techniques in use at 1.5 T to be applied at 3.0T with some modification and with some advantages and disadvantages.

References

Carlsson M, Töger J, Kanski M, Markenroth Bloch K, Ståhlberg F, Heiberg E, Arheden H. Quantification and visualization of cardiovascular 4D velocity mapping accelerated with parallel imaging or k-t BLAST: head to head comparison and validation at 1.5 T and 3 T. J Cardiovasc Magn Reson. 2011;13:55. doi:10.1186/1532-429X-13-55.

Fischer SE, Wickline SA, Lorenz CH. Novel real-time R-wave detection algorithm based on the vectorcardiogram for accurate gated magnetic resonance acquisitions. Magn Reson Med. 1999;42(2):361–70. doi:10.1002/(SICI)1522-2594(199908).

Lotz J, Döker R, Noeske R, Schuttert M, Felix R, Galanski M, Gutberlet M, Meyer GP. In vitro validation of phase-contrast flow measurements at 3T in comparison to 1.5T: Precision, accuracy and signal-to-noise ratios. J Magn Reson Imaging. 2005;21:604–10. doi:10.1002/jmri.20275.

Schar M, Kozerke S, Fischer SE, Boesiger P. Cardiac SSFP imaging at 3 tesla. Magn Reson Med. 2004;51(4):799–806. doi:10.1002/mrm.20024.

Further Reading

Kelle S, Nagel E. Cardiovascular MRI at 3.0T. Eur Radiol Suppl. 2007;17 Suppl 6:F42–7. doi:10.1007/s10406-007-0227-4.

Korosoglou G, Stuber M. High field cardiovascular magnetic resonance. In: Manning WJ, Pennell DJ, editors. Cardiovascular magnetic resonance. 2nd ed. Philadelphia: Saunders; 2010. p. 170–8.

Lee VS, Hecht EM, Taouli B, Chen Q, Prince K, Oesingmann N. Body and cardiovascular MR imaging at 3.0T. Radiology. 2007;244(3):692–705. doi:10.1148/radiol.2443060582.

Nael K, Fenchel M, Saleh R, Finn JP. Cardiac MR imaging: new advances and role of 3T. Magn Reson Imaging Clin N Am. 2007;15:291–300. doi:10.1016/j.mric.2007.08.002.

Oshinski JN, Delfino JG, Sharma P, Gharib AM, Pettigrew RI. Cardiovascular magnetic resonance at 3.0T: Current state of the art. J Cardiovasc Magn Reson. 2010;12:55. doi:10.1186/1532-429X-12-55.

Soher BJ, Dale BM, Merkle EM. A review of MR physics: 3T versus 1.5T. Magn Reson Imaging Clin N Am. 2007;15:277–90. doi:10.1016/j.mric.2007.06.002.

Part II

How CMR Is Performed

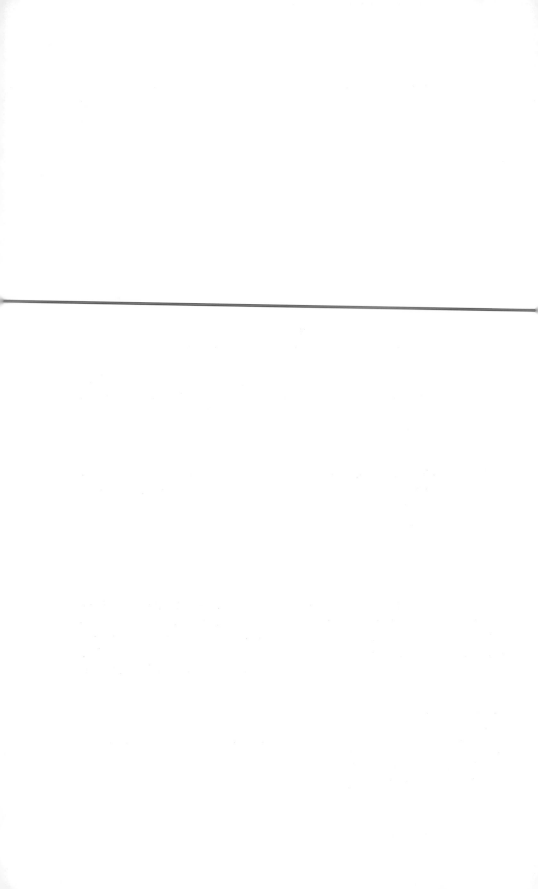

The Basics of a CMR Study

19

Sven Plein

Abstract

A good CMR study requires a good referral that provides the relevant background information about the patient and any previous investigations and clearly states which information is required from the test. Screening for contraindications such as implantable devices prior to the scan is mandatory. Common indications for CMR include assessment of congenital heart disease, phenotyping of cardiomyopathies, diagnosis of and risk stratification in ischaemic heart disease and vascular applications.

Keywords

Cardiovascular • Magnetic resonance imaging • Indications • Contraindications • Safety • Screening • Nephrogenic systemic fibrosis • Contrast agent • Vectorcardiogram • Pacemaker

The Referral

A good referral is a key prerequisite for a clinically useful CMR study, providing relevant clinical background information, placing the scan in the appropriate context and allowing the CMR department to optimally plan the examination ahead of time (e.g. the acquisition protocol, scan duration, special requirements such as the need for an interpreter or sedation). The referral is also an important first step in the

S. Plein, MD, PhD
Division of Biomedical Imaging, Leeds Institute of Cardiovascular and Metabolic Medicine,
University of Leeds and Leeds Teaching Hospitals,
Clarendon Way, Leeds LS1 9JT, UK
e-mail: s.plein@leeds.ac.uk

© Springer International Publishing 2015
S. Plein et al. (eds.), *Cardiovascular MR Manual*,
DOI 10.1007/978-3-319-20940-1_19

safety screening by identifying patients with potential contraindications to MR imaging. All too often, request forms are filled out poorly or incompletely. A well-designed request form will help to ensure all relevant information is provided.

The request form should include information about

1. Patient demographics
2. Patient height and weight
3. Possible absolute or relative contraindications to CMR imaging
4. Information on allergies, especially reactions to MR contrast media
5. Pregnancy status
6. Results of other imaging tests
7. Relevant clinical information
8. Recent renal function test results
9. Presence of arrhythmia
10. The clinical questions to be answered by the CMR study

An example of a CMR referral form is given in Fig. 19.1.

Key Points
The CMR referral form

1. Is key to a clinically useful study
2. Can identify patients that may be unsuitable for CMR
3. Should contain detailed clinical information and formulate specific clinical questions

Tips and Tricks for Referrals
1. In patients with poorly controlled arrhythmia (such as atrial fibrillation), consider deferring referral for CMR until rhythm and/or rate are controlled.
2. In obese patients it is useful to note weight AND height to determine if they are likely to fit in the magnet bore.
3. Claustrophobia is not necessarily a contraindication to CMR. Inform the department of possible claustrophobia on the referral form so that special arrangements (scanning prone or using sedation) can be made in advance.
4. If the patient has any implanted medical devices, indicate type, model, year of implantation on the referral form. This saves time on the day of the examination and may avoid the patient being cancelled.

Referral form for Cardiovascular Magnetic Resonance scan
Institution details

Patient Name: _ _ _ _ _ _ _ _ _ _ _ _ _ _ Date of Birth _

Address: _ _ _ _ _ _ _ _ _ _ _ _ _ _ _ _ _Identification Number: _ _ _ _ _ _ _ _ _ _ _ _ _ _

Height _ _ _ _ _ _ _ _ _ _ _ _ _ _ _ _ _ _ Weight _

Please tick if the patient has:

_ Pacemaker/Implanted defibrillator   _ Pregnancy
_ Any implants   _ Allergies
_ Metal in eyes (consider orbital x ray)   _ Reaction to MR contrast agents
_ Asthma   _ Claustrophobia
_ Aneurysm clip   _ brain surgery
_ Arrhythmia
_ Renal failure (Result of latest Creatinine _ _ _ _ eGFR: _ _ _ _)

Clinical details:

_ _
_ _
_ _
_ _

Details of other investigations:
ECG: _
Echocardiogram: _
Nuclear Perfusion scan: _
CT scan: _
Coronary angiography: _

Specific clinical question(s) this scan should answer:

_ _
_ _

Fig. 19.1 Typical CMR referral form

Indications for CMR

CMR has become a highly versatile imaging modality with a wide range of clinical indications. These range from assessment of congenital heart disease to the pheno-typing of cardiomyopathies, diagnosis of and risk stratification in ischaemic heart disease and vascular applications. Clinical indications for CMR have been appraised by European and North American societies (Pennell et al. 2004; ACCF/ACR/AHA/

NASCI/SCMR 2010) and several international practice guidelines include CMR. In this book, we will make reference to these guidelines in the disease-specific chapters in Part III.

Common Indications for CMR
1. Heart failure
2. Ischaemia detection – mostly vasodilator stress perfusion
3. Congenital heart disease – initial assessment and follow-up
4. Diseases of the aorta – especially aneurysm and coarctation
5. Cardiomyopathy – in particular ARVC, DCM, HCM and iron overload
6. Suspected myocarditis
7. Viability assessment – for example post MI
8. Pericardial disease
9. Cardiac masses
10. Course of anomalous coronary arteries
11. Heart valve disease

Contraindications/Safety

CMR, like all MR imaging, is a generally safe and harmless imaging procedure that is non-invasive and does not involve the use of ionising radiation. However, a CMR scanner produces a very strong magnetic field (>10.000 times the strength of the Earth's magnetic field!). The scanner's magnetic field and other forces can have important biological effects on patients and health care workers. Effects of medication administered during the scan may also cause side effects. Therefore, strict regulations have to be observed in the CMR environment to avoid injury or death. At least 15 reports of patient deaths due to MR scanning have been published, mostly associated with pacemakers and other implanted devices, but also including a case in which an oxygen cylinder caused fatal injuries in an MR scanner. Much more frequent than fatal incidents are device malfunctions, burns from wires and injuries from ferromagnetic projectiles. It is important to remember that the scanner's magnetic field is *always* on, even if the scanner is not in operation and that the magnetic field extends beyond the physical outline of the scanner.

It is therefore essential that

• Patients undergo a thorough and effective safety assessment and screening procedure before entering the MR environment.
• Patients with contraindications are identified and do not enter the MR scanner room or its fringe field.
• Health care providers involved in MR imaging understand the relevant risks and that this understanding is regularly assessed and documented.

- Procedures and guidelines are in place in an institution to control access to the MR environment and to prevent personal items and other potentially problematic objects being brought into the scanner room.

Screening

Information on potential contraindications to CMR or special circumstances such as pregnancy, disability, or metallic foreign body or implantable device should be obtained from the referral form. This preliminary screening helps to ensure efficient running of the MR list and allows patients to be listed for further investigations e.g. orbital X-ray imaging, ahead of their MR appointment.

Upon arrival in the MR department, patients complete a detailed safety questionnaire, in communication with a trained healthcare worker. This means they may need to be accompanied by an interpreter. No MR scan should be undertaken if the safety form cannot be filled in. In unconscious patients, information may need to be obtained from relatives, the family physician, the attending clinical team and the case notes. An example for a screening form is given in Fig. 19.2.

Contraindications to CMR Scanning

The contraindications to CMR scanning are equivalent to contraindications for general MR imaging. The CMR scanner can have the following effects on a person in the scanner:

1. Missile effects: The scanner will attract any ferromagnetic objects with enormous force. This force is higher the closer one gets to the middle (isocentre) of the scanner. Non MR-compatible metallic objects like scissors or oxygen cylinders can become deadly missiles.
2. Displacement: Metallic objects in the body such as shrapnel, aneurysm clips etc. may be moved by the magnetic field and cause injury.
3. Internal devices: The magnetic field can have torque effects on implanted active devices such as cardiac pacemakers or insulin pumps, causing them to malfunction.

Medical Devices
The most common reason why a patient cannot undergo an MR scan is the presence of a non-MR compatible implanted device. Thousands of medical devices are in use that contain ferromagnetic materials and may therefore be potentially unsuitable for MR scanning, making it impossible to give a meaningful representation of this subject in a textbook. There are large databases that contain information on the MR compatibility of most medical devices (most prominently www.mrisafety.com) and

manufacturers will usually have relevant safety information about their devices in the 'instructions for use'. A joint statement has summarised the MR safety of cardiovascular devices (Levine et al. 2007).

PRE-MRI PROCEDURE SCREENING FORM
MR Facility

Date____/_____/_____   MR# _____

Name _____ Height _____ Weight _____
        Last name   First name   M.I.
Birthdate_____   Social Security # _____/_____/_____
Address_____ City_____
State_____   Zip Code_____   Phone (H)(_____)_____   (W)(_____)_____
Physician's name & address_____

1. Have you ever had surgery or any other invasive procedures?   ☐ Yes   ☐ No
   If yes, please list:
      Type:_____   Date: _____/_____/_____
      Type:_____   Date: _____/_____/_____

2. Have you had any previous studies? ☐ Yes   ☐ No   If yes, please list below.

	Body part	Date	Facility Location
MRI:	_____	___/___/_____	_____
CT/Computed Tomography:	_____	___/___/_____	_____
X-Ray:	_____	___/___/_____	_____
Ultrasound:	_____	___/___/_____	_____
Nuclear Medicine:	_____	___/___/_____	_____

3. Have you ever:
   - worked as a machinist, metal worker, or in any profession or hobby grinding metal?
   - had an injury to the eye involving a metallic object (e.g., metallic slivers, shavings, or foreign body)?
   - been injured by a metallic foreign body (e.g., bullet. BB, buckshot, or shrapnel)?
      ☐ Yes   ☐ No   If yes, please describe:_____
   _____

4. Are you pregnant, experiencing a late menstrual period, or having fertility treatments?☐ Yes   ☐ No

5. Are you breast feeding?   ☐ Yes   ☐ No   6. Date of last menstrual period:_____/_____/_____

7. Are you taking oral contraceptives or receiving hormone treatment?   ☐ Yes ☐ No

8. Are you currently taking or have recently taken any medication?   ☐ Yes ☐ No
   If yes, please list:_____

9. Do you have anemia, diseases affecting your blood, history of kidney disease or seizures? ☐ Yes ☐ No
   If yes, please describe:_____

10. Do you have drug allergies? ☐ Yes   ☐ No If yes, please list: _____
    _____

11. Have you ever had asthma, an allergic reaction, respiratory disease, or a reaction to a contrast medium
    used for an MRI or CT exam?   ☐ Yes   ☐ No   If yes, please describe: _____
    _____

Fig. 19.2 Screening form (From: (Sawyer-Glover and Shellock 2000))

Some of the following items may be hazardous to your safety and some can interfere with the MRI examination. Please check the correct answer for each of the following.

☐ *Yes* ☐ *No*	*Cardiac pacemaker*	
☐ *Yes* ☐ *No*	*Implanted cardiac defibrillator*	
☐ *Yes* ☐ *No*	*Aneurysm clip*	
☐ *Yes* ☐ *No*	*Carotid artery vascular clamp*	
☐ *Yes* ☐ *No*	*Neurostimulator*	
☐ *Yes* ☐ *No*	*Insulin or infusion pump*	
☐ *Yes* ☐ *No*	*Implanted drug infusoin device*	
☐ *Yes* ☐ *No*	*Spinal fusion stimulator*	
☐ *Yes* ☐ *No*	*Cochlear, otologic, or ear implant*	
☐ *Yes* ☐ *No*	*Ear tubes*	
☐ *Yes* ☐ *No*	*Prosthesis (eye/orbital, penile, etc.)*	
☐ *Yes* ☐ *No*	*Implant held in place by a magnet*	
☐ *Yes* ☐ *No*	*Heart valve prosthesis*	
☐ *Yes* ☐ *No*	*Artificial limb or joint*	
☐ *Yes* ☐ *No*	*Other implants in body or head*	
☐ *Yes* ☐ *No*	*Electrodes (on body, head or brain)*	
☐ *Yes* ☐ *No*	*Intravascular stents, filters, or coils*	
☐ *Yes* ☐ *No*	*Shunt (spinal or intraventicular)*	
☐ *Yes* ☐ *No*	*Vascular access port and/or catheters*	
☐ *Yes* ☐ *No*	*Swan-Ganz catheter*	
☐ *Yes* ☐ *No*	*Transdermal delivery system (Nitro.)*	
☐ *Yes* ☐ *No*	*IUD or diaphragm*	
☐ *Yes* ☐ *No*	*Pessary or bladder ring*	
☐ *Yes* ☐ *No*	*Tattooed eyeliner or eyebrows*	
☐ *Yes* ☐ *No*	*Body piercing(s)*	
☐ *Yes* ☐ *No*	*Metal fragments (eye, head, ear, skin)*	
☐ *Yes* ☐ *No*	*Internal pacing wires*	
☐ *Yes* ☐ *No*	*Aortic clips*	
☐ *Yes* ☐ *No*	*Venous umbrella*	
☐ *Yes* ☐ *No*	*Metal or wire mesh implants*	
☐ *Yes* ☐ *No*	*Wire sutures or surgical staples*	
☐ *Yes* ☐ *No*	*Harrington rods (spine)*	
☐ *Yes* ☐ *No*	*Metal rods in bones, joint replacements*	
☐ *Yes* ☐ *No*	*Bone/joint pin, screw, nail, wire, plate*	
☐ *Yes* ☐ *No*	*Hearing aid (**Remove before scan**)*	
☐ *Yes* ☐ *No*	*Dentures (**Remove before scan**)*	
☐ *Yes* ☐ *No*	*Breathing or motion disorders*	
☐ *Yes* ☐ *No*	*Claustrophobia*	
☐ *Yes* ☐ *No*	*Other: _____*	

Please mark on the figure below, the location(s) of any implants or metal inside or on your body.

Right   Left

Please remove all metallic objects before MRI including: keys, hair pins, barrenttes, jewelry, watch, safety pins, paperclips, money clip, credit cards, coins, pens, belt, metal buttons, pocket knife, & clothing with metal in the material.

YOU ARE REQUIRED TO WEAR EARPLUGS OR EARPHONES DURING THE MRI EXAMINATION.

_____   _____ / _____ / _____

Signature of Person Completing Form   Date

Form Completed by: ☐ Patient ☐ Relative: _____

Name & relationship to patient

☐ Physician or other: _____

Name & relationship to patient

To Be Completed By MRI Department Medical Record number: _____ Completed by: _____

Procedure: _____ Clinical History: _____

Fig. 19.2 (continued)

Over the past years, MR conditional pacemakers and other implanted cardiac devices have been introduced. See Chap. 33 for details of scanning patients with pacemakers.

MR Safe - an item that poses no known hazards in all MRI environments. MR safe items include non-conducting, non-metallic, non-magnetic items such as a plastic Petri dish.

MR Conditional - an item that has been demonstrated to pose no known hazards in a specified MRI environment with specified conditions of use. The MRI environment is defined by static magnetic field strength, spatial gradient, dB/dt (time varying magnetic fields), radio frequency (RF) fields, and specific absorption rate (SAR). For MR Conditional items, the item labeling includes results of testing sufficient to characterize the behavior of the item in the MRI environment.

MR Unsafe - an item that is known to pose hazards in all MRI environments. MR Unsafe items include magnetic items such as a pair of ferromagnetic scissors.

Fig. 19.3 Classification for MR compatibility as proposed by the American Society for Testing and Materials International

It is essential that at the time of referral, detailed information is given about the exact specifications of any implanted device or material in a patient, including model specification and implant date, as the MR compatibility of devices can differ between models and editions. The classification in common use, proposed by the American Society for Testing and Materials International. Distinguishes between "MR safe", "MR conditional" and "MR unsafe" devices. Many devices fall into the category of "MR conditional", which means that the device is safe under certain conditions (Fig. 19.3).

Heating Effects

As outlined in Part I, MR systems generate high frequency radiofrequency (RF) pulses to create the MR signal. These electrical currents can be concentrated in conducting materials within the RF field resulting in heating. Conducting material of certain geometrical shapes such as loops of tens of centimeters are particularly liable to heating effects. Other conducting materials like tattoos may also warm up during the MR scan. Several steps can be taken to prevent excessive heating and possible burns in association with MR procedures, including ensuring that there are no unnecessary metallic objects contacting the patient's skin, preventing skin-to-skin contact points and the formation of "closed-loops" of conducting materials and using only electrically conductive materials that are MR safe.

Contrast Agents and Nephrogenic Systemic Fibrosis

The safety of MR contrast agents is tested in drug trials and they have a high compatibility with very few side effects. The variations of the side effects and possible contraindications are similar to X-ray contrast medium, but very rare. In general, an adverse reaction increases with the quantity of the MR contrast medium and also with the osmolarity of the compound.

There is also an established association between some MR contrast media and a condition called Nephrogenic systemic fibrosis (NSF) or Nephrogenic fibrosing dermopathy. This is a rare condition that leads to fibrosis of the skin, but in the later stages can involve joints, eyes, and internal organs and can be fatal. It is now assumed that this reaction occurs only in patients with advanced renal failure, in particular those undergiong haemodialysis, in whom clearance of gadolinium-based contrast agents is delayed. No cases have been reported in patients with normal renal function. NSF also seems to depend on the specific gadolinium chelate, with non-ionic linear agents being particularly associated with NSF. It is assumed that these agents release $Gd3+$ ions in the body, leading to a toxic effect in patients with advanced renal failure and reduced clearance of these ions. The European Medicines Agency has classified the gadolinium-containing contrast agents in three groups:

- high risk: gadoversetamide (OptiMARK), gadodiamide (Omniscan) and gadopentetic acid (Magnevist, Magnegita, and Gado-MRT-ratiopharm);
- medium risk: gadofosveset (Vasovist), gadoxetic acid (Primovist) and gadobenic acid (MultiHance);
- low risk: gadoteric acid (Dotarem), gadoteridol (ProHance) and gadobutrol (Gadovist).

In the United States, the US Food and Drug Administration introduced a class ban and warned about the use of gadolinium-based contrast agents in patients who have reduced renal function.

Importantly, since the introduction of these recommendations, no cases of NSF have been reported worldwide.

Performing Stress Examinations in CMR

If stress studies are to be performed, an additional level of safety consideration needs to take place. Haemodynamic monitoring of patients with an MR compatible blood pressure machine needs to be available. Heart rate has to be monitored either from the scanner display or a stand-alone MR-compatible physiological monitoring station. Emergency recovery procedures of patients from the MR environment must be in place and rehearsed. Arrangements for resuscitation in an appropriate area outside the magnet room must be made. Staff need to be trained in basic and advanced life support. Further details on stress CMR studies can be found in Chap. 29.

Other Safety Issues

Other safety concerns are related to the acoustic noise of the scanner and the cryogenic liquids. The noise generated by the MRI scanner is an important occupational hazard and European guidelines regulate exposure to noise as well as magnetic field exposure. The outflow from cryogens like liquid helium is improbable during normal operation and not a real danger for patients.

Key Messages CMR Safety
MRI is very safe, but there are important health and safety considerations.

1. The magnetic field requires careful screening of patients for contraindications to prevent injuries
2. The magnetic field is *always* on, even if no scans are performed
3. If in doubt whether a device/impant is MR safe – check www.mrisafety.com
4. Some MR contrast agents should be avoided in renal failure, but MR contrast agents in conventional doses are not nephrotoxic

Common devices that are NOT contraindications for MR imaging (considered as "MR conditional")
1. Most metallic heart valves
2. Intracoronary stents
3. Prosthetic joints etc.
4. Sternal wires
5. Dentures
6. Cardiac closure devices

Common devices that are ABSOLUTE contraindications to CMR
1. Most pacemakers – but MR conditional generation pacemakers are now available
2. Implanted cardioverter/defibrillators – but MR conditional devices are becoming available
3. Insulin pumps
4. Metal foreign bodies in the eye

Setting up a CMR Study

Equipment

In addition to the basic equipment of a general purpose MR scanner, performing cardiac MR examinations requires some additional software and hardware. The MR vendors offer software packages that provide the functionality (such as ECG gating) and pulse sequences needed for CMR studies. In addition, physiological monitoring is required, i.e. ECG monitoring (ideally on a screen in the MR room as well as in the control room), MR compatible blood pressure monitoring with remote activation from the control room and an Oxygen saturation monitor. A automated injector should be used to administer contrast agents for perfusion studies. If stress studies are to be performed, several additional requirements should be met.

- Emergency medication should be available on site. This includes all basic emergency drugs such as Adrenaline and Atropine, as well as specific medication for pharmacological stress studies: Aminophylline, inhaled bronchodilators and intravenous beta blockers, GTN.
- A suitable resuscitation area needs to be identified that is close to but separate from the magnet room. This should hold a resuscitation trolley and a defibrillator, access to emergency medication, high flow oxygen and suction.

It is essential that all staff are trained in basic cardiac life support and that during stress studies staff trained in advanced life support are present. Emergency procedures such as removal of patients from the magnet room need to be regularly rehearsed.

ECG Signals

In order to allow ECG gating and ECG triggering (see sections "Triggering versus gating for cine imaging" and "Prospective versus retrospective ECG gating"), which are essential for almost all CMR acquisitions, a reliable ECG trace must be obtained. This is complicated by the fact that the MR environment interferes with the ECG in many ways and that the potential risk of heating from ECG electrodes needs to be considered. The static, gradient, and RF electromagnetic fields of the MR scanner all distort the ECG. In addition, the so-called magneto-hydrodyamic effect occurs when a conductive fluid such as blood flows in the presence of a strong static magnetic and induces a biopotential. This effect typically distorts the T-waves of the received ECG. Further distortion can occur with respiration, in particular if the skin contact of electrodes is poor.

As a consequence of these difficulties, manufacturers have developed specialised algorithms that maximise the received ECG signal and filter out some of the described interferences. In addition, special electrodes and leads have been developed for use in the MR environment that reduce the risk of heating effects and optimise signal reception. Most CMR systems now use fibre-optic or wireless ECG transmission. Manufacturers also recommend optimal positioning of the ECG electrodes. With these specialised tools, reliable ECG signals can be obtained in virtually all patients. Still, at times repositioning of ECG electrodes is required to obtain an optimal signal. Often, the effects of the magnetic field can only be fully appreciated once the patients is positioned in the isocentre of the magnet, making repositioning of electrodes a small challenge. This is particularly the case at higher field strengths (e.g. 3 T) where all of the effects described above are more prominent than at 1.5 T.

Despite all improvements in ECG technology, it has to emphasised that the ECG obtained in the MR environment cannot be used as a diagnostic tool. This becomes particularly relevant, when CMR stress studies are performed.

Tips and Tricks for ECG Positioning
1. Use only ECG electrodes that are recommended by MR manufacturers
2. Follow manufacturer's recommendation for positioning of electrodes
3. Ensure good skin contact of electrodes by shaving chest hair where necessary and prepare skin with specialised gels
4. When repositioning electrodes test effects in the magnet bore
5. Test the stability of the signal during respiration
6. Avoid forming loops with ECG leads that could induce heating.

Patient Preparation

- Following the completion of the screening form, patients will usually be asked to change into hospital clothing to ensure no metallic objects are inadvertently brought into the scanner room. They should then be shown the MR scanner and introduced to its basic operation. Most CMR studies are performed in the supine position, but sometime patients are positioned prone (e.g. ARVC protocols or in case of claustrophobia). Often, a knee support is provided to improve patient comfort.
- If required, i.v. cannulae are inserted for administration of contrast and stress agents. This can be performed outside the scanner in a preparation area.
- Next, MR-compatible ECG electrodes are placed on the patient's chest (see notes above). A good ECG tracing is essential for a high quality CMR study and care should be taken to optimise the signal.
- The phased-array receiver coil is the placed on the front of the chest. The coil designs vary widely between vendors.
- Frequently a respiratory motion sensor is placed on the anterior chest wall.
- A blood pressure cuff should be placed on the patient for stress studies. Consideration needs to be given to which side the cuff is placed relative to contrast injection sites.
- Headphones and if required earplugs are provided. The headphones are also used for communication with the patient form the control room and often to play music to the patient.
- It should now be explained to the patient that the scan is about to begin and what to expect. Mention that the scanner is noisy when it acquires images and that this is perfectly normal. Explain breath-holding instructions you will use and consider a practice run while the patient is outside the magnet bore.

Commencing the Scan

The patient is now moved into the magnet bore. Be careful not to injure the patient as the table slides into the bore and that cables do not get trapped. Consider asking the patient to close their eyes as they move into the scanner to reduce the sensation of claustrophobia. The area of interest is placed in the isocentre of the magnet where signal uniformity is highest. All scanners have automatic guidance systems to position the patient. For cardiac studies, this means that the chest is in the middle of the scanner and the head usually remains within the scanner bore. Patients may find this claustrophobic, in which case removing a pillow or offering eye cover may help.

References

ACCF/ACR/AHA/NASCI/SCMR 2010 expert consensus document on cardiovascular magnetic resonance: a report of the American College of Cardiology Foundation Task Force on Expert Consensus Documents. J Am Coll Cardiol. 2010;55(23):2614–62.

Levine GN, Gomes AS, Arai AE, et al. Safety of magnetic resonance imaging in patients with cardiovascular devices: an American Heart Association scientific statement from the Committee on Diagnostic and Interventional Cardiac Catheterization, Council on Clinical Cardiology, and the Council on Cardiovascular Radiology and Intervention: endorsed by the American College of Cardiology Foundation, the North American Society for Cardiac Imaging, and the Society for Cardiovascular Magnetic Resonance. Circulation. 2007;116:2878–91.

Pennell DJ, Sechtem UP, Higgins CB, et al. Clinical indications for cardiovascular magnetic resonance (CMR): Consensus Panel report. Eur Heart J. 2004;25:1940–65.

Sawyer-Glover A, Shellock FG. Pre-MRI procedure screening: recommendations and safety considerations for biomedical implants and devices. J Magn Resonan Imag. 2000;12(3):510.

Components of CMR Protocols

20

John P. Greenwood and David P. Ripley

Abstract

CMR is an advanced imaging modality with important clinical applications and has become an established technique for both the anatomical and functional assessment of cardiovascular disease. There are specific technical challenges when imaging the cardiovascular system, notably the rapid and complex movement of the heart, the effects of respiratory motion and fast/high volume blood flow. Techniques such as ECG triggering/gating, breath-hold image acquisition, respiratory navigation and advanced accelerated pulse sequences help to overcome these challenges.

In the CMR exam numerous pulse sequences can be applied to interrogate different aspects of the cardiovascular system (e.g. volume and function, viability, perfusion, tissue characterisation). To select a comprehensive protocol the user should understand the basic pulse sequences and their clinical applications, as well as be able to optimise the parameters depending on patient considerations (e.g. patient size and ability to breath-hold).

In this chapter we describe the commonly used pulse sequences, scan protocols and methods of interpretation that are used in everyday clinical CMR protocols. For each component, there is a brief description of the pulse sequence, how it is planned & optimised, an example image and finally tips and tricks for the novice user.

J.P. Greenwood, MBChB, PhD, FRCP (✉) • D.P. Ripley, BSc (Hons), MBChB, MRCP
Division of Biomedical Imaging, Leeds Institute of Cardiovascular and Metabolic Medicine, University of Leeds and Leeds Teaching Hospitals, Clarendon Way, Leeds LS1 9JT, UK
e-mail: j.greenwood@leeds.ac.uk, d.ripley@leeds.ac.uk

© Springer International Publishing 2015
S. Plein et al. (eds.), *Cardiovascular MR Manual*,
DOI 10.1007/978-3-319-20940-1_20

Keywords

Cardiovascular magnetic resonance components • Cardiovascular magnetic resonance protocols • Cine imaging • Coronary artery imaging • Parametric mapping
• Myocardial tagging • Myocardial perfusion imaging • Phase contrast velocity
encoding • Pulse sequence • T1-weighted imaging • T2-weighted imaging • T2*
imaging • Contrast enhanced MR angiography • Early gadolinium enhancement
imaging • Late gadolinium enhancement imaging • Coronary artery imaging

**Core Components of Commonly Applied CMR Protocols for the Diagnosis
of Cardiovascular Disease**
1. Localising images and simple planning
2. Anatomical & morphological imaging
    (a) T1-weighted (black blood) imaging
    (b) T2-weighted (black blood) imaging
    (c) T2* relaxometry
3. Cine imaging (including real time cine imaging)
4. Myocardial tagging
5. Phase contrast velocity encoding
6. Contrast enhanced MR angiography
7. Myocardial stress/rest perfusion imaging
8. Early and late gadolinium enhancement
9. Mapping techniques (T1, T2 & T2* mapping)
10. Coronary artery imaging

Introduction

Cardiac magnetic resonance (CMR) imaging has become a fundamental technique
for the evaluation of cardiovascular disease. With improvements in both hardware
(e.g. coils and higher static field strength) and software (pulse sequences), CMR
image acquisition has now become very fast, often requiring just short breath holds
of only a few seconds. With an ever growing range of pulse sequences it is possible
to perform detailed anatomical, functional and tissue characterisation imaging of
the cardiovascular system. This ability to undertake a multi-parametric approach to
diagnosis is one of the unique strengths of CMR.

This chapter will take the reader step-by-step through each of the commonly
used components that are used in everyday clinical CMR protocols. For each component, there will be a brief description of the pulse sequence, how it is planned/
optimised, an example image and finally tips and tricks for the novice. These

individual components will be referred to frequently in Part III of this book, where a disease orientated approach to CMR imaging will be presented.

Localising Images and Simple Planning

Localiser or scout scans are the first part of any imaging protocol. Using either a gradient or spin echo technique (see Chap. 11), a set of low resolution images are acquired in the three standard orthogonal planes, sagittal, coronal and transverse (Fig. 20.1). These images are acquired during free breathing and are not gated to the ECG (so they are prone to artefacts). This first image set is used to confirm that the patient is positioned correctly on the table (with the heart in the isocentre of the magnet), the RF receiver coil is correctly positioned and that the appropriate array coil elements are turned on. These basic images can also be used to help plan the position and orientation of future standard imaging planes.

The next step for most imaging protocols is to acquire a transaxial spin echo or gradient echo stack, from the level of the diaphragm to just above aortic arch, often at low resolution, and planned from the coronal and sagittal localiser images (Fig. 20.2).

The resultant stack of images is then used to plan the main cardiac axes. There are several ways to derive the standard views and we present our typical approach: Choose a mid ventricular image to plan the vertical long axis (VLA) cine acquisition by orientating an orthogonal slice along the long axis of the LV (Fig. 20.3,

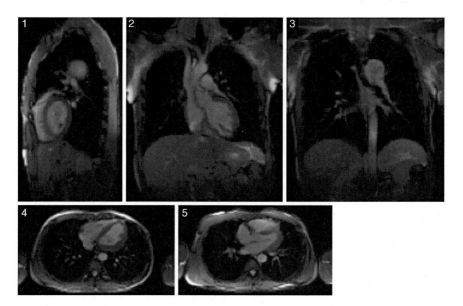

Fig. 20.1 Localiser scans demonstrating the three standard imaging planes (sagittal, coronal and transverse)

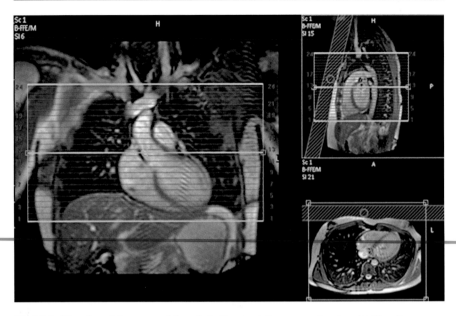

Fig. 20.2 Planning of the trans-axial stack (*yellow box*) from coronal and sagittal localisers

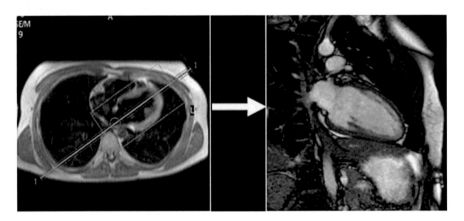

Fig. 20.3 Planning of the VLA cine from the trans-axial T1-w image (*orange line*)

orange line), bisecting the mitral valve and the apex (not necessarily completely parallel to the septum).

Using the end diastolic phase of the VLA cine acquired in the previous step, plan the next slice orthogonal to this and bisecting the mitral valve and apex to produce a horizontal long axis (HLA) cine image (Fig. 20.4).

To plan the true short axis (SA) cine, use the VLA and HLA cines just acquired, and plan the next slice(s) parallel to the atrio-ventricular (AV) ring (Fig. 20.5).

Finally, to plan the true 4-chamber (4ch) geometry, use the VLA and the SA cine images just acquired, and plan the next slice through the apex and the maximum lateral dimensions of both ventricles, avoiding the LVOT (Fig. 20.6).

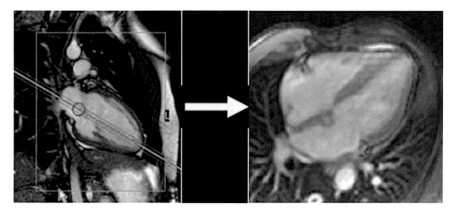

Fig. 20.4 Planning of the HLA cine from the VLA cine (*orange line*)

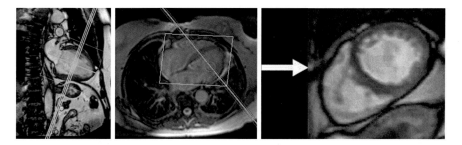

Fig. 20.5 Planning of the SA cine from the VLA and HLA cine images

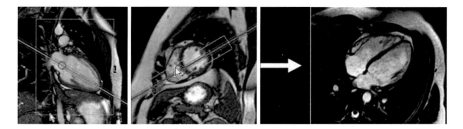

Fig. 20.6 Planning of the 4ch cine from the VLA and SA cine images

It is now just one final simple step to plan a full LV short axis cine stack for quantitative analysis of LV and RV volumes and ventricular mass. Use the end-diastolic frames from the VLA and 4ch cines to plan the first slice through the AV groove seen on both views. Then acquire parallel slices, typically 7 mm slice thickness with a 3 mm gap (or 8+2 mm or 10+0 mm) until you have covered the entire ventricle (Fig. 20.7).

It is now possible to complete a simple functional assessment of the left and right ventricles by examining the left and right ventricular outflow tracts (LVOT and RVOT). Using the end-diastolic frame from the basal slice of the SA stack, rotate

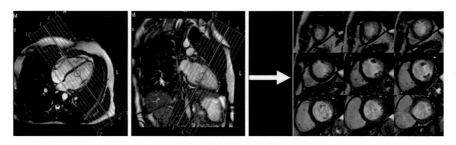

Fig. 20.7 Planning of the LV short axis cine stack (typically 10–12 slices) from the VLA and 4ch cine images

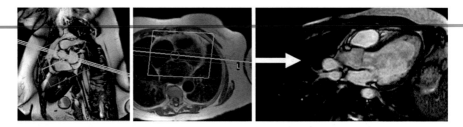

Fig. 20.8 Planning of the LVOT view

Fig. 20.9 Planning of the LVOT coronal view from the original LVOT cine image

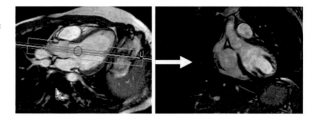

the next orthogonal imaging plane so that it passes through the aortic valve and up into the ascending thoracic aorta. This can be confirmed on the trans-axial stack. This will produce an LVOT cine which is equivalent to the parasternal long axis view on echocardiography (Fig. 20.8). A second LVOT view (LVOT coronal) can be piloted perpendicular to the initial LVOT view (Fig. 20.9).

To get the RVOT view, use the trans-axial T1-w BB stack and plan a sagittal plane directly through the main pulmonary artery, checking by scrolling through the slices, that it also passes through the pulmonary valve and cavity of the right ventricle (Fig. 20.10).

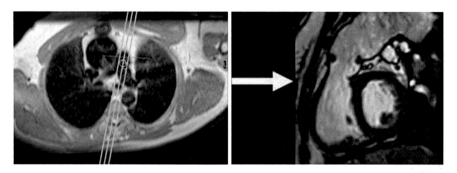

Fig. 20.10 Planning of the RVOT view from the original trans-axial T1-w stack

Interactive Planning

All vendors now offer software that allows planning of these standard imaging planes in an interactive mode that uses real-time cine acquisition to provide instant feedback on chosen imaging planes. The defined planes can then be saved for use in subsequent imaging protocols. Recently, tools have been developed that perform these tasks semi-automatically based on anatomical landmarks in an attempt to simplify CMR scanning.

Anatomical & Morphological Imaging

Spin echo imaging is one of the most basic and commonly applied pulse sequences used in all forms of general MR imaging. As seen in Part I, there are many different variations that can be applied to the basic spin echo pulse sequence, either to accelerate the acquisition (section "Turbo (or fast) spin echo") and to produce T1-weighted and T2-weighted images (section "Black blood FSE/TSE (double inversion)"). Different body tissues have different T1 and T2 relaxation times due to the different molecular environments of the hydrogen nuclei (section "Relaxation: what happens after the RF excitation pulse?"). Because fat has very constant T1 and T2 values it is often used as a reference tissue. On T1 weighted images, fat has a very high signal intensity, muscle has intermediate signal intensity and blood has low signal intensity. On T2 weighted images, tissues with high water content (e.g. cysts, effusions) have the highest signal intensity. A particular advantage of spin echo sequences are their relative insensitivity to local magnetic field inhomogeneity, produced for example by metallic implants such as sternal wires, prosthetic valves and arterial stents.

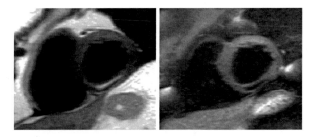

Fig. 20.11 T1-weighted spin echo short axis images, with and without fat suppression. In the first image fat is 'bright' in the inferior wall, in the second image the signal from fat has been suppressed so that it appears '*black*'; thus the presence of intra-myocardial fat is confirmed

T1-weighted (Black Blood) Imaging

T1-weighted spin echo sequences provide excellent tissue contrast between the myocardium and adjacent structures (e.g. epicardial fat or intra-cavity blood). As such they are a fundamental part of morphological cardiac imaging and also for tissue characterisation (e.g. tumour assessment). One important feature of spin echo images is that blood flowing rapidly through the image plane will appear dark (black), whereas slow flowing or stationary blood will have some residual signal. This can produce characteristic artefacts that can catch out the uninitiated (See section "Black blood (spin echo pulse sequence)"). The use of Black-Blood preparation schemes reduces this tendency (See section "Black blood – double inversion preparation pulses").

For high resolution T1-weighted images free from artefact, it is usual to acquire 1 or 2 slices per breath hold. This can be performed as a stack of contiguous images (typically 8–10 mm thick to get adequate SNR) in any slice orientation depending on the anatomical structure of interest. Although they are ECG triggered, the resultant image is from a single time point approximately mid way through the cardiac cycle. Thus it is not ideal to make measurements of vascular structures from static T1-weighted images, as they are not acquired at end-diastole.

T1-weighted spin echo sequences can also be performed using a frequency-selective fat suppression technique (e.g. SPIR, Fat SAT, or CHESS) to produce a 'fat suppression' image (section "Frequency selective fat suppression"). This can be useful to help in tissue characterisation (e.g. the identification of a lipoma) or to delineate abnormal presence of fat within a tissue (e.g. fatty infiltration of the myocardium in ARVC). Frequency selective fat suppression is now widely used in CMR imaging (Fig. 20.11).

To further aid tissue characterisation, T1-weighted imaging is often repeated after the administration of a gadolinium based contrast agent. This can be particularly useful in highlighting infiltrative or inflammatory myocardial disease.

Fig. 20.12 T1-weighted spin echo images pre- and post-contrast showing increased signal intensity in the 'mass lesion' in the inferior septum (*arrow*)

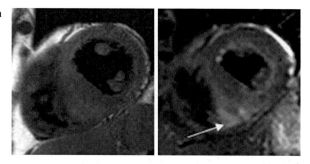

The presumed cause of the increased signal intensity in the pathological area is a combination of increased inflow (hyperaemia), altered interstitial contrast kinetics (capillary leakage and oedema) and diffusion into cells (necrosis) (Fig. 20.12).

Tips and Tricks
1. Generally scan in diastole when there is less cardiac motion and a greater amount of blood in the left ventricle.
2. If patient is poor at breath holding only acquire one slice per breath hold or try a respiratory navigator.
3. Adjust the trigger delay so that in combination with the TI, the Black Blood preparation and the data acquisition both occur when the heart is in a similar position.
4. If there is loss of signal from the basal region of the RV, LV or septal wall, increase the thickness of the Black-Blood inversion pulse.
5. Note that the Black Blood Inversion time on Siemens systems is called the 'TR'.

T2-weighted (Black Blood) Imaging

T2-weighted MR imaging has become established in the diagnosis of a number of cardiac inflammatory conditions, in particular acute myocarditis and myocardial infarction (Fig. 20.13). This in part relates to the known correlation between T2 relaxation times and myocardial water content; the higher the water content the greater the signal intensity on T2-weighted images. However T2-weighted imaging is hampered by the requirements for relatively long breath holds (producing respiratory motion artefacts) and low SNR ratios. This is because in order to increase the TR as required for T2-weighting, data acquisition is performed only on every 2nd or 3rd

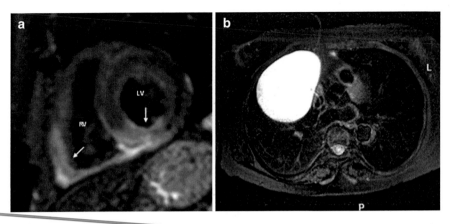

Fig. 20.13 (**a**) T2-weighted triple inversion recovery short axis image demonstrating marked oedema in the inferior wall of the LV and RV. (**b**) T2 weighted transaxial image demonstrating the very high signal intensity seen in a fluid filled pericardial cyst

heart beat. Increasing the slice thickness can improve signal and signal-to-noise ratio (SNR), but the trade off is a reduction is spatial resolution. There are also issues regarding the choice of surface coils or body coils to receive the image, with the former there is a progressive loss of signal moving away from the surface coil, leading to a drop in the sensitivity of T2-weighted imaging to detect oedema in the posterior LV; with the latter there is the general issue of low SNR. T2-weighted imaging has been improved by short tau inversion recovery (STIR) techniques, using segmented fast spin echo (FSE) acquisition with dark blood preparation (triple inversion recovery) (see section "Black blood turboSTIR (triple inversion recovery)").

Oedema Module
1. Perform imaging prior to contrast administration!
2. Body coil should be used or alternatively functional surface coil intensity correction algorithms.
3. Breath hold, segmented fast spin-echo imaging (double inversion recovery).
4. Adjust readout to mid-diastole.
5. Slice thickness at least 10 mm.
6. The slice thickness of the dark blood pre-pulse should be greater than the longitudinal shortening of the LV.

Tips and Tricks
1. T2-w imaging must be performed prior to contrast administration.
2. Aim for a slice thickness of at least 10 mm to ensure good SNR.
3. The slice thickness of the dark blood pre-pulse should be greater than the longitudinal shortening of the LV.

T2* Relaxometry

CMR has become a standard clinical technique for the quantitation of cardiac and liver siderosis (iron loading), both for diagnosis and disease/treatment monitoring. Iron has very strong paramagnetic properties, and deposits will considerably shorten the decay constant T2* as a result of increased inhomogeneity in the magnetic field. T2* is typically quantified using a single breath hold spoiled gradient multi-echo T2* sequence (or modified black blood sequence with blood signal suppression using a double inversion recovery pulse).

A single mid ventricular short axis slice is acquired using the above bright blood or black blood sequence (the latter of which may be more reproducible). From this, using dedicated software (e.g. Thalassaemia Tools, CMRtools, Cardiovascular Imaging Solutions, London) a region of interest (ROI) can be planimetered in the inter-ventricular septum, and the signal intensity for each image is plotted against the echo time (TE) to give a decay curve, from which T2* can be derived after solving the equation $y = Ke^{-TE/T2*}$ (Fig. 20.14). The same pulse sequence is also performed in a transaxial orientation at the level of the liver, and the same software used to plot the liver decay curve and hence derive the liver T2* value. There are now well established normal ranges for liver and cardiac iron loading, such that this has now become the preferred technique for guiding chelation therapy in cardiac/liver iron loading conditions.

T2* Module
1. T2* quantitation is now a standard CMR technique for disease monitoring and guiding chelation therapy in cardiac iron loading conditions.
2. Use a single breath hold, multi echo, T2* sequence (gradient echo or modified black blood sequence).
3. Acquire a single mid ventricular slice (and a single transaxial slice of the liver). Ensure good patient breath holding by coaching, as the scan duration is quite long.
4. Repeat the scan if there is respiratory artefact as this will compromise quantitation.

Tips and Tricks
1. Make sure the septum is of good image quality as this is where the ROI for quantitation is placed.
2. If not repeat scan to with strict breath hold instructions to avoid respiratory motion artefacts.
3. Position the transverse liver slice at a location so as to avoid large hepatic vessels so that an ROI can be easily defined in the liver tissue.

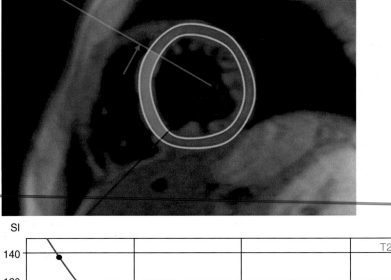

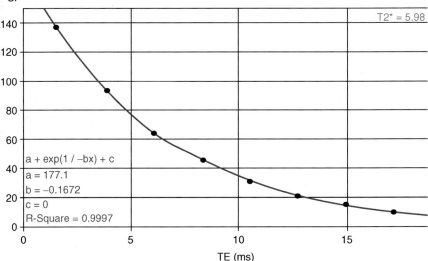

Fig. 20.14 Region of interest placed in the inter-ventricular septum and the corresponding decay curve in a patient with cardiac iron loading

Cine Imaging

Many different pulse sequence approaches are used for rapid cine imaging which will depend in part on the local availability of the MR system manufacturer. Cine imaging is performed using gradient echo pulse sequences; examples include turbo gradient echo (TGE), and balanced SSFP techniques (see section "Spoiled gradient echo versus bSSFP"). Images are typically acquired during short breath hold periods (although it is also possible to perform acquisition during free breathing, but respiratory motion artefacts will spoil image quality). To account for cardiac motion during the cardiac cycle, ECG triggering, ECG gating or real-time imaging is required (see Chap. 19).

ECG triggering is the most basic form of cardiac synchronisation and can be used in almost all forms of CMR image acquisition (see section "Triggering versus gating for cine imaging"). The QRS complex of the ECG is detected and then after a short delay the pulse sequence is initiated. In this way, over repeated cardiac cycles an image is formed at a particular time point in the cardiac cycle. If the delay time after the QRS complex is varied then different time points within the cardiac cycle can be imaged, and in this way a cine image can be built up, usually from a minimum of 20–25 different time points or phases. The other commonly used cardiac synchronisation technique is retrospective gating (see section "Prospective versus retrospective ECG gating"). This involves repeating the sequence at a constant repeat time over many R-R intervals. After all the data have been acquired, the information is sorted according to where it was collected from within the cardiac cycle. The advantages of this technique are that variations in the heart rate can be corrected for (retrospectively), and that more of the cardiac cycle can be acquired (i.e. late diastole, which can be difficult from a prospective gating technique).

Real-Time Cine Imaging

Most real-time imaging techniques are faster versions of SSFP or turbo gradient echo cine sequences. Methods such as parallel imaging and half Fourier imaging are part of the approach used to accelerate the acquisition (sections "Reducing the total number of phase encoding steps acquired for each image" and "Parallel imaging"). To gain a sufficient level of acceleration, so that all data can be acquired in real-time (i.e. a full set of images every single heart beat) typically requires sacrifices in both spatial and temporal resolution. Temporal resolution can be as low as 50–70 ms with a spatial resolution of ~3 mm × ~3 mm (reconstructed). Although this generally does not satisfy requirements for good quality cine imaging, the advantage is that ECG triggering is not required and nor is breath holding. Thus this can be a very useful technique in patients with arrhythmias (e.g. poorly controlled atrial fibrillation) or in those that cannot breath hold at all (e.g. young children). Furthermore, real-time acquisition can be used to acquire information on dynamic variability of cardiac morphology and function, for example in constrictive pericarditis.

Quantitation

CMR is the most accurate and reproducible method for both LV and RV mass and volume calculations, as it provides a 3D volume dataset avoiding the need for mathematical models and geometric assumptions of the shape of each ventricle. Several commercial software packages are available to perform these calculations. Typically, end diastolic and end systolic contours are drawn on each slice of the short axis stack. Many software packages provide automatic or semi-automatic

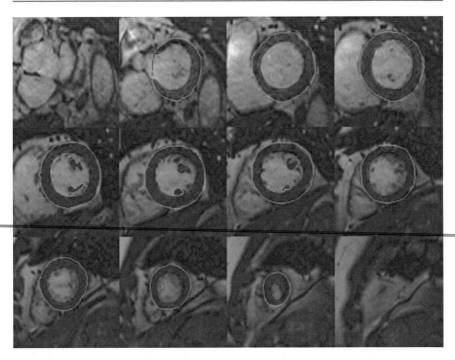

Fig. 20.15 Multi-phase multi-slice SSFP short axis cine stack showing endocardial (*red*), epicardial (*green*) and papillary muscle (*orange and pink*) contours at end diastole

algorithms for this task, but not all are reliable. In most cases, outlining only the diastolic and systolic images is sufficient, but all phases need to be tracked if more detailed analysis of ventricular filling and contraction is sought. In the analysis of an LV short axis stack, care needs to taken at the base of the heart, where the left ventricular and left atrial borders may overlap. Within a centre, it is essential to define an objective approach to dealing with these partial volume effects. In many centres, slices are considered to be within the LV if the blood volume is surrounded by 50 % or more of ventricular myocardium. Importantly, the most basal slice and its shape typically differ between diastole and systole because of the longitudinal shortening of the heart, which needs to be considered when outlining LV contours. Towards the apex of the LV, trabeculations within the LV cavity are typically excluded from the LV wall and the papillary muscles are planimetered separately. Once all slices are planimetered, the EDV, ESV, SV, EF% and mass for both the LV and RV can be calculated by the analysis software using the summation of disks method (Fig. 20.15). For the calculation of RV volumes many centres prefer a cine stack acquired in the transaxial orientation, due to its relative ease in delineating the tricuspid valve annulus. For the purposes of reporting ventricular volumes and mass, it is important to use pulse sequence specific normal ranges as there may be a systematic difference between traditional fast, segmented k-space, gradient echo (TGE) and the balanced steady-state free precession techniques

Table 20.1 Normal ranges for short axis orientation (two standard deviations above and below the mean) for TGE and SSFP sequences, with adjustment to BSA and height

	TGE		SSFP	
	Male	Female	Male	Female
LV EDV (ml)	84–221	84–162	102–235	96–174
LV EDV/BSA (ml/m^2)	45–104	48–94	53–112	56–99
LV EDV/HT (ml/m)	50–122	54–97	60–130	61–104
LV EF%	57–74	58–76	55–73	54–74
LV Mass (g)	108–211	82–132	85–181	66–114
LV Mass/BSA (g/m^2)	60–96	47–77	46–83	37–67
LV Mass/HT (g/m)	65–115	50–80	51–100	41–69
RV EDV (ml)	95–226	71–164	111–243	83–178
RV EDV/BSA (ml/m^2)	50–106	42–93	58–114	48–103
RV EDV/HT (ml/m)	56–124	45–99	66–133	52–108
RV EF%	47–68	51–72	48–63	50–70

LV left ventricle, *RV* right ventricle, *EDV* end diastolic volume, *ESV* end systolic volume, *SV* stroke volume, *EF* ejection fraction, *BSA* body surface area, *HT* height

(SSFP) (see Table 20.1). The cine data sets can also be used to derive regional contractile function. Short axis sections can be divided into segments and their diastolic to systolic thickening and inward motion calculated from segmental endocardial and epicardial contour displacement.

LV Function Module
1. Use SSFP pulse sequence (parallel imaging as required).
2. Acquire VLA, 4-chamber, short axis and LVOT cine images.
3. Plan the short axis stack from the mitral valve plane through the apex; slice thickness 6–8 mm, with 2–4 mm inter-slice gaps to equal 10 mm.
4. Keep temporal resolution ≤45 ms between phases.
5. LVOT cines in 2 orthogonal planes.

RV Function Module
1. Use SSFP pulse sequence (parallel imaging as required).
2. Acquire transaxial cine stack from the level of the diaphragm to the pulmonary artery bifurcation.
3. To assess subtle RV wall motion abnormalities it can help if the slice thickness is kept at 6–8 mm, with no inter-slice gap.
4. Keep temporal resolution ≤45 ms between phases.
5. Long axis images should include an RV vertical long axis view aligned with tricuspid valve inflow and a RV outflow tract view.

Tips and Tricks

1. If it is necessary to shorten breath hold times, reduce the number of slices or phases acquired for each breath hold (section Cine gradient echo), reduce spatial resolution or use parallel imaging.
2. Segmented k-space gradient echo techniques (e.g. TFE, TurboFLASH) are more flow/velocity sensitive than SSFP sequences, and so may be useful for the evaluation of valvular pathology or shunts (section "Flow-related signal loss and flow jets").
3. Remember that the heart contracts towards the apex in systole so that usually at least one basal slice is lost.
4. Use the movie function of the analysis software to check position of contours.

Myocardial Tagging

Myocardial tagging is a CMR technique that allows the visualisation of intra-myocardial contraction (see section "Myocardial tagging (binomial pulses)"). It is typically performed using a breath hold, ECG-gated, spoiled gradient echo technique (although SSFP pulse sequences may permit better tag-line contrast and reduced tag-line fading). Triggered from the ECG R wave, radiofrequency and gradient pulses are applied that saturate or 'tag' the tissue magnetisation in a linear or grid pattern. These alternate bands of saturation/desaturation persist for a short period of time, typically through systole and into early diastole (Fig. 20.16). Different techniques have been used to generate tagged images, such as SPAMM

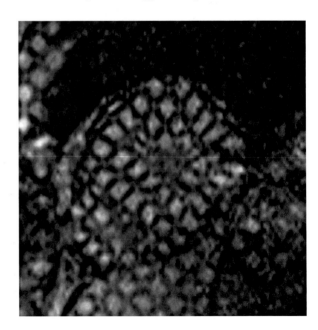

Fig. 20.16 Myocardial tagged cine image (in short axis) showing deformation of the tagging grid during systole

(spatial modulation of magnetisation), CSPAMM (complementary spatial modulation of magnetisation), which improves tag persistence and DANTE (delays alternating with nutations for tailored excitations). More recently, full 3D data sets of tagged images can be acquired allowing full cardiac coverage, as opposed to conventional single 2D slices.

Analysis of tagged images can either be by simple visual interpretation or by quantitative software techniques. At present routine clinical applications of tagged images are limited to visual analysis. Quantitative techniques are particularly time consuming and are currently a focus of research. In the future, standard tagging acquisitions may be superseded by 'feature tracking' which is a post-processing technique that can be performed on standard SSFP cine images to give comparable information on myocardial wall mechanics and strain.

Tagging Module
1. Scout imaging as per LV structure and function module.
2. Choose line tagging or grid tagging pattern.
3. Chose slice orientation from cine study.
4. Acquire data in breath hold.

Tips and Tricks Tagging
1. Linear tags are more useful if you are interested in contraction of the RV free wall; grid tags are well suited to the study of the LV.
2. Linear tag orientation is usually by personal choice as is tag-line spacing.
3. Acceleration techniques used to shorten the breath hold time are the same as for cine imaging.
4. Use a low flip angle to reduce tissue saturation and prolong the tagging pattern throughout the cardiac cycle.

Phase Contrast Velocity Encoding

Techniques for measuring blood flow have greatly enhanced the utility of CMR (analogous to Doppler measurements by echocardiography). The unique advantage of CMR is that as well as measuring accurately the velocity at pixel locations in any imaging plane, the area of the vessel of interest is also measured simultaneously. This allows volume of flow to be measured. This is particularly useful for calculating regurgitant fraction through a leaking valve or for comparing left and right heart cardiac outputs to assess cardiac shunting.

A phase-contrast acquisition is made up of two acquisitions with different flow sensitivities that produce the images in magnitude (i.e. anatomical) and in phase (quantitative for flow direction and velocity) (Fig. 20.17 and section "Velocity

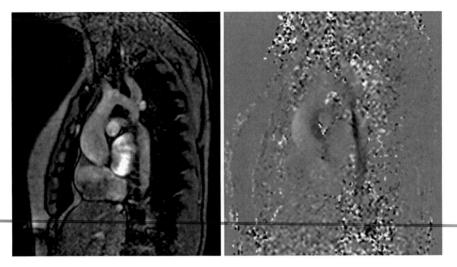

Fig. 20.17 Magnitude and phase images acquired from the thoracic aorta showing a high velocity jet (*dark*) in the descending thoracic aorta associated with aortic coarctation

encoded cine gradient echo (velocity mapping)"). An appropriate encoding speed (VENC: velocity encoding) must be chosen by the operator before running the sequence so as to avoid aliasing errors from high velocity flow measurements. This can either be predicted by an experienced operator, or a short breath hold acquisition can be performed with a particular VENC and the image checked afterwards for aliasing. If this occurs then the VENC is increased by an appropriate amount. This type of acquisition is typically performed during free breathing (as many cardiac cycles are needed); cardiac gating is retrospective, with continuous gradient echo acquisition and phase encoding changes for each R wave.

Phase-contrast images are analysed off-line using commercial software (or the vendor supplied workstation). The vessel of interest is manually planimetered at each phase of the cardiac cycle to correct for motion and change in diameter of the vessel lumen between systole and diastole. From this the absolute forward and reverse flow volumes can be calculated and the peak forward low velocity (Fig. 20.18).

Phase Contrast Velocity Encoding Module
1. Choose appropriate imaging plane (typically orthogonal to the expected direction of flow).
2. Set required direction of flow.
3. Choose appropriate VENC (start with 150 cm/s for normal systemic flow and 100 cm/s for right-sided flow. Adjust in pathological situations).
4. Choose between free breathing and breath hold techniques. For flow/volume calculations use a free breathing phase-contrast acquisition; a breath hold acquisition is acceptable if just peak velocity is required.

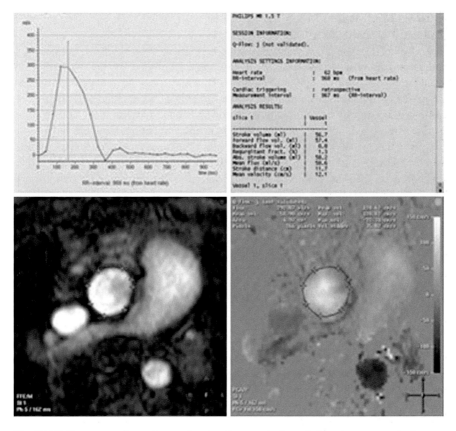

Fig. 20.18 Post processing software showing the magnitude and phase images acquired transverse to the thoracic aorta. Contours have been drawn around the ascending thoracic aorta and a volume-time curve plotted showing aortic flow (volume and direction) throughout the cardiac cycle

Tips and Tricks Velocity Encoded Imaging

1. Do not set the VENC too high above the maximum predicted velocity otherwise error will be introduced (ideally should be within 25 % of the true peak velocity).
2. Always check that you have set the correct direction of flow to be measured, whether you are scanning in-plane or through-plane.
3. For peak velocity measurements always make sure that the true jet axis has been well defined and perform in-plane imaging using this geometry. Ideally a thin slice should be acquired and rotate the field of view so that it is orthogonal to the direction of flow. Make sure there is adequate temporal resolution so that velocity is not underestimated (e.g. for free breathing acquisition use 30 phases; for breath hold use 20–25 phases).

Contrast Enhanced MR Angiography (Excluding Coronary Arteries)

MR angiography has become a widely accepted technique for the evaluation of vascular abnormalities in all areas of the body. It has many advantages over X-ray angiography in that it is minimally invasive (no arterial access required), uses safer contrast agents (non-iodinated) and is free of ionising radiation.

The technique involves a peripheral venous bolus injection of gadolinium based contrast agent which shortens the T1, providing increased vascular signal, avoidance of blood signal saturation, and better turbulent flow imaging. Typical pulse sequences are fast 3D spoiled gradient echo sequences, with short TR and a short TE. A parallel imaging technique can be used to speed up the image acquisition duration. A 3D acquisition is used to obtain high spatial resolution and a good signal-to-noise ratio, and the imaging volume can be acquired in any desired orientation. The sequence does not require ECG triggering (so is unaffected by arrhythmias) and can be performed in a single breath hold (20+ seconds).

To routinely obtain high quality images, it is important to have the correct timing between intravenous contrast injection and image acquisition. Central filling of k-space needs to occur at the moment of peak intravascular contrast, otherwise if too late there is the risk of contamination by the venous signal. The optimal timing between contrast injection and imaging can be determined in several ways:

- Test bolus technique: injection of a small dose of contrast (2 ml) and saline flush (20 ml) whilst acquiring a 2D gradient echo slice through the region of interest every 1–2 s. The contrast arrival time can then be calculated visually and used for the main acquisition.
- Automatic triggering: this involves monitoring signal intensity in the vascular territory of interest. The arrival of the contrast produces a sharp increase in signal intensity which is used to automatically trigger the 3D gradient echo sequence.
- Time resolved ce-MRA: This technique is independent of the exact contrast arrival time. Rapid collection of successive 3D data sets is performed immediately after contrast injection (10 ml, 3–5 ml/s), such that at least one is timed at the arterial phase after contrast injection. With this technique multiple vascular phases are acquired (arterial, tissue perfusion and venous).

Sophisticated post processing software is now available to allow viewing of the 3D data set from any desired angle / orientation. Maximum intensity projections and surface rendered image projections (Fig. 20.19) can be manipulated off line to display specific vascular anatomical features.

MR Angiography Module
1. Prepare contrast infusion pump with contrast agent and flush
2. Define 3D target region; unlike most other CMR applications, a very large volume is usually selected.
3. Define required timing of acquisition (arterial or venous phase)

4. Determine best timing parameters for data acquisition (pre-bolus or auto-matic triggering)
5. Perform a dummy acquisition
6. Perform acquisition with contrast administration

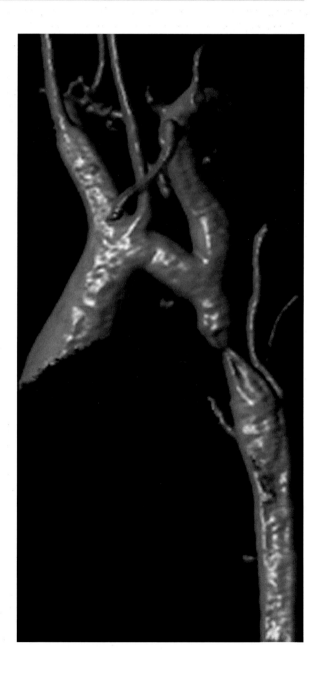

Fig. 20.19 Surface rendered image of the thoracic aorta showing a tight aortic coarctation

Tips and Tricks MR Angiography
1. Make sure that chosen your timing technique ensures that the centre of k-space is acquired at the same time as the bolus of contrast arrives in the vessel of interest.
2. Ensure that when you plan the volume it covers the whole area of interest including any collateral or aberrant vessels (if unsure you could acquire a 'dummy' scan without contrast to check the positioning of the volume).

Myocardial Perfusion CMR

Assessment of myocardial blood flow using contrast-enhanced dynamic first pass myocardial perfusion CMR has become a routine clinical application. Perfusion studies are predominantly performed to detect reduced myocardial perfusion reserve in suspected or known coronary artery disease; other applications include the interrogation of the vascularity of both cardiac and extracardiac masses. For the detection of reduced myocardial perfusion reserve, perfusion imaging needs to be combined with either physiological or pharmacological stress. Although performed in some research centres, physiological exercise is not practical in the MR environment and coronary vasodilator (e.g. adenosine) stress is the primarily used pharmacological stress agent. Under conditions of maximal hyperaemia (vasodilatation), regions of myocardium supplied by a stenotic artery will demonstrate relative hypoperfusion during 1st pass perfusion imaging.

The optimal imaging pulse sequence for stress perfusion MR is still open to debate and therefore individual choice generally comes down to local experience/preference. The three most commonly used methods are described below, with some potential advantages and disadvantages of each (see also section "Saturation recovery, single-shot fast gradient echo for dynamic, contrast-enhanced myocardial perfusion imaging"):

Spoiled Gradient Echo

- Short time between radiofrequency pulses so lower flip angles must be used, which can lead to lower signal to noise (SNR) and contrast to noise (CNR) ratios relative to other sequences.
- Relatively long acquisition time per image, which limits the maximum heart rate at which perfusion imaging may be performed. Can be combined with acceleration techniques such as parallel imaging to speed up image acquisition.

Balanced Steady State Free Precession (bSSFP)

- Highest CNR of all three sequence types
- Sequence type most prone to artefacts

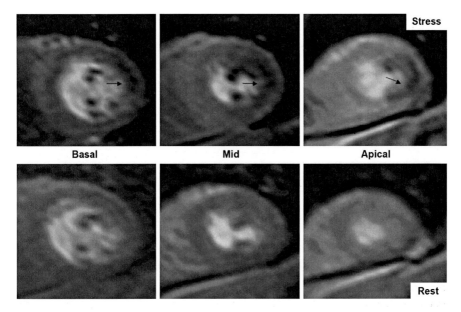

Fig. 20.20 1st pass MR perfusion study. Three slices are acquired during adenosine stress (*upper row*) and at rest (*lower row*). A lateral wall perfusion defect is demonstrated at stress (*arrows*), but no abnormality is seen at rest. Coronary angiography revealed subtotal occlusion of a large obtuse marginal branch of the circumflex artery

Echo Planar Imaging (EPI)

- Multiple data lines acquired per radiofrequency pulse.
- Potentially higher flip angles than gradient echo, which can translate into a higher CNR.
- Shorter acquisition time per image, allowing imaging at higher heart rates than gradient echo.
- Similar level of artefacts to gradient echo.

Whatever pulse sequence is chosen, ideally it should permit the acquisition of at least 3 short axis slices (apical, mid and base), every heart beat, with an in plane spatial resolution of less than 3×3 mm (to minimise 'dark rim' artefacts) (Fig. 20.20).

Reproducible Planning of Three Short Axis Slices

It is important to position the three short axis slices correctly. If they are too basal, the LVOT will appear in the slice and make some segments uninterpretable. If they are too apical, then you will only image the apical cap. In addition, if serial studies are planned it is important to 'individualise' the slice positioning for that patient so that future studies can be performed in exactly the same location. The '3 of 5' technique allows this to be achieved:

The "3 of 5" Technique

1. Use the 4 chamber and VLA localiser views for planning. Advance both of these scans into end-systole (maximal LV contraction).
2. Plan **five** 10mm thick short axis slices (Stage A).
3. Alter slice gap to achieve coverage from the mitral valve plane to the apex of the LV cavity (Stage B).
1) Reduce the number of slices to **three**, leaving optimally positioned apical, mid and basal slices (Stage C).

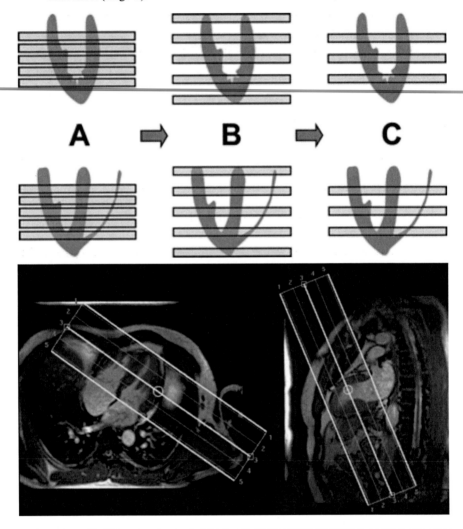

Perfusion Module

1. Scout imaging as per LV structure and function module.
2. Saturation-recovery imaging with gradient echo-echo planar (GRE-EPI) hybrid, GRE, or SSFP readout.

3. Parallel imaging, two-fold acceleration, if available.
4. Readout temporal resolution ~100–125 ms or shorter as available.
5. Short-axis view imaging (at least 3 slices per heart beat); preferably obtain data every heart beat.
6. Slice thickness 8–10 mm; in-plane resolution, <3×3 mm.
7. Contrast is given (0.05–0.1 mmol/kg, 3–7 ml/s) followed by at least 30 ml saline flush (3–7 ml/s).
8. Breath hold starts during early phases of contrast infusion before contrast reaches the LV cavity.
9. Image for 40–50 heart beats by which time contrast has passed through the LV myocardium.

'Dark Rim Artefact'

The 'dark rim artefact' is a common abnormality seen during perfusion imaging. A number of factors contribute to its existence, including magnetic susceptibility effects, Gibbs ringing, cardiac motion and spatial resolution. It may mimic a subendocardial perfusion defect in its location but has certain characteristics that allow it to be differentiated from a genuine perfusion defect (Fig. 20.21):

- The artefact is usually most intense when signal intensity reaches a peak in the LV cavity. As this is before the arrival of contrast in the myocardium, it cannot be attributed to a blood supply issue
- The artefact is generally short-lived, often lasting only 5–10 dynamic frames in duration
- The location of the artefact is often determined by the pulse sequence design. If a consistent design is used for all of your studies, the experienced observer will learn to recognise where the artefact occurs and not misread it as a perfusion abnormality

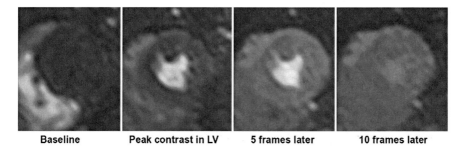

Baseline   Peak contrast in LV   5 frames later   10 frames later

Fig. 20.21 A typical subendocardial dark rim artefact is seen in the septal wall of a healthy volunteer. Characteristically, it is of maximal intensity when contrast levels peak in the LV cavity and fades as contrast enters the myocardium

Interpretation of CMR Myocardial Perfusion Images

MR perfusion images may be assessed by either visual or semi-quantitative/fully quantitative means. In a clinical setting, visual assessment is generally preferred, as this requires no additional post-processing.

Visual Assessment

As all CMR perfusion sequences are T1-weighted to maximise the signal generated by a gadolinium-based contrast agent, the principles of visual assessment are identical irrespective of the pulse sequence design used. Contrast agents shorten T1 and so increase signal intensity. If the coronary blood supply is normal, the myocardium should develop a homogenous grey appearance after 1st pass. However, where there is a functionally significant obstruction to myocardial blood flow, the entry of contrast agent will be impaired. This manifests as a darker area, "a perfusion defect", in the poorly perfused myocardium.

Perfusion should be assessed and recorded in accordance with the 17-segment American Heart Association model. However, a three short axis slice acquisition strategy will not provide views of segment 17 (true apex) so typically only 16 segments are reported. Perfusion defects should be graded according to their transmurality. Stress perfusion images should be compared with late gadolinium enhancement (+/- rest perfusion images if acquired) to identify inducible ischaemia, infarction, artefacts and normal areas of perfusion.

Semi-Quantitative Assessment

The 1st pass of contrast into the myocardium can be assessed objectively by semi-quantitative and fully quantitative means. However, this is a time-intensive process, which currently lends itself better to research rather than normal clinical practice.

- Contours are drawn around the epicardial and endocardial surfaces of the left ventricular myocardium and an area of interest is drawn within the LV cavity using a dedicated software package (Fig. 20.22).
- The myocardium is divided into six segments and the signal intensity in each region is calculated.
- A graph of signal intensity versus time can be generated for each myocardial segment and for the LV blood pool (Fig. 20.23).

A semi-quantitative assessment of perfusion is undertaken by calculating the myocardial perfusion reserve index (MPRI). This is undertaken as follows:

- The maximal upslope of the signal intensity-time curves for the myocardium and left ventricular blood flow are calculated by the software using a 'line of best fit'.
- The myocardial upslope at stress and rest are divided by the corresponding LV blood pool upslope, to correct for differences in the arterial input function at stress and rest.
- The MPRI is then calculated by dividing the corrected upslope value at stress by the value at rest. This value correlates with myocardial blood flow but does not represent absolute flow.

Fig. 20.22 Perfusion contours. Epicardial (*green*), endocardial (*red*) and LV blood pool (*yellow*) contours are drawn on each phase of every slice of both the rest and stress perfusion images to allow an objective assessment of first pass myocardial perfusion

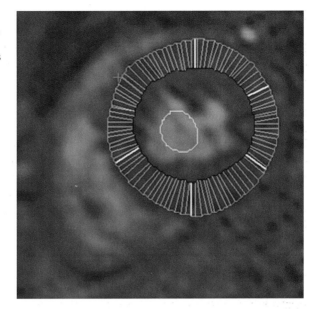

Fig. 20.23 1st pass CMR myocardial perfusion curve from a normal individual. Each coloured line represents the signal intensity/time profile in a different myocardial segment, as indicated by the legend on the right hand side of the graph

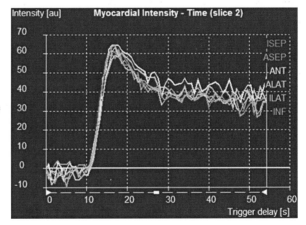

Quantitative Assessment

It is also possible to use the signal intensity profiles to estimate absolute myocardial blood flow (MBF) quantitatively in ml/g/min. Through manual or semi-automatic contouring techniques, following rigid motion correction, a circular region of interest is drawn in the LV cavity to derive arterial input function; epicardial and endocardial contours are carefully drawn, excluding any dark rim artefact. These allow the depiction of signal intensity-time profiles, which chart the passage of contrast through the blood pool (AIF) and myocardium. Several model-dependent or model-independent analysis methods have been proposed involving complex mathematical processes to generate the absolute myocardial blood flow quantification (e.g. Fermi function deconvolution). This technique also allows the generation of a transmural endocardial to epicardial perfusion gradient. Quantitative perfusion assessment, however, is time consuming and its moderate reproducibility means that it is rarely used in clinical practice.

Arterial spin labelling is an alternative approach to determine myocardial blood flow, and has the advantage of not requiring an exogenous contrast agent; currently this is only utilised as a research tool.

> **Tips and Tricks**
> 1. Always run a 'dummy' scan to ensure correct slice positioning and that there are no parallel imaging (wrap) artefacts. Ensure on the dummy scan that triggering really does occur every single heart beat; if necessary reposition the ECG and repeat the dummy.
> 2. When heart rate is too high (e.g. during stress) switch to alternate heart beat acquisition (some systems may do this automatically).
> 3. Keep the field of view as small as possible (without wrap) to maximise in-plane spatial resolution.
> 4. Angle the field of view so that it is parallel to the anterior chest wall to minimise the chance of getting wrap.
> 5. Make sure that both IV lines are patent and that 3-way taps are open correctly and all lines are attached before you start.
> 6. Make sure you know what to do in the event of serious arrhythmia or complications during stress perfusion imaging!
> 7. If there are triggering or breath hold problems during 1st pass, consider repeating the stress study after 15–20 min in place of rest perfusion (i.e. a stress-stress protocol rather than stress-rest).

Early and Late Gadolinium Enhancement (LGE)

Following animal and clinical validation in the late 1990's, this technique has become established as one of the most fundamental in CMR clinical practice. Often referred to as delayed enhancement imaging (or delayed hyper-enhancement imaging), it is used principally for the detection of irreversible myocardial damage (infarction or fibrosis) typically seen in ischaemic, infiltrative (e.g. sarcoid, amyloid) and other forms of cardiomyopathy (e.g. DCM, HCM, Fabrys disease). The technique is also used as an adjunct to tissue characterisation, for example imaging of tumours and their differentiation from simple thrombus (see Chap. 27).

As the name suggests, this technique involves the use of a gadolinium-based intravenous contrast agent. The gadolinium is bound to a chelate so as to avoid toxicity (e.g. gadolinium diethylene triamine penta-acetic acid (Gd-DTPA)), which limits its distribution to the extracellular space. As cell membrane integrity is preserved in normal and viable myocardium the extracellular space is minimal, such that the volume of distribution of gadolinium is small. The sharp demarcation of myocardial necrosis by LGE relates to the increased concentration of

Fig. 20.24 Mid ventricular short axis LGE images from the same patient showing the standard 2D IR-GRE sequence and the PSIR sequence

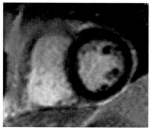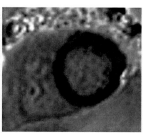

contrast material within necrotic tissue. The disruption of cell membranes in acute myocardial infarction allows gadolinium to passively diffuse into the intracellular space. This increases the distribution volume of gadolinium and in combination with slower washout kinetics, leads to relative hyper-enhancement compared to normal myocardium, which can be detected in the late washout phase. However, LGE also highlights chronic myocardial infarction and this is thought to be due to accumulation of gadolinium in the collagen matrix of the infarcted tissue.

Gadolinium shortens T1 relaxation and therefore increases the signal intensity on T1-weighted images. The contrast between normal myocardium and infarcted tissue should be optimized by manually setting the inversion time delay so that normal myocardium appears black and infarcted myocardium is bright. This can be determined by performing a "Look-Locker" or "TI scout" sequence. Most commonly a 2D segmented inversion recovery (IR) gradient echo sequence is used, timed to read out at mid diastole (to reduce motion artefact) with a single slice acquired per breath hold (see section "Inversion recovery fast/turbo gradient echo"). For a more rapid assessment (but lower spatial resolution) a 3D acquisition can be used to cover the entire left ventricle in a single (but longer) breath hold. A more recent alternative is the phase sensitive IR-GRE (PSIR) sequence, which avoids the need for precise 'nulling' of normal myocardium (Fig. 20.24). The practicalities of performing early and late gadolinium enhancement imaging (EGE & LGE) are described below.

Protocol for Early & Late Gadolinium Enhancement (LGE) Imaging

- Administer a bolus IV injection of gadolinium-based contrast agent at a dose of 0.1–0.2 mmol/kg.
- For the early gadolinium enhancement technique (detection of microvascular obstruction or intra-cardiac thrombus), imaging is performed immediately after contrast administration (and usually no later than 5 min) with a fixed long inversion time (TI), often 400–500 ms. Typically images are acquired in the VLA, SA and 4ch orientations. This produces images whereby normal myocardium has an intermediate signal intensity (grey) and areas of microvascular obstruction or thrombus appear black as contrast has not been able to permeate into them due to their lack of blood supply (Fig. 20.25).

Fig. 20.25 EGE image acquired in the 4CH orientation showing intermediate signal intensity (*grey*) in normal myocardium and a large apical thrombus (*black*)

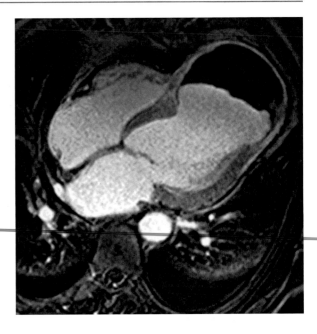

- For the late gadolinium enhancement technique, imaging typically starts at around 10 min post-contrast injection. For this to be performed correctly the optimal TI to 'null' the signal from normal myocardium must be determined. This can be done by performing a 'Look Locker' or 'TI scout' sequence. This is a breath hold sequence whereby a series of images are acquired each with a progressively longer TI. These images can then be examined by the operator to decide which TI depicts normal myocardium as black, i.e. nulled (Fig. 20.26).

- A full stack of SA slices are then usually acquired using this TI. As the TI for correct myocardial 'nulling' changes with time, typically the TI is increased by 10–15 ms before the VLA and 4CH slices are acquired. The Look Locker TI scout can be repeated at any point if the chosen TI appears to be incorrect. The technique of LGE applied according to this convention produces images whereby normal myocardium appears black and areas of infarction or fibrosis appear white (hence the well used phrase *"white is dead"*).

Early and Late Gadolinium Enhancement Module

1. Use 2D segmented inversion recovery GRE imaging during diastolic stand-still.
2. Same views as for cine imaging (short axis, VLA, 4chamber).
3. In-plane resolution ~1.4–1.8 mm.
4. For EGE, image immediately after contrast with a set TI of 440 ms.
5. For LGE wait 10 min after gadolinium injection (0.1–0.2 mmol/kg). Note – The delay may be shorter than 10 min if lower doses are used.

6. Inversion time set to null normal myocardium (use a T1 scout or Look Locker sequence). Alternative is to use fixed TI with a phase-sensitive sequence.
7. Read-out is usually every other heart beat but could be modified to every heart beat in the setting of bradycardia, and every third heart beat in the setting of tachycardia.

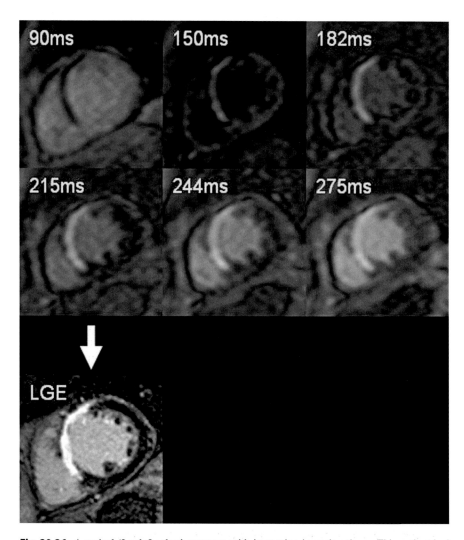

Fig. 20.26 A typical 'Look-Locker' sequence with increasing inversion times. This patient had suffered an anterior MI. The normal myocardium appeared 'nulled' (i.e. *blackest*) with a TI of 215 ms and this produced clear demarcation of the infarction (*white* appearance of the anterior wall and septum) on LGE imaging

Tips and Tricks

1. When acquiring LGE images, help in determining the optimum inversion time (TI) can be gained from the performance of a 'Look Locker' or 'TI scout' sequence.
2. Once determined, the correct TI for 'nulling' of normal myocardium slowly changes over time, therefore every couple of minutes the TI needs to be increased by 10–15 ms.
3. Images should generally be acquired in mid or late diastole to minimize cardiac motion artefact.
4. Saturation (section "Selective tissue saturation") bands can be applied across the spinal column and the anterior chest wall to reduce ghosting artefacts across the heart.
5. If you are not sure whether there is an artefact or true abnormality on an image then 'phase swapping' (i.e. changing the phase encoding direction) and repeating the scan should always be performed.
6. Using a respiratory navigator and performing the scan during free breathing can help in those few patients that cannot perform an adequate breath hold.
7. Acquiring the images during every second or third heart beat can help if there are problems with arrhythmia (e.g. atrial fibrillation).

T1, T2 and T2* Mapping Techniques

A key unique advantage of CMR is the ability to directly perform tissue characterisation by non-invasively interrogating the fundamental structure of the myocardium. Paramagnetic mapping techniques with T1, T2 and T2* offer a robust and reproducible quantitative assessment of the myocardium which may be utilised in the evaluation of both focal or diffuse myocardial disease. There is growing evidence to suggest that mapping may be sufficiently accurate and reproducible to translate into the clinical pathway.

T1 Mapping

The myocardium has an inherent longitudinal relaxation time constant (T1) which may be altered in various disease processes. This is based on the composite of the cellular and interstitial components (i.e. water, protein, fat and iron contents). Pre-contrast T1 mapping (or native T1) can be used to demonstrate intrinsic myocardial contrast (Fig. 20.27) and the T1 value of normal myocardium falls within a predictable range (940–1000 ms at 1.5 T). T1 changes are large in some disease processes and detectable even in early subclinical disease. T1 is measured in milliseconds and is higher where the extracellular compartment is increased such as focal or diffuse

Fig. 20.27 Pixel by pixel T1 map of the normal myocardium

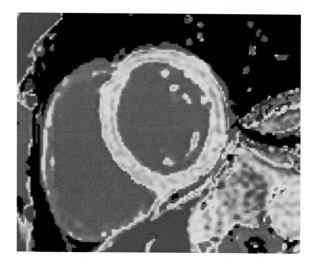

fibrosis, oedema and amyloidosis. T1 is lower in lipid storage disorders (Anderson Fabrys disease) and iron accumulation.

Mapping techniques may employ various pulse sequences which are either based on inversion recovery (MOLLI, ShMOLLI), saturation recovery (SASHA) or a combined approach (SAPPHIRE). Early T1 measurement techniques were multi-breath hold, although current methods use single breath hold protocols with single shot 2D imaging. The original scheme was the Modified Look-Locker Inversion Recovery (MOLLI) approach which involved acquiring 11 separate images at multiple time points on the recovery curve, and pixel-wise curve fitting was performed to estimate the relaxation time, to produce a pixel by pixel map of T1 relaxation values. T1 mapping images are acquired at the same cardiac phase and respiratory phase in order to eliminate tissue motion. These maps may be displayed in colour to aid interpretation.

The use of extracellular contrast agent shortens the T1 relaxation time by several hundred milliseconds and adds an extra dimension to T1 mapping. The acquisition of post-contrast T1 maps allows quantification of the extracellular volume (ECV) by subtracting the pre- and post-contrast T1 maps and correcting for haematocrit.

T1 Mapping & ECV Technique Module
1. Scout imaging as per LV structure and function module.
2. Choose appropriate mapping sequence (e.g. MOLLI / ShMOLLI etc.)
3. Short-axis view imaging with either a single mid-ventricular slice or 3 slices planned using '3 of 5' technique for Native T1 images. Acquire one slice per breath hold.
4. Wait until contrast equilibrium (at least 15 min post contrast injection) to acquire post contrast T1.
5. Take full blood count for haematocrit to calculate extracellular volume.

T2 and T2* Mapping

The T2 relaxation time is altered by the water content within that tissue (Chap. 16). Traditional T2-weighted images are challenging both to acquire and interpret. T2 parametric maps are generated on a similar basis to that of T1 mapping, a series of images obtained to calculate a T2 decay curve. A T2 preparation pulse is applied to obtain T2 signal contrast and readout performed with SSFP allowing a pixel-wise map to be generated. As with T1 mapping, T2 maps may be used to identify global myocardial disease such as pan-myocarditis, rheumatological diseases and detecting early transplant rejection, although T2 mapping has received less clinical focus than T1 mapping.

Segmented T2* measurement is the clinical standard for both the detection and serial assessment of diseases involving cardiac and liver siderosis, and is used to guide management and monitor treatment (Chap. 16). T2* mapping is an emerging technique with the benefit of short acquisition time, high SNR and the benefit of global quantitative assessment of the myocardial iron content.

> **Tips and Tricks**
> 1. Whilst absolute native T1 values are reproducible they vary by magnet strength (with 3 T resulting in longer native T1 times), vendor platform and the mapping sequence employed in the acquisition.
>   - Use normal ranges that are specific for the mapping method and field strength used.
> 2. Acquire post-T1 maps at least 15 min post-contrast injection to achieve equilibrium state.
>   - In diffuse myocardial diseases, take measurements in the interventricular septum.

Coronary Artery Imaging

Although techniques for coronary MR angiography have improved over the last 10 years, it is still fundamentally limited by low spatial resolution and problems with cardiac and respiratory motion. As such this technique has only limited clinical applications in the setting of ischaemic heart disease. Its main clinical use is in the detection and determination of aberrant coronary arteries and their anatomical course, for which CMR is the investigation of choice (due to its accuracy in classification and lack of ionising radiation).

There are a variety of techniques available for coronary artery imaging by CMR, which will be summarised into two broad types:

1. *"Whole Heart Technique"* – a 3D volume of the heart is acquired from transverse slices at isotropic spatial resolution. Data can be reformatted off-line in any desired plane using post-processing software.
2. *"Targeted Technique"* – left & right coronary arteries are imaged separately using a smaller 3D volume specifically adapted for each coronary artery.

In general, a *navigator-gated free breathing technique* is preferred (see section "Navigator-gated 3D fast/turbo gradient echo (coronary artery imaging)"). This method has the benefit of allowing much longer acquisitions with subsequently better SNR and resolution. This is the preferred method in the vast majority of patients, assuming a regular breathing pattern can be achieved. It is possible to acquire a 3D data set in a long breath hold, especially when using multi-channel coil arrays and parallel imaging. However the achievable spatial resolution and SNR are limited.

Whole Heart Technique

- Perform a 4-chamber cine acquisition with 50 phases (for coronary artery motion tracking). *Tip* – use a parallel imaging technique to reduce breath hold duration.
- Perform a low resolution 3D coronary survey. Position a "navigator" on the dome of the right hemi-diaphragm, approximately 2/3 into the liver. Coverage should include the inferior border of the heart up to the pulmonary artery bifurcation (Fig. 20.28). Set 'longest trigger delay' for optimal diastolic imaging. Then check for 'navigator efficiency' (Fig. 20.29).

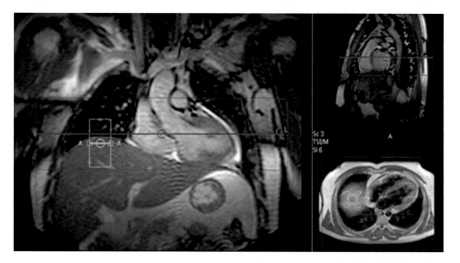

Fig. 20.28   Position of the respiratory navigator

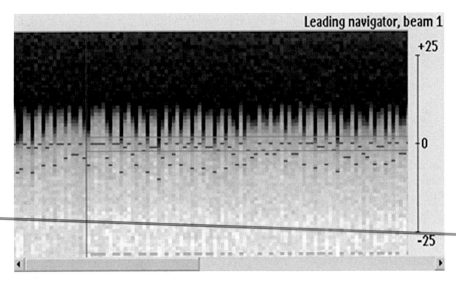

Fig. 20.29 Real-time navigator tracking. *Blue bars* represent data acceptance window for image reconstruction (all other data outside of this window rejected)

Fig. 20.30 Example of coronary artery rest periods

	Left Coronary	Right Coronary	Over-lap Range
Early Diastole	550ms	500ms	From ~ 550ms
Late Diastole	1100ms	900ms	Up to ~ 900ms

- If poor:
  - practise breathing patterns with the patient
  - reposition the navigator to avoid vascular structures or fat planes below the diaphragm

- Whilst the coronary survey is acquiring, scroll through the phases of the 4 chamber cine and note the time points in the cardiac cycle when each coronary artery is stationary. Note, this is different for the LCA and RCA
- Note the stationary over-lap range for the left and right coronary arteries (see example in Fig. 20.30). The optimal timing range for imaging the left and right coronary arteries in this example is between 550–900 ms. If the overlap between left and right coronary arteries is small (<50 ms), a timing range suited to the more important artery is selected. Remember, the left artery is usually more dif-

ficult to image and therefore timings chosen should favour imaging of the left coronary artery.

• To plan a 3D Whole Heart acquisition adjust the number of slices to cover left ventricular apex to pulmonary artery bifurcation by checking coverage on the 3D coronary survey images. Select a "trigger delay" that corresponds to, or slightly after, the start point of the optimal timing range. Adjust the "shot" or "acquisition" duration to fit in the optimal timing range (best results are obtained below 100 ms). Reduce the rectangular field of view (RFOV) to reduce the scan time. The resultant 3D coronary dataset can be manually reformatted to delineate course of individual coronary arteries (Fig. 20.31).

Targeted Technique

This technique relies on the patient being able to perform a reasonably long breath hold. Perform a low resolution 3D Coronary Survey as described above. Then use the '3-Point Plan Scan' facility to plan the optimal imaging plane for either left or right coronary artery imaging. Typically points are placed at the ostium, mid vessel and at the distal vessel. If the whole of the left coronary needs to be imaged in a single acquisition then points will need to be chosen in both the LAD and LCx (Figs. 20.32 and 20.33).

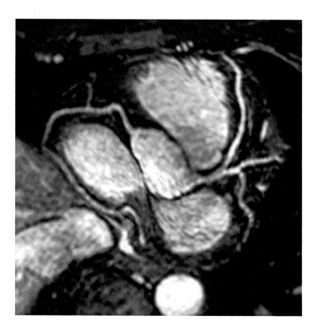

Fig. 20.31 Reformatted 3D coronary MRA dataset using SoapBubble™ software

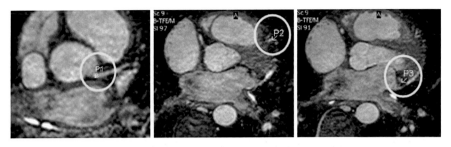

Fig. 20.32 The targeted technique: Left Coronary Artery using '3-Point Plan Scan'. *Point 1 –* origin of left main stem; *Point 2 –* mid-distal portion of left anterior descending artery; *Point 3 –* mid-distal portion of circumflex artery

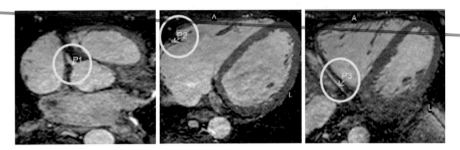

Fig. 20.33 The targeted technique: Right Coronary Artery using '3-Point Plan Scan'. *Point 1 –* origin of RCA; *Point 2 –* mid portion of RCA; *Point 3 –* distal portion of RCA

Coronary Artery Imaging Module
1. Repeat horizontal long axis with high temporal resolution (50 phases) to accurately determine quiescent period of RCA.
   Navigator-gated, 3D, free-breathing, MRA sequence:
2. Transaxial slices spanning from level of proximal main pulmonary artery down to the middle of the right atrium (entire cardiac coverage if desired). Slice thickness 1–1.5 mm; acquired spatial resolution in-plane of 1.0 mm or less.
3. Slices – typically 50–80, as needed to encompass vessels of interest.
4. Adjust trigger delay and acquisition window according to observed coronary artery rest period.
5. Parallel acquisition preferred; Navigator placed over the right hemi-diaphragm.
6. Optional – consider contrast to increase vessel conspicuity
7. Breath hold techniques if poor image quality or navigators unavailable or they are of poor quality.
8. T2-prepared sequence may be useful.

Tips and Tricks

1. If no rest period between systole/diastole is seen, repeat high temporal resolution 4ch cine scan at the correct cardiac frequency and reassess for rest periods. Hint: timings are more accurate when this is performed just before the actual coronary artery acquisition. Consider cine scan during free breathing if heart rate changes during breath hold. Correct input of the heart rate (for the 4Ch cine) ensures that the full cardiac cycle is captured to allow accurate identification of the rest periods.

2. Still no rest period seen. Solution 1, check for early rest period during systole and scan with a tight window (<50 ms). It is sometimes possible and necessary to scan during systole if there is a short natural rest period. A short acquisition duration is necessary to avoid blurring.

3. Still no rest period seen in systole or diastole. Solution 2, select longest trigger delay and scan with a tight window (<50 ms). In some cases there are no natural coronary artery 'rest periods' in the cardiac cycle. Scanning at the longest trigger delay with a short acquisition duration is a compromise that may be useful in some cases.

4. Heart rate is 90 bpm or above. The solution is to scan with the tightest scan window possible. This will minimise blurring of the coronary arteries and due to the high heart rate, the scan will be completed in a faster time.
   - Remember:
     - Coronary blurring occurs with the slightest movement
     - Keep scan times to a sensible limit
     - Higher spatial resolution equals longer scan times.
     - Longer scan times can lead to more patient movement

Key Points

1. CMR protocols are made up of a number of core components, carefully selected to highlighted and/or differentiate specific pathological features.

2. CMR therefore allows a multi-parametric approach to cardiovascular imaging.

3. One must be aware of how to plan and perform these core components so that image quality can be optimised.

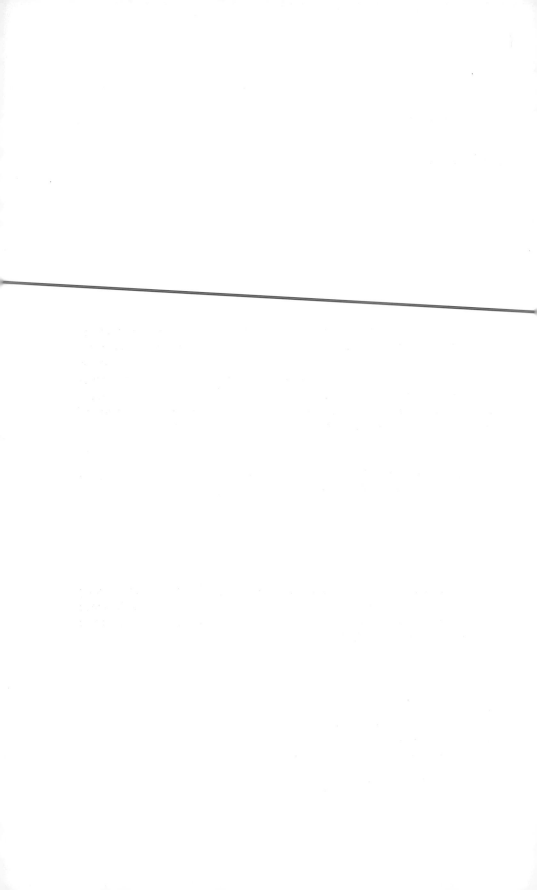

Anatomy by CMR

21

Charles Peebles

Abstract

An understanding of normal cardiac and extra-cardiac thoracic anatomy is essential for the performance and interpretation of CMR studies. This chapter describes the normal anatomy, and common variations, seen on a CMR study. The focus is on the interpretation of the standard axial, coronal and sagittal imaging planes as well as the specific cardiac imaging planes. In clinical practice the ability to scroll through imaging planes greatly enhances the identification of both normal and abnormal anatomy.

Keywords

Cardiac anatomy • Cardiac MR • Left ventricle • Right ventricle • Left atrium • Right atrium • Pericardial anatomy • Cardiac imaging planes

Cross-Sectional Anatomy

A basic understanding of anatomy is a prerequisite for performing and interpreting a CMR examination. A detailed discussion of cardiac anatomy is beyond the scope of this text but this section will provide an introduction to the essentials of cardiac and thoracic anatomy as applied to CMR.

C. Peebles, MBBS, MRCP, FRCR
Department of Cardiothoracic Radiology,
University Hospital Southampton,
E level, North wing, Tremona Rd, Southampton,
Hampshire SO16 6YD, UK
e-mail: charles.peebles@uhs.nhs.uk

© Springer International Publishing 2015
S. Plein et al. (eds.), *Cardiovascular MR Manual*,
DOI 10.1007/978-3-319-20940-1_21

One of the strengths of MRI is the unique ability to acquire images in any cross-sectional plane. Whilst this allows visualisation of complex structures in the optimal orientation it does demand a 3 dimensional understanding of relevant anatomy.

The standard imaging planes are axial, coronal and sagittal. All CMR examinations will include a localising scan which uses these orientations. In addition most studies will also obtain a stack of images, usually in an axial plane, as a prelude to planning the specific views along the cardiac axis. These images are often acquired with a 'black blood' sequence. Figures 21.1, 21.2, and 21.3 demonstrate standard

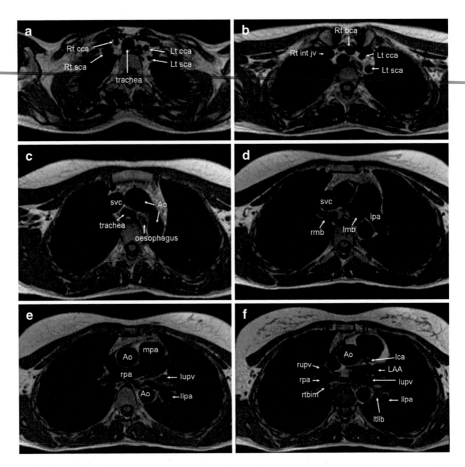

Fig. 21.1 Axial views. Axial Black blood images. *Rt cca* right common carotid artery, *Rt sca* right subclavian artery, *Lt cca* left common carotid artery, *Lt sca* left subclavian artery, *Rt int jv* right internal jugular vein, *Rt bca* right brachiocephalic artery, *SVC* superior vena cava, *Ao* aorta, *rmb* right main bronchus, *lmb* left main bronchus, *lpa* left pulmonary artery, *rpa* right pulmonary artery, *mpa* main pulmonary artery, *lupv* left upper pulmonary vein, *llpa* left lower pulmonary artery, *rupv* right upper pulmonary vein, *rtbim* right bronchus intermedius, *lca* left coronary artery, *LAA* left atrial appendage, *ltllb* left lower lobe bronchus, *RAA* right atrial appendage, *rca* right coronary artery, *rvot* right ventricular outflow tract, *lad* left anterior descending coronary artery, *cx* circumflex coronary artery, *llpv* left lower pulmonary vein, *ct* crista terminalis, *LA* left atrium, *lvot* left ventricular outflow tract, *RA* right atrium, *RV* right ventricle, *LV* left ventricle, *pap m* papillary muscle, *TV* tricuspid valve, *mb* moderator band, *IVC* inferior vena cava, *PV* pulmonary valve

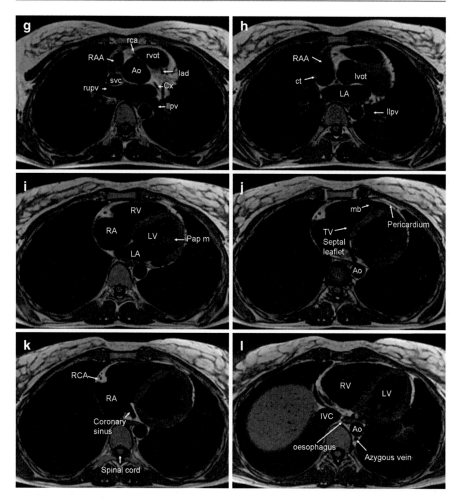

Fig. 21.1 (continued)

anatomy in the axial, coronal and sagittal planes respectively. Axial images are conventionally viewed as though from the feet and ordered from top to bottom. Coronal images are viewed as though from the front and ordered front to back. Sagittal images are viewed as from the patients left side and ordered right to left.

Customised Views

The variable orientation of the heart and great vessels within the thorax necessitates further imaging in specific planes to allow accurate and reproducible assessment of the cardiac structures. These customised views are largely comparable with the echocardiographic views of the heart and great vessels and are planned from the axial images obtained earlier in the examination. They are

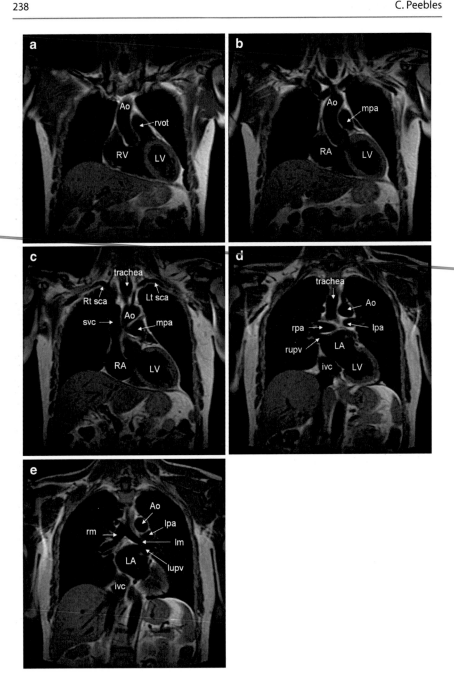

Fig. 21.2 Coronal views. Coronal Black blood images. *Lt sca* left subclavian artery, *Rt int jv* right internal jugular vein, *Rt bca* right brachiocephalic artery, *SVC* superior vena cava, *Ao* aorta, *rmb* right main bronchus, *lmb* left main bronchus, *lpa* left pulmonary artery, *rpa* right pulmonary artery, *mpa* main pulmonary artery, *lupv* left upper pulmonary vein, *llpa* left lower pulmonary vein, *rupv* right upper pulmonary vein, *lca* left coronary artery, *rvot* right ventricular outflow tract, *llpv* left lower pulmonary vein, *LA* left atrium, *lvot* left ventricular outflow tract, *RA* right atrium, *RV* right ventricle, *LV* left ventricle, *mv* mitral valve, *IVC* inferior vena cava

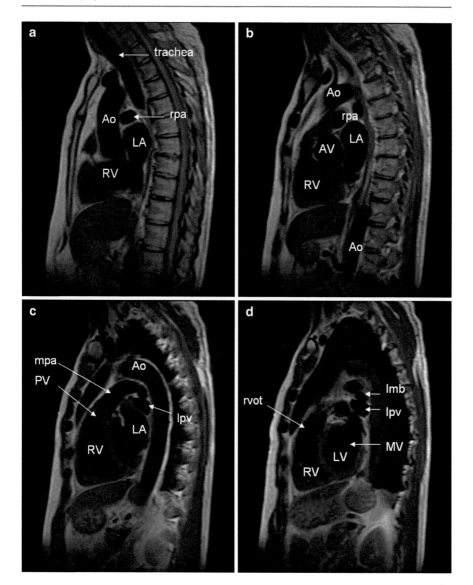

Fig. 21.3 Sagittal views. Sagittal Black blood images. *SVC* superior vena cava, *Ao* aorta, *rmb* right main bronchus, *lmb* left main bronchus, *lpa* left pulmonary artery, *rpa* right pulmonary artery, *mpa* main pulmonary artery, *rpv* right pulmonary vein, *rvot* right ventricular outflow tract, *llpv* left lower pulmonary vein, *LA* left atrium, *lvot* left ventricular outflow tract, *RA* right atrium, *RV* right ventricle, *LV* left ventricle, *TV* tricuspid valve, *MV* mitral valve, *IVC* inferior vena cava

generally designed to assess the intracardiac structures and because of their complex obliquities in a number of planes can cause confusion if looking at extra cardiac structures.

Comparison with Other Imaging Modalities

Echocardiographic imaging planes resemble the customised CMR views. Cardiac CT acquires an axial stack of data, which then during post-processing can be reformatted in any plane like CMR.

> **Tips and Tricks**
> 1. If unsure about anatomy always scroll up and down through the image stack following the relevant structure – this will almost always answer the question.
> 2. When acquiring the scan images always obtain views in orthogonal planes if there is a difficult anatomical question to be answered.
> 3. Three-dimensional data sets such as MR angiograms will often give optimal anatomical views particularly of great vessels and extracardiac structures.
> 4. On black blood images, it can be difficult to differentiate between air-containing (bronchi) and fluid-filled (blood vessels) structures. Compare with bright blood (cine) images in cases of uncertainty.

The CMR Report

22

Sven Plein

Abstract

A structured approach to reporting a CMR study considers the information given in the referral, from other investigations and the scan itself. Standard reporting templates are available.

Keywords

Cardiovascular • Magnetic resonance imaging • Indications • Report

A typical CMR study generates hundreds of images and consists of many different image types. Reporting a CMR study therefore requires a comprehensive and structured approach.

S. Plein, MD, PhD
Division of Biomedical Imaging, Leeds Institute of Cardiovascular and Metabolic Medicine,
University of Leeds and Leeds Teaching Hospitals,
Clarendon Way, Leeds LS1 9JT, UK
e-mail: s.plein@leeds.ac.uk

© Springer International Publishing 2015   241
S. Plein et al. (eds.), *Cardiovascular MR Manual*,
DOI 10.1007/978-3-319-20940-1_22

A Structured Approach to Reporting a CMR Study

In this chapter an outline of a structured approach to reporting a CMR study is given. This is complemented by indication-specific suggestions for reporting in Part III of this book.

1. Identify the key clinical questions from the referral letter.
2. Review if possible original data from relevant related procedures such as echocardiography or angiography.
3. Identify the correct CMR study on the patient database by checking patient name, date of birth, unique identification number and study date.
4. Check that all CMR data are available for reporting.
5. Take note of any particular circumstances affecting the CMR study (such as ECG-gating problems, arrhythmia, breath-holding problems etc.).
6. Start the data review by gaining an overview of the gross cardiovascular anatomy. This overview can use localiser or other data that cover the largest section of the heart and great vessels. A stack of axial black blood or cine images is an ideal source. This overview can be quick or may need to be more detailed, for example in patients with congenital heart disease. It is useful to focus on the vascular morphology and connections and the extracardiac findings separately. Every CMR report should include an assessment of
   (a) The connection of the great vessels and heart chambers
   (b) global LV and RV dimensions and function
   (c) the pericardium
   (d) any other incidental findings (e.g. valve regurgitation)
   (e) incidental extracardiac findings. However, when reporting potential extracardiac findings, recognise and indicate in your report that CMR images are optimized for the cardiovascular system and not for assessment of abnormalities outside of the cardiovascular system.
7. Depending on the specific indication now look at the acquired data in a logical order. For example, in a study indicated for assessment of myocardial ischaemia, one might want to assess the components of the scan in the following order:
   (a) Global and regional LV function from cine images
   (b) Presence and extent of scar from late gadolinium enhanced images

(c) Presence and extent of inducible perfusion defects outside scar from stress perfusion images

(d) If applicable, comparison of stress with rest perfusion images to identify artefacts.

8. Describe these findings (without interpretation) in the general report section.

9. Relating the scan findings to the clinical indication and any previous imaging reports, an overall summary and conclusion(s) should complete the report. Be mindful that this is the part of the report that referring clinicians will often read first – or indeed the only part they will read at all. Thus be sure to include all relevant information, while keeping the content concise. Be sure to answer specifically the clinical questions in the referral letter. Here, findings can be interpreted for example as 'significant inducible ischaemia'.

10. Images or Bulls's eye plots may be added to the report to illustrate specific findings.

In Part III of this book, specific additional items that should be reported on for particular CMR indications are listed.

The Report

The Society of Cardiovascular Magnetic Resonance has published guidelines for reporting of CMR examinations Hundley et al. (2009). The recommendation is that the report includes information pertaining to

(a) site and equipment information
(b) patient demographics
(c) indications for study
(d) study performance
(e) cardiovascular imaging features of the examination
(f) concluding statements that synthesize the study results into a comprehensive diagnosis that can be used for planning therapy or determining prognosis.

Figure 22.1 shows a sample CMR report, modified from the SCMR recommendation in Hundley et al. (2009).

Cardiovascular Magnetic Resonance Report

Cardiac MRI Unit, The Hospital

Patient details: *Name:* **Anthony Nonymous**   *Patient ID:* **111111**
                      Date of Birth: 01/01/1950   *Gender:* male   *Height:* 175cm
                      Weight: 80kg

CMR Study: *Date and time of procedure:* 01/01/2015. 10:00am
                      Personnel involved in procedure: A. Consultant, B. Radiographer
                      Scanner details: Vendor 1.5T, 32 channel receiver coil

                      Primary indication for test:
                      Previous anterior MI in 2001, now recurrent chest pain, ?ischaemia

                      Listing of sequences used:
                      • Non-contrast T1 weighted dark blood (axial stack)
                      • Cine SSFP imaging
                      • Adenosine stress and rest first pass perfusion
                      • Late gadolinium enhancement

                      Contrast agent: XX, 24ml, i.v. right antecubital fossa.
                      Stress agent: Adenosine i.v., 140mcg/kg/min for 5 minutes.
                      Haemodynamics: BP rest: 130/80mmHg, HR rest: 60bpm, BP stress: 140/80, HR stress: 73bpm.

CMR findings: *General findings:*
                      The gross vascular anatomy and connections are normal.

                      Specific findings:
                      The left ventricle is dilated, with a LVEDD of 68mm (measured in the ap direction at the tip of the
                      papillary muscles). Global LV systolic function is mildly impaired. Volumetric measurements by
                      summation of discs from a SAX stack are as follows:

EDV	ESV	SV	EF	LVmass	LVmass/BSA
228ml	114ml	114ml	50%	125g	63g/m2

                      The mid anterior and basal anterior and septal segments are hypokinetic, all other segments are
                      normokinetic.

                      The right ventricle is of normal size and function.

                      Late gadolinium enhanced images demonstrate transmural (>75%) infarction of the mid anterior and
                      basal anterior and septal segments. All other segments are viable.

                      Adenosine stress provoked marked symptoms of chest tightness. The first pass perfusion images show
                      an extensive perfusion defect in all anterior and septal segments.

                      Normal appearance of the pericardium. Valves appear normal.

Summary: 1. Mildly dilated LV (EDV 228ml) with mildly impaired systolic function (EF 50%).
                      2. Transmural anterior myocardial infarction in the mid anterior and basal anterior and septal segments
                      3. Inducible peri-infarct ischaemia in the LAD territory affecting 4 viable segments.

                      Signature of interpreting physician   Date and time of signature

Fig. 22.1 A sample CMR report (Modified from the SCMR recommendation in Hundley et al.
(2009))

Reference

Hundley WG, Bluemke D, Bogaert JG, Friedrich MG, Higgins CB, Lawson MA, McConnell MV, Raman SV, van Rossum AC, Flamm S, Kramer CM, Nagel E, Neubauer S. Society for Cardiovascular Magnetic Resonance guidelines for reporting cardiovascular magnetic resonance examinations. J Cardiovasc Magn Reson. 2009;11(1):5.

Tips and Tricks
1. When reporting aortic dimensions, describe how measurements were obtained (for example 'from diastolic cine images'). This helps when comparisons are made between serial scans.
2. Normal values found in the literature vary and depend on the acquisition and analysis method used. Ensure to use the correct normal values.

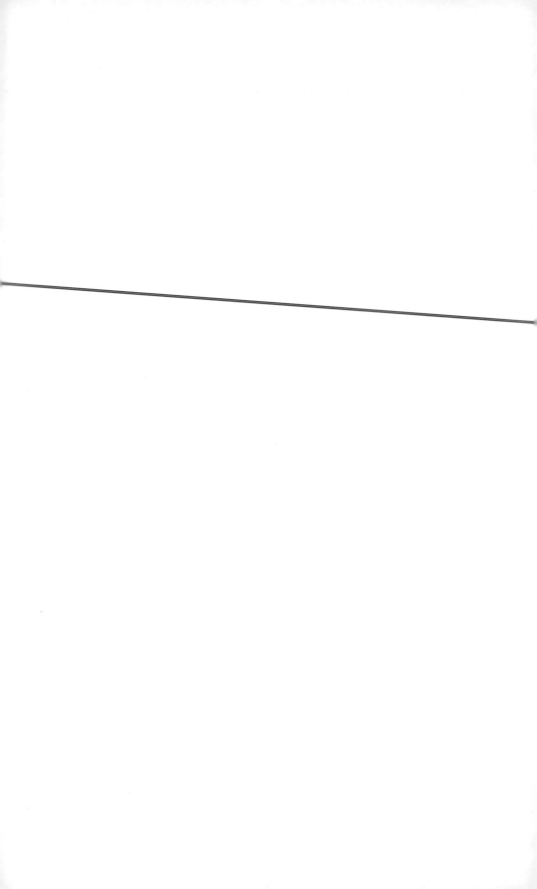

Part III

Clinical Indications for CMR Imaging

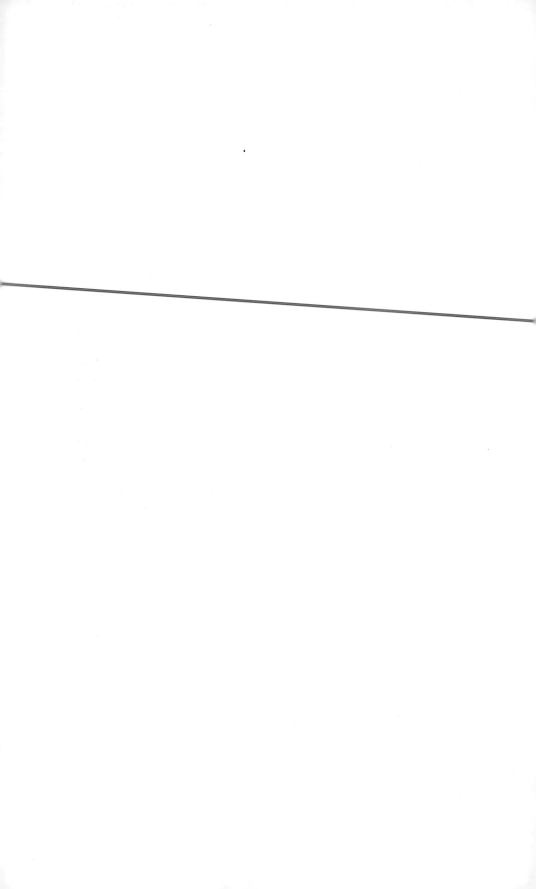

Aortic Disease

23

Andrew M. Crean

Abstract

Aortic disease is common and consists of pathologies that are both congenital and acquired in later life. Although often considered as a simple conduit between the heart and the end organs, the aorta may be afflicted by a myriad of processes including constrictive, degenerative, vasculitic, inflammatory and haemorrhagic conditions. These pathologies may have effects that are silent but harmful (e.g. chronic hypertension in coarctation) at one end of the spectrum with acute life threatening presentations (e.g. aortic dissection) at the other end. Although the ascending aorta is seen relatively well by echocardiography, the arch and descending aorta are relative blind spots where significant disease may be overlooked. CMR is the ideal tool for aortic scrutiny because of its large unobstructed field of view, multiplanar reprocessing capabilities and the range of techniques using both exogenous and endogenous contrast techniques for producing excellent 3D models which are readily understood by non specialists. Finally since the aorta is not an isolated tube but a structure with important ventricular interactions, the degree and consequences of aortic valve disease may be readily assessed at the same examination.

Keywords

Aorta • Aortic dissection • Intramural haematoma • Penetrating atherosclerotic ulcer • Aortic aneurysm • Coarctation • Vasculitis • Takayasu • Atherosclerosis • Familial thoracic aortic aneurysm • Turner syndrome • Loeys-Dietz syndrome

A.M. Crean, BSc, BM, MRCP, MSc, MPhil, FRCR
Department of Cardiology,
University of Cincinnati Medical Center and Cincinnati Children's Hospital,
222 Piedmont Avenue #4300, Cincinnati, OH 45219, USA
e-mail: andrewcrean@gmail.com

© Springer International Publishing 2015
S. Plein et al. (eds.), *Cardiovascular MR Manual*,
DOI 10.1007/978-3-319-20940-1_23

The Role of CMR in Aortic Disease
1. To establish the location, size and patency of the aorta and its major branches
2. To assess the aortic wall and its components
3. To demonstrate inflammatory, vasculitic or atherosclerotic lesions
4. To follow non-invasively chronic aortic disease (e.g. type B dissection) and the post-operative aorta (e.g. following coarctation repair)

CMR Protocol in Aortic Disease
1. Anatomy module
2. Flow module where relevant e.g. dissection, coarctation, valvular lesions
3. Contrast module i.e. thoracic MRA
4. Post contrast T1 weighted imaging module where relevant e.g. arteritis
5. Special views – sagittal oblique SSFP imaging of aorta 'candy cane view' (Fig. 23.1)

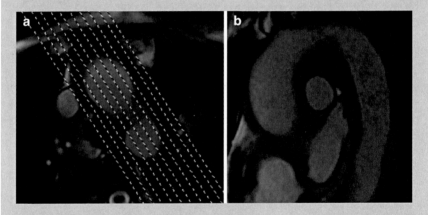

Fig. 23.1 'Candy cane view' of the aorta. (**a**) Multiple slices are acquired parallel to the long axis of the aortic arch. (**b**) The resulting image is often referred to as the candy-cane view. (**c**) Example of a breath held cine SSFP slice in a patient post Bentall procedure – the replaced aortic root and ascending aorta is indicated (*asterisks*). (**d**) Same patient as (**c**) but this image was acquired using a free breathing navigated sequence. The site of surgery is clearly assessed (*asterisks*). Note that the signal is intrinsic to the pulse sequence – no gadolinium was administered to produce this image

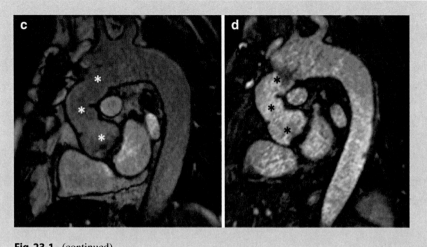

Fig. 23.1 (continued)

Introduction

Thoracic aortic disease is one of the commonest indications for performing a CMR study. The technique is particularly suited to examination of the aorta since it facilitates a wide field of view which – when employed in magnetic resonance angiography – allows the entire length of the vessel to be studied. The lack of ionising radiation is a distinct advantage also since many of the conditions for which MR is employed are chronic and will require multiple examinations over an individual's lifetime.

CMR in the Assessment of Aortic Atherosclerosis and Dissection

Atherosclerosis is the dominant cause of mortality in the western world, largely from coronary arterial disease. However there are a number of pathological manifestations of aortic atherosclerosis which also account for significant morbidity and mortality. The entities of penetrating atherosclerotic ulcer (PAU), acute intramural haematoma (IMH) and acute aortic dissection are inter-twined pathologically, yet have relatively individual CMR appearances.

Acute Intramural Haematoma

This condition is regarded as a *forme fruste* of aortic dissection. The initiating event is believed to be a spontaneous rupture of one of the vasa vasorum within the media of the aortic wall. The clinical presentation is similar to that of a standard aortic dissection (although often without differential BP if the great vessels are uninvolved). The resulting collection of blood is readily appreciated as localised, circumferential aortic wall thickening on either SSFP or black blood imaging (Fig. 23.2a). However, the majority of these cases are diagnosed by CT, since this modality is readily available out of hours and the scan time much shorter – a major safety consideration with a potentially unstable patient. It is also one of the few conditions in which CT provides a degree of tissue characterisation (usually the sole province of MR) (Fig. 23.2b). The main role of CMR therefore is to follow up the acute lesion to ensure that it stabilises/resolves and that progression to chronic dissection does not occur.

Penetrating Atherosclerotic Ulcer

This entity often occurs on the background of generalised atherosclerosis and may also be a precursor to dissection. Just as in the coronary tree, the reason some plaques erode and fissure and some do not remains obscure. CMR readily identifies the site of focal erosion into the media (Fig. 23.2c), defines the extent of the abnormal collection and identifies any associated thrombus formation. Volume-rendered imaging displays only the enhanced portion of an MR angiogram and aortic thrombus may be missed if only an early angiographic phase is acquired (Fig. 23.2d, e).

Aortic Dissection

For reasons given above the diagnosis of acute aortic dissection is appropriately more often sought by CT imaging (although CMR is equally accurate). However if CMR is performed acutely, the principal aim is to confirm the diagnosis and establish whether there is ascending aortic involvement (Stanford Type A) since this usually predicates immediate surgery. Ancillary signs – other than the presence of an intimal flap – include pericardial effusion and aortic valvular regurgitation. Identification of extension into head and neck vessels also pre-warns the surgeon that hemi-arch replacement may be required.

CMR is ideally suited to the follow up of chronic aortic dissection (Fig. 23.3). The main points to consider in the examination are shown in Table 23.1. Acute CT imaging is often performed and reported in a necessarily hurried manner prior to transfer of the patient to a cardiothoracic centre. On occasion outside studies are not archived on the tertiary centre image vault. It is vital therefore that the first MR is thorough and answers all of the questions listed. Magnetic resonance angiography (MRA) should **always** be performed on the first occasion. **This is ideally done in the sagittal**

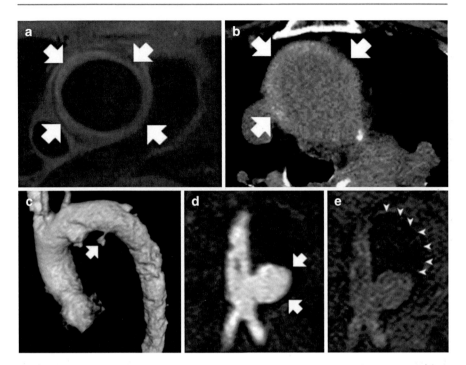

Fig. 23.2 Acute aortic syndromes. (**a**) Double inversion recovery MR image shows circumferential thickening of the ascending aorta (*arrows*). This appearance is non specific and may also be seen in active vasculitis. However in the setting of acute chest pain it represents acute intramural hematoma. (**b**) Non contrast acute CT image (same patient) demonstrates a crescenteric ring of increased density compared to the aortic lumen (*arrows*) – this is due to the presence of haematoma in the aortic wall and confirms the diagnosis of IMH. (**c**) A volume-rendered reconstruction of a thoracic aortic MRA demonstrates a focal collection of contrast (*arrow*) beyond the arterial lumen. Note also the marked irregularity of the descending thoracic aorta due to widespread atherosclerosis. (**d**) A different patient with PAU and a large atherosclerotic ulcer which has transformed into a pseudoaneurysm (*arrows*) is clearly seen above the aortic bifurcation on this arterial phase MRA. (**e**) A second venous phase permits better visualization of the associated thrombus within the aneurysm cavity (*arrowheads*)

oblique plane to minimise coverage, allow for thinner slices and maximise spatial resolution. Follow-up imaging can reasonably be performed without gadolinium contrast if cine imaging or navigated whole heart MRA of the aorta is substituted.

Aortic Aneurysm

Weakening of the medial layer of the aortic wall leads to progressive fusiform or focal enlargement of the aorta over time. Several congenital disorders, most importantly Marfan disease, are associated with life-threatening progressive dilatation and rupture. Other conditions in which aortic dilatation, dissection and rupture are a major risk are familial thoracic aortic aneurysm (FTAA), Turner syndrome and

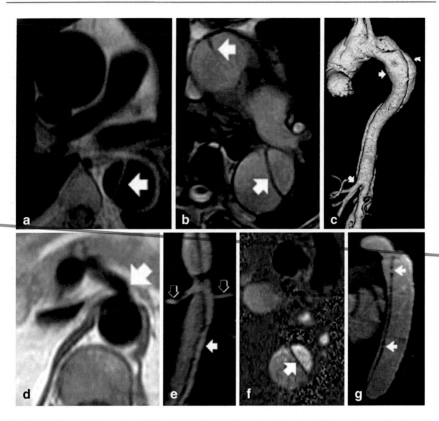

Fig. 23.3 Dissection imaging. Either black blood (**a**) or cine imaging (**b**) may be used to identify dissection flaps (*arrows*). A volume rendered MRA (**c**) is a visually attractive method of demonstrating both true lumen (*straight arrow*) and false lumen (*curved arrow*) as well as the origin of major branch vessels – in this example the mesenteric vessels arise from the true lumen (*oblique arrow*). Thin slice axial imaging (different patient) also allows evaluation of vessel origin – here the celiac trunk arises from the smaller more anterior true lumen (**d**). Contrast MRA (**e**) demonstrating origin of both renal arteries (*black arrows*) from true lumen (*white arrow*). Phase velocity mapping of the descending thoracic aorta (**f**) demonstrates faster flow and thus a more intense white in the true lumen (*arrow*). Sagittal reconstruction from an MRA (**g**) demonstrates several fenestrations (*arrows*) in the intimal flap allowing exchange of blood between true and false lumens

Table 23.1 Principal points to address in the CMR follow up of aortic dissection

Key imaging features of aortic dissection
Extent of dissection
Head and neck vessel involvement
Renal involvement
Mesenteric involvement
Extension into the legs
Relative luminal size
Partial, complete or no thrombosis of false lumen
Progressive enlargement of the false lumen.
Follow up of surgical repair of type A dissection to exclude complications

Loeys-Dietz syndrome (LDS). Susceptible individuals require close monitoring at least every 2 years whilst the aorta remains of normal size and more frequently once enlargement is established. A sinus of Valsalva measurement greater than 5.5 cm or one that changes diameter rapidly between serial scans is an indication for root replacement in most institutions (less if pregnancy is anticipated). Note that the surgical threshold is usually considerably lower for both Turner syndrome and LDS patients who may dissect even at normal aortic dimensions. Turner syndrome patients are especially vulnerable since the absolute measurement of the root may fall within the 'normal' range but represent significant enlargement when indexed to body surface area. Examples of the predisposing conditions for aneurysm formation are given in Table 23.2 and Fig. 23.4.

Patients with unoperated but dilating aortic aneurysms are a source of considerable clinical anxiety. This should not be unduly heightened by inaccurate or inappropriate measurements of the aorta. The advantage of using a cine sequence for this is that the maximum diameter can be tracked throughout the cardiac cycle and thus subsequent examinations may be easily compared for genuine change. An MRA is less ideal for comparative measurements since it is usually performed ungated and as such represents the pulsating aorta averaged over multiple cardiac phases. Nevertheless an MRA should be part of every initial assessment and ought to be repeated if the aneurysm is significantly enlarging, since a volume render of this data set is often the most effective method of 'accelerating' surgical assistance. When an MRA is performed, reconstructed double oblique imaging planes should be used to ensure accurate aortic dimensions are reported. 'Whole heart' navigated and gated steady state free precessions (SSFP) MRA sequences are a good alternative for patients who cannot hold their breath (performed free breathing with diaphragmatic motion tracking) or who are needle-phobic (intrinsic high signal from SSFP sequence).

As with aortic dissection, MRA may miss sizeable aortic thrombus layering within an aneurysm unless a second acquisition is performed in the early venous phase following the initial contrast bolus.

Table 23.2 Conditions which predispose to aortic aneurysm formation

Conditions in which aortic aneurysm may occur
Familial thoracic aortic aneurysm (MYH11 mutation)
Loeys-Dietz syndrome (TGFBR1 and TGFBR2 mutations)
Aneurysms-osteoarthritis syndrome (SMAD3 mutation) – Loeys Dietz subtype
Marfan (FBN1 mutation)
Turner syndrome (45, X karyotype)
Atherosclerotic
Congenital e.g. tetralogy of Fallot, bicuspid aortic valve, Sinus of Valsalva aneurysm
Post-infective e.g. endocarditis, syphilis
Post-surgical e.g. coarctation with subclavian flap repair, neo-aortic valve post Ross or arterial switch procedures
Vasculitic e.g. SLE, Takayasu, giant cell arteritis
Valvular (e.g. aortic stenosis)

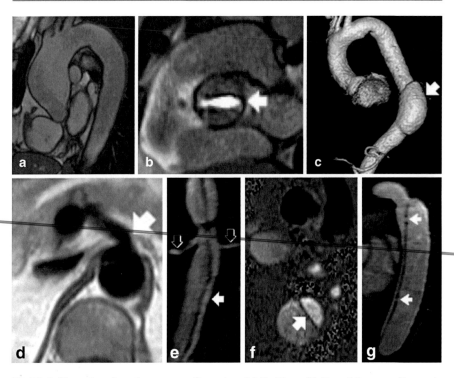

Fig. 23.4 Examples of aortic aneurysm formation. (**a**) Fusiform dilation of the ascending aorta may occur as an aortopathy associated with bicuspid aortic valve. (**b**) Bicuspid aortic valve with reduced systolic opening. (**c**) Aneurysm following penetrating atherosclerotic ulcer. (**d**) Aneurysm arising at site of previous subclavian flap patch repair of coarctation. (**e**) Aneurysm arising due to aortic vasculitis – SLE in this example. (**f**) Aortic dissection flap in cross section (*arrow*). (**g**) Aortic dissection (*arrows*)

Aortic Coarctation

This is discussed in greater detail in the chapter on basic adult congenital heart disease. The points to consider when imaging repaired coarctation are given in Table 23.3.

Aortic Vasculitis

There are several vasculitic processes which may affect the aorta. The commonest is Takayasu arteritis, which frequently affects the arch and great vessels but can also involve the pulmonary and coronary arteries. Imaging is usually prompted by clinical findings (new pulse deficit, reduced unilateral blood pressure) or biochemical deterioration (rising erythrocyte sedimentation rate despite treatment). Giant cell arteritis may present with similar imaging findings and both conditions can cause quite significant thoracic and abdominal aortic stenosis, sometimes at multiple levels. Angiography is the mainstay of CMR imaging in these conditions, with the

Table 23.3 Considerations in imaging coarctation of the aorta

Potential findings in coarctation to include in CMR report
Repaired or unrepaired? (will probably not have had sternotomy – thoracotomy more usually)
Evidence of prior subclavian flap repair? (Absent subclavian origin from arch)
Evidence of restenosis
Evidence of hypoplastic arch?
Evidence of collateral flow (large internal mammary or intercostal arteries)
Peak velocity across narrowing
Bicuspid aortic valve? Stenotic?
Evidence of aortopathy (associated with bicuspid valve)
Patch aneurysm? (if subclavian flap or Dacron patch repair)
Left ventricular hypertrophy if stenosis tight/longstanding (measure LV mass)
Multiple levels of left heart and aortic obstruction (Shone complex)?

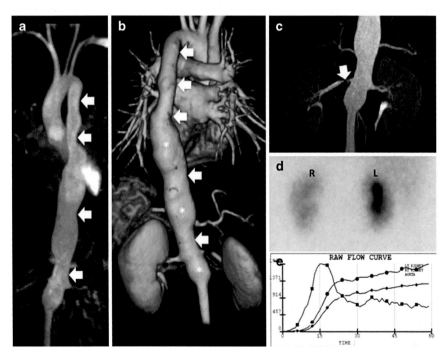

Fig. 23.5 Takayasu aortitis. (**a**) Full volume MIP image demonstrating multiple sites of stenosis (*arrow*) involving the descending thoracic and abdominal aorta. (**b**) Volume rendered image of same patient. Note the diffuse long segment stenosis of the upper descending thoracic aorta. The thoraco-abdominal stenoses are again evident (*arrows*) and also apparent are the intervening areas of relative aortic ectasia (*asterisks*). This pattern of stenosis and ectasia is common when Takayasu arteritis involves the aorta. (**c**) Right sided renal artery stenosis (*arrow*). (**d**) Reduced blood flow to the right kidney. (**e**) Reduced dynamic flow to right kidney

focus on demonstrating new or worsening stenotic disease (Fig. 23.5). Demonstration of disease 'activity' by demonstrating edema or enhancement of the vascular wall has not proven reliable in most clinical centers.

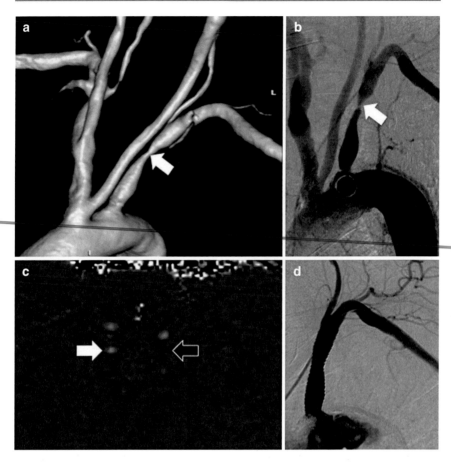

Fig. 23.6 Atherosclerotic arterial disease. (**a**) Volume rendered image from a 64 year old vasculopath with new onset left arm claudication and decreased left radial pulse. A focal stenosis is present in the proximal left subclavian artery (*arrow*). (**b**) Invasive angiography demonstrates good correlation with MR angiogram. (**c**) Phase velocity mapping at the level of the upper thorax shows normal cranial flow in the right vertebral artery (*white arrow*) but reverse flow in the left vertebral artery (*black arrow*) – this is the imaging appearance of subclavian steal syndrome where antegrade flow through a proximal subclavian stenosis is sufficiently poor that flow is maintained distal to the lesion by reversal of flow within the adjacent vertebral artery. In the absence of an intact cerebral circle of Willis this can lead to symptoms of transient cerebral ischemia. (**d**) Same patient following endovascular stenting of subclavian lesion

Chronic Atherosclerotic Disease

Older patients, smokers and diabetics all have an increased incidence of atherosclerosis which may affect not only the coronary arteries but also the cervical and abdominal branches. Carotid, subclavian, renal and mesenteric vessels may all be evaluated using both gadolinium and non-gadolinium enhanced techniques. Phase velocity mapping may also be a useful supplement to provide functional flow data relating to severity of stenosis (Fig. 23.6).

Summary

Aortic disease is one of the commonest indications for a CMR examination. Acquisition is relatively straightforward and both non-gadolinium and gadolinium-enhanced techniques are available. When imaging the aorta to evaluate for increase in size, it is important to acquire data in the same way as previously in order to facilitate direct comparison and accurate measurements.

Key Points CMR in Aortic Disease

1. CMR is the method of choice for diagnosis and follow-up of non acute aortic disease.
2. All aortic imaging for an individual patient should be performed at a single centre to allow for reproducible techniques and measurements.
3. Optimum assessment results from a combination of anatomical and cine imaging.

Tips and Tricks

1. Always perform a second breath held venous phase MRA after the initial arterial phase study (free data set without re-injection).
2. Standardise protocols so that the same technique, imaging plane and slice thickness are used for each follow up examination to facilitate meaningful comparison.
3. In an MR intolerant, restless or needle-phobic patient, a sagittal oblique cine acquisition ('candy cane view') of the aorta provides most of the necessary information in approximately 10 min from start to finish. Free breathing navigated whole heart angiography is a rapid alternative.

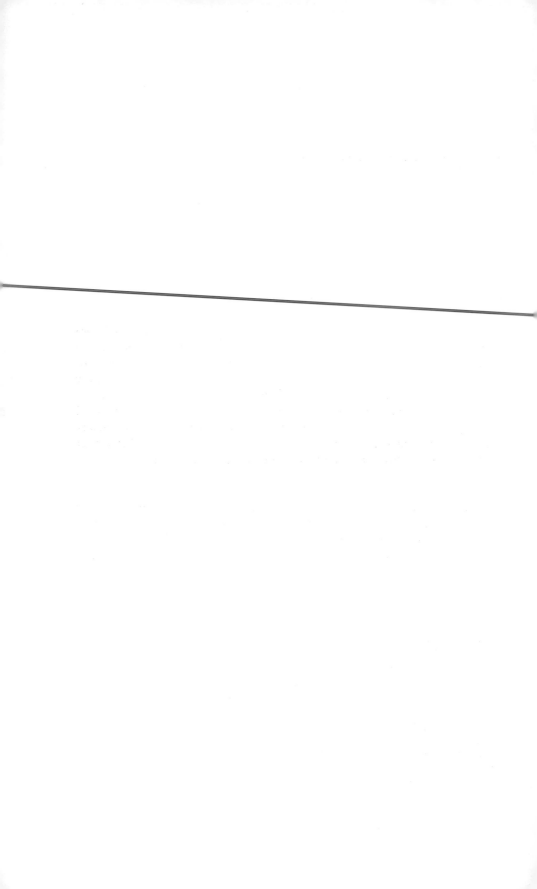

Cardiomyopathies

24

Daniel R. Messroghli and Sven Plein

Abstract

Primary and secondary cardiomyopathies are important causes of heart failure and arrhythmia. CMR is regarded as the non-invasive reference method to establish the diagnosis and stratify risk in cardiomyopathies by means of comprehensive phenotyping including the assessment of bi-ventricular morphology, function, and tissue characteristics. For hereditary forms, CMR screening of family members of index patients might be indicated. LGE represents an established tool to identify patients at elevated risk for cardiovascular events. T1 mapping adds quantitative information on tissue signal, allowing for assessing diffuse myocardial fibrosis and detecting storage diseases.

Keywords

Cardiomyopathy • Dilated cardiomyopathy • DCM • Hypertrophic cardiomyopathy • HCM • Arrhythmogenic right ventricular cardiomyopathy • ARVC • Non-compaction cardiomyopathy • LVNC • Myocarditis • Sarcoidosis • Amyloidosis • Siderosis • Tako-Tsubo • Apical ballooning • Tissue characterisation

D.R. Messroghli, MD (✉)
Internal Medicine – Cardiology, Deutsches Herzzentrum Berlin,
Augustenburger Platz 1, Berlin 13353, Germany
e-mail: dmessroghli@dhzb.de

S. Plein, MD, PhD
Division of Biomedical Imaging,
Leeds Institute of Cardiovascular and Metabolic Medicine,
University of Leeds and Leeds Teaching Hospitals,
Clarendon Way, LS1 9JT Leeds, UK
e-mail: s.plein@leeds.ac.uk

© Springer International Publishing 2015
S. Plein et al. (eds.), *Cardiovascular MR Manual*,
DOI 10.1007/978-3-319-20940-1_24

General Overview

In 1995, the World Health Organization (WHO) defined five classes of cardiomy-opathies: Dilated cardiomyopathy (DCM), hypertrophic cardiomyopathy (HCM), restrictive cardiomyopathy, arrhythmogenic right ventricular cardiomyopathy (ARVC), and unclassified cardiomyopathies. According to the 'contemporary definitions and classification of the cardiomyopathies' published in 2006 by the American Heart Association (AHA), cardiomyopathies are "a heterogeneous group of diseases of the myocardium associated with mechanical and/or electrical dys-function that usually (but not invariably) exhibit inappropriate ventricular hyper-trophy or dilatation and are due to a variety of causes that frequently are genetic. Cardiomyopathies either are confined to the heart or are part of generalized sys-temic disorders, often leading to cardiovascular death or progressive heart failure–related disability". This new definition acknowledges the wide range of myocardial diseases, some of which are primary (predominantly involving the myocardium), others secondary (due to a systemic disease affecting other organs).

CMR has emerged as the most powerful clinical imaging tool to detect and dif-ferentiate cardiomyopathies, except for those that primarily cause electrical rather than morphological changes of the heart (e.g. Brugada Syndrome). CMR is also the most sensitive method to screen family members of affected individuals. While it is impossible to cover all cardiomyopathies in this text, the CMR features of the most common primary and secondary disorders will be discussed.

General CMR approach to the patient with suspected cardiomyopathy:

With the exception of ARVC, CMR protocols for patients referred for evaluation of cardiomyopathy should contain the following elements:

- Anatomy module
- LV function module
- T1 mapping/ECV module
- Late Gadolinium Enhancement module

Further additions to the protocol and specific findings are discussed in the dis-ease specific sections below.

References:
Maron et al. (2006)

Dilated Cardiomyopathy (DCM)

CMR Protocol in DCM
1. Anatomy module
2. LV function module
3. Oedema module
4. LGE module

Introduction

DCM represents a heterogeneous group of disorders characterized by a dilated LV with impaired systolic function in the absence of CAD and other non-myocardial causes of dilatation such as valvular heart disease. A family history of sudden cardiac death or congestive heart failure at an early age is common in genetic forms, while a history of chronic alcohol abuse might be suggestive for an ethanol-induced form. However, in the clinical setting, patient and family history can be unclear and the aetiology remains inconclusive. A residual state of sub-clinical myocarditis has been considered as a potential mechanism for dilatation in such cases.

CMR Versus Other Imaging Modalities in DCM

CMR is the most accurate test for the measurement of left and right ventricular volumes and function. Echocardiography can be unreliable in the setting of abnormally shaped ventricles. CMR is therefore recommended for baseline volumetric measurements. Cine CMR can also delineate mitral valve annulus dimensions and combined with phase contrast velocity encoded imaging can be used to measure mitral regurgitant fraction (see Chap. 30). LGE-CMR is uniquely able to detect myocardial scar from (often silent) myocardial infarction, a common differential diagnosis of DCM with important implications on patient management. LGE-CMR may also be used to guide lead placement in resynchronisation therapy, in particular by avoiding areas with transmural scar. Similar information may be obtained from SPECT or in the future cardiac CT, but CMR is at present the most reliable test for identifying scar. In many cases, CMR can detect midline scar especially in the interventricular septum. The presence of scar and increased values of ECV as a marker for diffuse myocardial fibrosis may be an important predictor of arrhythmic complications (McCrohon et al. 2003; Leyva et al. 2011; Wong et al. 2012) Some speculate that the presence of midline scar suggests that DCM is an endstage of myocarditis.

The Role of CMR in DCM
1. Confirm DCM morphology
2. Provide precise measurement of LV dimensions and EF
3. Exclude ischemic aetiology
4. Exclude acute problem: signs of myocardial oedema?
5. Risk assessment: Arrhythmogenic substrate?

Findings on CMR
- Global LV dilation, wall thinning, reduction of systolic function
- No myocardial oedema
- Diffuse hyperenhancement on LGE, most frequently in a midventricular pattern
- Concomitant dilation of RV and atria
- Mitral valve regurgitation secondary to LV dilation

Differential Diagnosis
- Acute (active) myocarditis: Diffuse or focal myocardial oedema on T2-weighted images, patchy hyperenhancement predominantly of subepicardial origin in the inferolateral wall on LGE images
- Chronic myocarditis: Hyperenhancement on LGE as in acute myocarditis, without signs of oedema
- CAD: Regional rather than global wall motion abnormalities, subendocardial or transmural hyperenhancement on LGE that can be assigned to a coronary territory

Case Example
A 52 years male presented with heart failure. Cardiac investigations revealed normal coronary arteries and no significant valvular disease. CMR images showed a dilated left ventricle (LV end diastolic diameter 83 mn). Cine images showed globally impaired LV function with an ejection fraction of 13 %. LGE images suggested midwall enhancement (**see** Fig. **24.1**) consistent with a diagnosis of DCM.

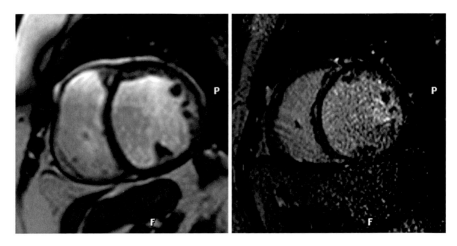

Fig. 24.1 Septal midwall hyperenhancement in DCM

Tips and Tricks
1. DCM patients are rarely good breath holders. Use parallel imaging techniques to keep the breath hold times short for cine imaging
2. If regional findings occur (marked regional wall motion abnormalities, subendocardial or transmural hyperenhancement) consider unrecognized CAD or thromboembolic myocardial infarction

Key Points of CMR in DCM
1. CMR can be used to differentiate acute myocarditis from the more chronic forms of DCM
2. LGE (presence of midwall sign) and ECV add prognostic value to exam

References:
Assomull et al. (2006)

CMR Report in DCM
Report dimensions of:
1. LV: EDV, ESV, SV, EF (all corrected for BSA), end-diastolic diameter
2. RV: EDV, ESV, SV, EF (all corrected for BSA)
3. Dimension of atria
Presence and severity of valvular regurgitation
Presence, location and extent (circumferential and transmural) of scar
Native T1 and ECV of left-ventricular myocardium
Presence of any abnormal vascular connections/shunts

Hypertrophic Cardiomyopathy (HCM)

CMR Protocol in HCM
1. Anatomy module
2. LV function module (consider tagging)
3. LVOT module
4. Long axis view through inferoseptal RV insertion point (para-VLA) to screen for myocardial crypts
5. Velocity encoded imaging in LVOT plane
6. LGE module

Introduction

In its primary form, HCM is a familial disease where genetic defects lead to malformation of contractile proteins such as myosin and troponin (Task Force members et al. 2014). While microscopic studies reveal myocardial disarray, the most prominent macroscopic feature is asymmetric hypertrophy, most frequently involving the septum. Narrowing of the LVOT or circular hypertrophy of the mid portion of the LV can lead to LVOT or intra-cavity obstruction (hypertrophic obstructive cardiomyopathy = HOCM), with haemodynamic consequences similar to those seen in valvular aortic stenosis. Clinical signs include malignant ventricular arrhythmias and heart failure (diastolic dysfunction in the early stages progressing to systolic dysfunction later), with an increased risk of syncope in obstructive forms. In family members carrying the same genetic defect, phenotypes can range from normal micro- and macroscopic appearance to severe asymmetric hypertrophy; there is also an overlap with LV non-compaction and primary restrictive cardiomyopathy. The presence of multiple myocardial crypts, predominantly affecting the inferobasal parts of the interventricular septum, is frequently observed in gene carriers without full HCM phenotype (Germans et al. 2006).

CMR Versus Other Imaging Modalities

The diagnosis of HCM is usually made by echocardiography. However, sometimes the differential diagnosis of HCM versus concentric LVH can be difficult, in particular if image quality is suboptimal or in cases with atypical locations of the hypertrophy such as the apex or lateral wall. In addition, early changes of HCM or aberrant forms, for example in relatives of affected individuals, may be missed on echocardiography. CMR is therefore commonly requested for inconclusive cases. CMR can clarify the diagnosis by providing high quality cine images, accurate quantitative measurement of myocardial thickness and clear depiction of LVOT morphology. In addition, typical patterns of replacement fibrosis may be seen with LGE-CMR, which cannot be identified with any other imaging modality.

The Role of CMR in HCM
1. Confirm HCM morphology
2. Assess LVOT or intracavity obstruction
3. Assess myocardial fibrosis for risk stratification
4. Follow-up therapeutic effects of septal ablation in obstructive forms
5. Family screening

Findings on CMR
- Asymmetric hypertrophy of LV with different patterns (e.g. septal form, apical form)
- RV involvement
- LVOT obstruction with or without SAM phenomenon (mitral regurgitation caused by systolic anterior movement of the anterior leaflet of the mitral valve due to jet effects of blood leaving the narrowed LVOT)
- Abnormal contraction of the hypertrophied segments
- Multiple myocardial crypts (in mutation carriers)
- Intracavity obstruction
- Intramyocardial fibrosis

Differential Diagnosis
- Other conditions leading to (concentric) LVH: athletic training, arterial hypertension, aortic stenosis, cardiac involvement in amyloidosis
- Fabry's disease: causes typical hyperenhacement in the inferolateral segments that can be midwall and patchy.

Tips and Tricks
1. Typical locations of hyper-enhancement on LGE images are the insertion points of the RV to the LV
2. Presence of hyper-enhancement on LGE images might be associated with adverse prognosis
3. Presence of hyper-enhancement and abnormal contraction on tagged cine images are suggestive of HCM rather than LVH

Key Points of CMR in HCM
1. Frequent referral for evaluation of LVH
2. Best tool for morphologic screening of family members
3. LGE might be able to identify high-risk patients
4. LV and LVOT obstruction can be quantified without provocational tests

References:
Moon et al. (2004)

Case Example
A 75 year old female with HOCM diagnosed 8 years ago was referred for CMR for follow-up of LVOT obstruction. Six months earlier she had suffered from decompensated heart failure, and therapeutic microsphere embolisation of a septal coronary artery had been performed in order to reduce LVOT obstruction (pre-interventional pressure gradient at rest on echocardiography: 160 mmHg). While there was some relief of symptoms, the patient still reported significant dyspnoea on moderate exertion (NYHA II to III) and occasional episodes of chest pain (Figs. 24.2, 24.3, 24.4, 24.5, 24.6, and 24.7).

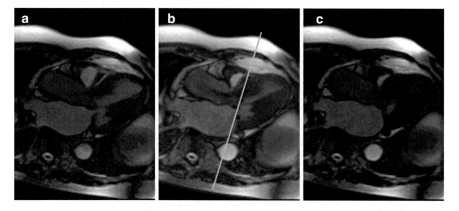

Fig. 24.2 Cine 3 chamber view demonstrating asymmetric hypertrophy of the septum, LVOT obstruction with turbulent flow and SAM phenomenon causing mitral regurgitation. (**a**) End-diastole, (**b**) mid-systole, and (**c**) end-systole

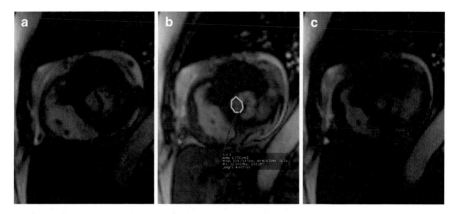

Fig. 24.3 Cine images of the LVOT perpendicular to the turbulent jet (positioning: see *line* in mid-systolic image of Fig. 24.2). The opening area of the LVOT is still reduced to 1.4 cm². (**a**) Enddiastole, (**b**) mid-systole, and (**c**) end-systole

Fig. 24.4 LGE 2 chamber view demonstrating patchy (inferior) and spotty (anterior) areas of hyperenhancement corresponding to myocardial fibrosis

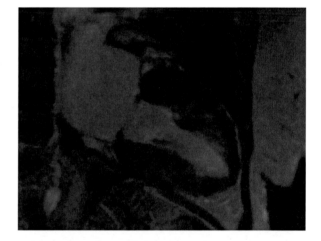

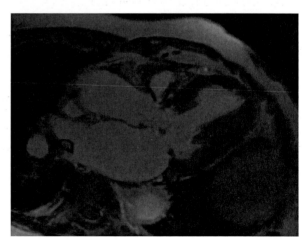

Fig. 24.5 LGE 3 chamber view without major signs of fibrosis

Fig. 24.6 LGE 4 chamber view showing bright area of hyper-enhancement in the mid-cavity level of the septum. This area was not present on pre-interventional images (not shown here) and represents the infarction induced by embolisation of the septal artery

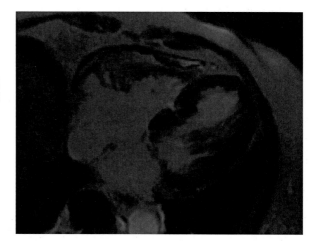

Fig. 24.7 LGE short-axis view with hyper-enhancement at the anterior and inferior insertions of the RV (typical for HCM) and in the inferior part of the septum (caused by therapeutic embolisation)

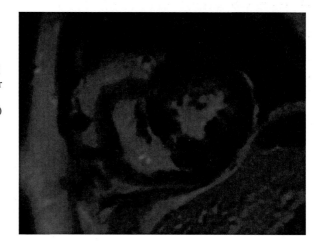

The area of therapeutic infarction appears to be located too apically to fully reduce LVOT obstruction in this patient. The location of the therapeutic infarct site on the RV side of the septum (as in this case) is common and does not lead to successful reduction of LVOT obstruction.

Case Example 2

In a 15 year old patient with recurrent syncope, HCM was diagnosed by echocardiography. Genetic analysis revealed a mutation in MYH6 (beta-myosin heavy chain). On subsequent family screening, the 49 y/o mother was found to have a normal echocardiogram but carry the same mutation (Fig. 24.8).

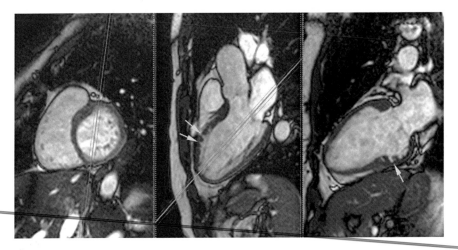

Fig. 24.8 *Left*: Short-axis cine image of a 15 y/o patient with HCM due to a mutation in MYH6 (beta-myosin heavy chain). *Mid* and *right*: 3-chamber view and para-VLA cine images of the patient's 49 y/o mother carrying the mutation. While there is no LVH, multiple deep myocardial recesses ("crypts") are found in the apical and mid-cavity parts of the anterior and in the basal part of the inferior septum of the inferior septum (see *arrows*)

CMR Report in HCM
Report dimensions of:
1. LV: EDV, ESV, SV, EF
2. LV mass
3. ECV
4. Thickness and function of myocardial segments
Presence of LVOT obstruction
Presence of SAM and mitral regurgitation
Presence of replacement fibrosis on LGE-CMR

Arrhythmogenic Right Ventricular Cardiomyopathy (ARVC)

CMR Protocol in ARVC
1. Anatomy module
2. LV function module
3. RV function module (axial SSFP cines, RVOT cines)
4. RV morphology module with and without fat suppression
5. Late gadolinium enhancement module in same orientations as above. Consider T1 nulling for RV.

Introduction

In contrast to other cardiomyopathies, ARVC is a familial disease that primarily affects the right ventricle. Clinical presentation is usually malignant arrhythmia or sudden cardiac death, equally affecting both sexes most frequently during the fourth decade. If patients survive these events, the disease might proceed towards heart failure. In later stages, the LV is usually also affected with varying degrees of LV dysfunction. From a cellular point of view, ARVC is a disease of the binding proteins that link the myocardial cells. Initially normal myocardium is infiltrated/replaced by fibrofatty tissue.

In 1994, the Task Force of the Working Group Myocardial and Pericardial Disease of the European Society of Cardiology and of the Scientific Society and Federation of Cardiology published a consensus statement, which listed criteria that should be used for the diagnosis of ARVC. According to this statement, two major, one major and two minor, or four minor criteria from five sections (history, imaging, pathology, ECG, rhythm) are necessary to establish the diagnosis ARVC, each section being allowed to contribute a maximum of one major and one minor criterion. In 2010, these criteria were further refined and quantitative cut-off values were added (see below) (Marcus et al. 2010).

CMR Versus Other Imaging Modalities

CMR is the optimal imaging modality for assessment of the right ventricle and has a very important role in the diagnosis and follow-up of ARVC and for screening of relatives. However, the ability of CMR to detect fatty infiltration of the RV free wall on T1-weighted images wall has been overestimated and was previously over-reported. It is now recognised that fatty infiltration is very difficult to conclusively identify and if present is usually associated with other clear abnormalities for example of contractile function. The ascent of LGE-CMR has added a further component to the CMR study of ARVC, which many centres now favour over T1-weighted imaging. It has to be recognised that ARVC cannot be diagnosed by CMR alone according to the Task Force criteria, and also that a normal CMR study does not exclude the presence of early "concealed" ARVC. CT has can show typical abnormalities in ARVC, but is not currently a first line investigation.

The Role of CMR in ARVC
1. Assess Task Force criteria (imaging section) for ARVC
2. Follow-up of patients with established ARVC
3. Assessment of fibrofatty infiltration/replacement
4. Assessment of LV involvement

Findings on CMR (according to Modified Task Force Criteria) (Marcus et al. 2010):

- Major criteria: Regional RV akinesia or dyskinesia or dyssynchronous RV contraction and 1 of the following:
    - Ratio of RV end-diastolic volume to BSA 110 mL/m^2 (male) or 100 mL/m^2 (female)
    - RV ejection fraction <40 %
- Minor criteria: Regional RV akinesia or dyskinesia or dyssynchronous RV contraction and 1 of the following:
    - Ratio of RV end-diastolic volume to BSA 100–110 mL/m^2 (male) or 90–100 mL/m^2 (female)
    - RV ejection fraction 40–45 %
- Additional features: Segmental RV aneurysms; signs of fibrofatty replacement/ infiltration (not part of the diagnostic criteria!)
- Thinning of LV wall, reduction of LV function, fibrofatty replacement/infiltration of LV myocardium

There is wide variance to RV morphology in healthy subjects. For example, relative end-systolic bulging of a thin but contractile region of the RV free wall adjacent to the moderator band can be a normal finding and basal short axis cines may give the impression of inferior wall dyskinesis due to normal through-plane motion. At the same time, ARVC is a rare disease. Therefore, CMR reports should always remain descriptive, and the diagnosis ARVC should never be based on CMR findings alone but rather be established using the combination of criteria recommended by the ESC task force.

- CMR has the ability to visualize fat with high sensitivity. However, it should be kept in mind that evidence of fat is not a recognized imaging criterion for the detection of ARVC. Therefore, reporting should not over-emphasize on the presence or absence of fat on CMR.
- Presence of hyper-enhancement on LGE images might be associated with impaired prognosis
- Presence of RV dilatation and impairment of RV function are often early imaging markers of disease.

Differential Diagnosis
- Normal variant
- RV dilation due to other cardiac condition (pulmonary hypertension, pulmonary valve regurgitation, atrial septal defect, partial anomalous pulmonary venous drainage)

Tips and Tricks
1. Since the RV wall is a very thin structure (~3 mm) even in normal subjects and since abnormalities might occur focally, high in-plane spatial resolution and thin slices without inter-slice gap should be used.
2. If there are no wall motion abnormalities or dilation of the RV seen on the RV function module, significant findings are very unlikely and the RV morphology module might be skipped in order to reduce scan time.
3. Hypokinesia at the insertion of the moderator band is a common finding in normals and should not be classified as pathologic.
4. In patients who are able, scanning should be performed in the prone position in order to optimize image quality of the RV.
5. Ventricular arrhythmia is a frequent finding in patients referred for ARVC and might severely affect image quality. In such cases, pre-treatment with anti-arrhythmic drugs should be discussed with the referring physician.
6. Typical locations of hyper-enhancement on LGE images are the insertion points of the RV to the LV but other parts of the LV can also be affected.

Key Points of CMR in ARVC
1. Frequent referral but rare disease
2. Diagnosis cannot be based on imaging criteria alone
3. Interest should be focussed on functional abnormalities of the RV

References:
McKenna et al. (1994), Tandri et al. (2004)

Case Example
A 65 year old female was referred with palpitations. There was no family history of cardiac arrhythmia or sudden cardiac death. A 24 h ECG recorded multiple episodes of non-sustained ventricular and supraventricular tachycardia. On echocardiography, enlargement and impaired function of the RV was noted. A CMR study was requested to further assess RV morphology and function (Figs. 24.9, 24.10, 24.11, and 24.12).

According to the Task Force criteria, this patient fulfilled two major criteria for ARVC (note that a maximum of only one major and one minor criterium from an imaging technique can be allowed according to the Task Force rules). Together with other clinical and ECG criteria, the diagnosis of ARVC with LV involvement was made and the patient received an internal cardioverter/defibrillator (ICD).

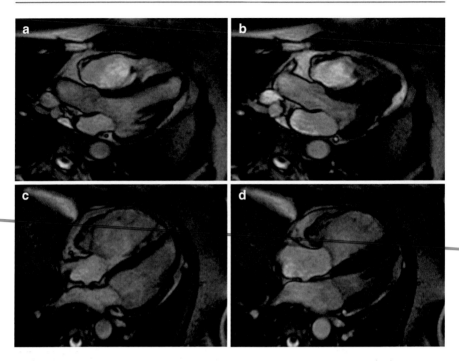

Fig. 24.9 Standard long-axis cine images showing enlargement and severe functional impairment of the RV. The LV is of normal size and function (EF 69 %) except for the lateral apex, where there appears to be depression of the myocardium by bulky epicardial fat. (**a**) 3 cv, end-diastole, (**b**) 3 cv, end-systole, (**c**) 4 cv, end-diastole, and (**d**) 4 cv, end-systole

CMR Report in ARVC
Identify major and minor criteria associated with ARVC:
1. Global right ventricular performance (RVEF)
2. RV dilatation
3. Location of regional RV wall motion abnormalities (infundibulum, body or apex of right ventricle).
Also comment on:
1. Fatty infiltration of the right ventricle
2. Occurrence of fibrosis by LGE in the RV or LV

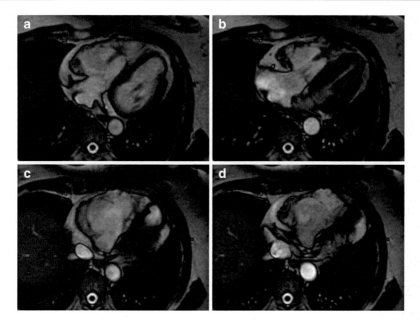

Fig. 24.10 Axial cine images at two different levels demonstrating marked enlargement of the RV (260 mL = 156 mL/m²), impairment of global RV function (EF 27 %), segmental aneurysm of the RV wall, and fatty infiltration of the lateral wall of the LV. Quantification of RV parameters was done using a full set of axial cine images covering the entire RV (not shown here). (**a**) Enddiastole, (**b**) end-systole, (**c**) end-diastole, and (**d**) end-systole

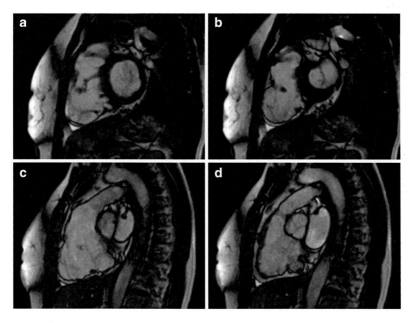

Fig. 24.11 Sagittal cine images at two different levels. The RV wall appears irregular and is dyskinetic in its anterior part. (**a**) End-diastole, (**b**) end-systole, (**c**) end-diastole, and (**d**) endsystole

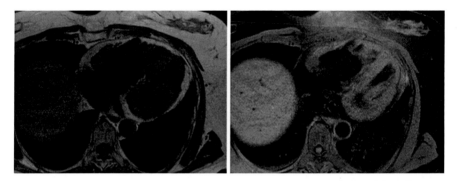

Fig. 24.12 Axial T1-weighted fast spin echo images without (*left*) and with (*right*) fat suppression. In the aneurysmal part of the anterior RV wall, there is severe thinning of the RV myocardium. The lateral apex of the LV appears infiltrated/replaced by epicardial fat. There is also a fatty streak within the basal inter-ventricular septum

Left Ventricular Non-compaction Cardiomyopathy (LVNC)

> **CMR Protocol in LVNC**
> 1. Anatomy module
> 2. LV function module
> 3. Consider first pass perfusion
> 4. Late Gadolinium Enhancement module

Introduction

LVNC is a congenital disease where the fetal process of compaction of the initially spongy myocardium is incomplete. Severe forms have been described as a frequent cause of early cardiac death in infants; its adult form has only been recognized recently with the technical advances in cardiac imaging. In the past, most cases might have been mis-diagnosed as LV hypertrophy due to poor image quality of early echocardiographic machines. Clinically, patients might present with congestive heart failure, malignant arrhythmia or thromboembolic complications such as stroke.

CMR Versus Other Imaging Modalities

LVNC is usually first suspected on a transthoracic echocardiogram. Echo contrast agents can be given to improve the diagnosis. However, LVNC is a difficult diagnosis to make and CMR may be requested for clarification because of its superior image quality and ability to visualise trabeculation. Cardiac CT may be used as an alternative investigation if CMR is contraindicated.

Role of CMR in LVNC:
1. Confirm diagnosis
2. Detect myocardial fibrosis
3. Detect LV thrombus

Findings on CMR
- Hyper-trabecularisation of the LV and thinning of the compact wall, particularly in apical segments
- LV dilation, reduced LV function
- Myocardial fibrosis
- LV thrombus

Differential Diagnosis
- HCM
- DCM
- Chronic myocardial infarction
- Normal variant

Tips and Tricks
- In contrast to echocardiography, where a ratio of 2.0:1 of trabecula diameter vs. compact wall thickness on end-systolic images is used as cut-off to make the diagnosis of LVNC, a ratio of 2.3:1 on end-diastolic images has been proposed for CMR. In either case, some normal subjects without signs or history of LVNC fulfil these criteria; so far it is not known whether these findings have any clinical value in these subjects or not. One or two segments with a ratio ≥2.3 are a common finding in healthy subjects. To avoid over-sensitivity, analysis should be performed on a segmental basis for apical/mid/basal slices, and the number of positive segments should be reported (e.g. 4 out of 16). LVNC is more probable in subjects with ≥3 positive segments (Kawel et al. 2012).
- Patients with congenital heart disease (e.g. VSD) might present with large areas of non-compacted myocardium. Whether this represents a concomitant primary defect or a secondary dysplasia remains unknown, as does the clinical impact of such findings. In order to account for this uncertainness, it might be more appropriate to describe these findings (e.g. "limited compaction of the myocardium") rather than making the diagnosis LVNC.
- Hyper-enhancement on LGE images has been found in a number of, but not all cases of LVNC. It is postulated that these cases represent severe or late forms of the disease.

Key Points of CMR in LVNC
1. CMR can identify hyper-trabecularisation that might have been under-diagnosed (taken for LV hypertrophy) in the past
2. Using quantitative standards (trabecula – compact ratio of 2.3:1) alone might lead to over-diagnosis of LVNC

References:
Petersen et al. (2005a)

Case Example
A 39 year old female was referred with a 5 years history of recurrent syncope. There was no family history of arrhythmia or sudden cardiac death. Holter monitoring documented repeated episodes of non-sustained ventricular tachycardia. Echocardiography raised the suspicion of LVNC, but was not conclusive due to poor acoustic windows (Figs. 24.13 and 24.14).

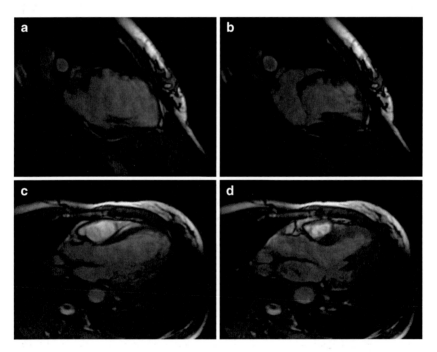

Fig. 24.13 Cine images. The compact LV wall is thin and irregularly shaped. There is excessive non-compaction/hyper-trabecularisation within the LV cavity. As a result, the LV wall appears "spongy". The ratio of non-compact to compact wall thickness at end-diastole was 4.1:1. (**a**) 2-chamber view end-diastole, (**b**) 2-chamber view end-systole, (**c**) 3-chamber view end-diastole, (**d**) 3-chamber view end-systole, (**e**) 4-chamber view end-diastole, (**f**) 4-chamber view end-systole, (**g**) short-axis end-diastole, and (**h**) short-axis endsystole

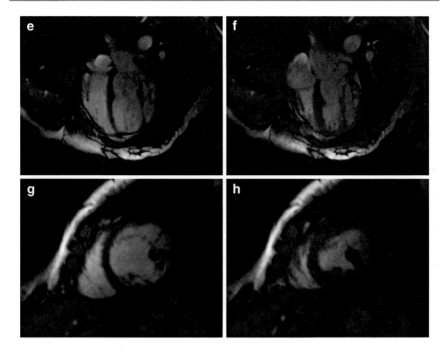

Fig. 24.13 (continued)

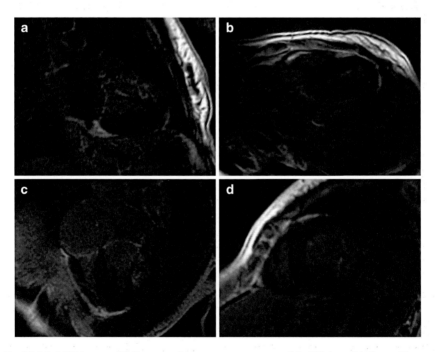

Fig. 24.14 LGE images. While some of the non-compact parts of the LV show thin lines of hyper-enhancement, none of the normal compact parts of the LV wall do. (**a**) 2-chamber view, (**b**) 3-chamber view, (**c**) 4-chamber view, and (**d**) short-axis

CMR showed no ischaemic scar DCM (irregular LV wall, hyper-trabecularisation) and myocarditis (no patchy or sub-epicardial hyper-enhancement) as cause of LV dilation and impairment of LV function, and established the diagnosis of LV non-compaction cardiomyopathy. The patient received heart failure therapy, was given an ICD, and anticoagulated.

CMR Report in LVNC
1. LV volumes and function
2. RV volumes and function
3. Location and number of abnormal segments
4. Ratio of trabeculated versus compacted myocardium

Inflammatory Diseases: Myocarditis

CMR Protocol in Myocarditis
1. Anatomy module
2. LV function module
3. Oedema module
4. T1 mapping/ECV module
5. Late gadolinium enhancement module

Introduction

Myocarditis is an inflammatory disease of the myocardium caused by viral infection and subsequent immunological response, with onset of symptoms (chest pain, arrhythmia, heart failure, fatigue) typically starting several days to 6 weeks after a respiratory or gastro-intestinal tract infection. While sub-clinical involvement of the myocardium is frequent and self-limiting, symptomatic myocarditis can lead to lethal arrhythmia and/or severe reduction of LV function especially if protection of the myocardium by pharmacological (ACE inhibitors, beta blockers) and physical (rest) measures is not initiated and maintained adequately. Acute myocarditis might be accompanied by (global) ST changes on ECG and elevation of troponin, creatine kinase and C-reactive protein levels.

CMR Versus Other Imaging Modalities

CMR is the currently best imaging modality to confirm a suspected diagnosis of myocarditis. Echocardiography can detect regional or global wall motion abnormalities, but CMR has the additional ability to detect focal inflammation and scarring. CMR is commonly requested in patients presenting with acute chest pain and raised myocardial biomarkers, but normal X-ray coronary angiograms. In these patients CMR can very accurately confirm or exclude the presence of myocardial infarction, which may have arisen from the rupture of a minor atherosclerotic plaque. This distinction has obvious implications for the management of patients with secondary prevention medication. In many patients, CMR can also identify characteristic positive features of myocarditis. In only approximately 1/3 of patients with Troponin-positive chest pain but normal coronary angiography can no conclusive answer be given by CMR. CMR is therefore widely regarded as mandatory in patients with suspected acute myocarditis.

Role of CMR in Myocarditis
1. Confirm diagnosis
2. Assess presence of 'inflammation'
   – Assess pericardial involvement
3. Assess pericardial involvement
4. Follow-up LV function

Findings on CMR
- Hyper-enhancement on late gadolinium enhancement images (not confined to specific coronary territory; typically sub-epicardial or intramural; less bright than myocardial infarction; most frequently in the infero-lateral wall)
- Myocardial oedema (not confined to coronary territory; might be used as marker for acute process) as detected by T2-weighted CMR T1 mapping, or T2 mapping
- Impairment of LV function
- Impairment of RV function
- Pericardial effusion/inflammation

Differential Diagnosis
- Thromboembolic myocardial infarction (subendocardial or transmural hyper-enhancement on late gadolinium enhancement images assigned to coronary territory)
- Dilated cardiomyopathy (global thinning of LV; differentiation between chronic myocarditis and DCM often impossible)
- Tako-Tsubo cardiomyopathy (apical ballooning or "inverted" pattern = basal ballooning; full recovery of LV function within 5–14 days)
- Other inflammatory diseases with myocardial involvement (e.g. sarcoidosis, systemic lupus erythematosus: no history of recent infection; additional non-cardiac symptoms)

Tips and Tricks

1. Most severe cases present with LGE hyper-enhancement in the acute stage. If present, hyper-enhancement is usually less bright than in myocardial infarction and might shrink or even disappear in some cases over time.
2. Late gadolinium enhancement imaging might be used to guide myocardial biopsy.
3. At first presentation, systolic function might not be impaired even in the presence of severe clinical symptoms and extensive myocardial lesions as demonstrated by late gadolinium enhancement. Nevertheless, these patients should not be allowed to exercise, and should be considered for ACE inhibitors ± beta blockers in order to avoid deterioration of LV function.
4. Both T1 mapping (Ferreira et al. 2013) and T2 mapping (Thavendiranathan et al. 2012) have been shown to detect acute myocarditis as reflected by myocardial oedema with better diagnostic accuracy than conventional T2-weighted CMR. Thus, T1 mapping or T2 mapping should be performed in addition to T2w MRI, if available. CMR techniques using the skeletal muscle as reference standard (early gadolinium enhancement, global T2 ratio) might be considered but suffer from limited reproducibility.

Key points CMR in Myocarditis:

- CMR can detect myocardial injury in the course of myocarditis
- The presence of hyper-enhancement on LGE images has a high specificity for a severe course of the disease
- The presence of focal myocardial oedema might be used as a marker for ongoing inflammatory activity

References:
Mahrholdt et al. (2004)

Case Example

A 28 year old male presented to the emergency department with acute chest pain. He had also suffered from diarrhoea for the last 3 days. On the ECG there was ST elevation in leads I, II, V4-V6. Blood tests showed elevated troponin T, creatine kinase, WBC, and CRP values. Coronary artery disease was excluded by X-ray coronary angiography. CMR was performed 2 days after onset of cardiac symptoms (Figs. 24.15, 24.16, 24.17).

The patient remained asymptomatic and after 1 month was re-studied by CMR. Oedema on STIR images had resolved (Fig. 24.18). Late gadolinium enhanced images showed a reduction in the hyperenhanced lesions (Fig 24.19). Regional wall motion abnormalities had resolved and ejection fraction improved to 63 % (images not shown).

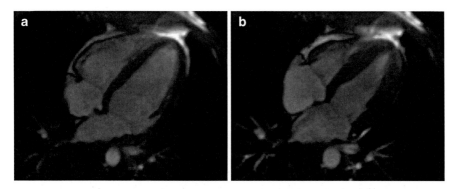

Fig. 24.15 Cine 4 chamber view at end-diastole (**a**) and end-systole (**b**) showing apical anterolateral wall motion abnormality; ejection fraction is mildly reduced (52 %)

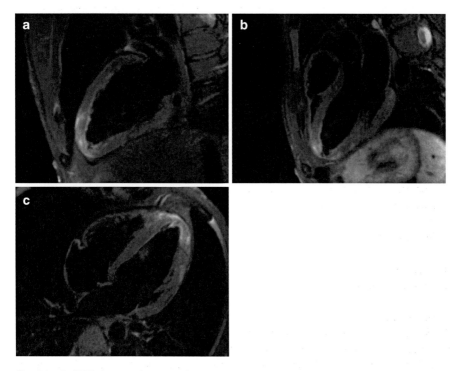

Fig. 24.16 STIR images demonstrating apical myocardial oedema. (**a**) 2-chamber view, (**b**) 3-chamber view, and (**c**) 4-chamber view

The initial CMR study excluded thromboembolic infarction and demonstrated multiple myocardial lesions typical of viral myocarditis. The follow-up study demonstrated regression of inflammatory activity, improvement in ventricular function and a reduction of lesion size during therapy.

CMR Report in Myocarditis
1. Presence and location of oedema
2. Presence and location of hyperenhancement on LGE
3. Regional and global LV function
4. Pericardial effusion or hyperenhancement

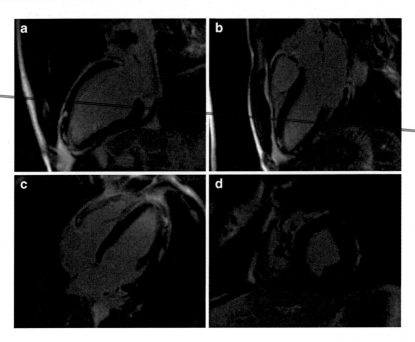

Fig. 24.17 LGE images showing multiple areas of hyper-enhancement in apical, anterolateral and inferolateral regions. The lesions are predominantly seen in the subepicardial layer. There is no pericardial effusion (which would indicate concomitant pericarditis). (**a**) 2-chamber view, (**b**) 3-chamber view, (**c**) 4-chamber view, and (**d**) short-axis view

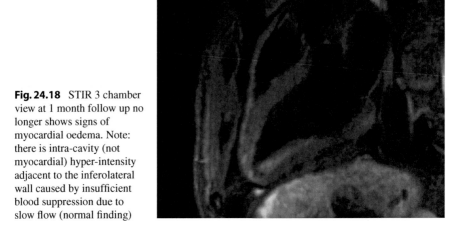

Fig. 24.18 STIR 3 chamber view at 1 month follow up no longer shows signs of myocardial oedema. Note: there is intra-cavity (not myocardial) hyper-intensity adjacent to the inferolateral wall caused by insufficient blood suppression due to slow flow (normal finding)

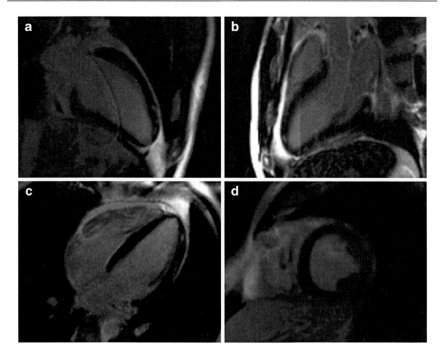

Fig. 24.19 LGE images at 1 month follow up still show myocardial lesions which appear smaller. (**a**) 2-chamber view, (**b**) 3-chamber view, (**c**) 4-chamber view, and (**d**) short-axis view

Inflammatory Diseases: Sarcoidosis

CMR Protocol in Sarcoidosis
1. Anatomy module
2. LV function module
3. Oedema module
4. T1 mapping/ECV module
5. Late gadolinium enhancement module

Introduction

Sarcoidosis is a granulomatous systemic disease most frequently involving lung and skin. Cardiac involvement is a rare (~5 %) but a severe complication which requires immunosuppressive therapy in order to prevent malignant arrhythmia and heart failure.

The Role of CMR in Sarcoidosis
1. Confirm cardiac involvement
2. Assess inflammatory activity and response to treatment
3. Follow-up LV function

Findings on CMR
- Hyper-enhancement on late gadolinium enhancement images.
- Elevated relative enhancement index on early gadolinium enhancement images
- Parametric mapping techniques (T1 or T2) might be helpful for follow-up of myocardial activity.
- Impairment of LV function.
- Pericardial effusion.
- Mediastinal lymphadenopathy.

Differential Diagnosis
- Other inflammatory diseases of the myocardium (e.g. myocarditis, systemic lupus erythematosus)
- Myocardial infarction (subendocardial or transmural hyper-enhancement on LGE images assigned to coronary territory)

Tips and Tricks
1. Hyper-enhancement is usually intramural, spotty and can be almost as pronounced as in myocardial infarction.
2. Lesions presenting as hyper-enhancement usually respond to immunosuppressive treatment.
3. Pure cardiac sarcoidosis is a rare condition. Hilar or mediastinal lymphadenopathy can be pronounced and is often visible on scout images.

Key points CMR in

1. Late gadolinium enhancement can be used to detect focal myocardial lesions that might disappear on follow-up after medical treatment.

References:
Smedema et al. (2005)

Case Example
A 31 year male with known pulmonary sarcoidosis developed acute chest pain accompanied by ST elevation in leads I and aVL and elevated levels of troponin T and creatine kinase. Initially he had been hospitalized for painful skin lesions and fever. CMR was performed on the day of onset of chest pain: (Figs. 24.20, 24.21, and 24.22)

A follow up CMR study was performed after treatment with prednisolone (100 mg/day) and after resolution of chest pain (Figs. 24.23, 24.24, and 24.25).

CMR detected acute cardiac involvement of sarcoidosis initially and showed good response to steroid therapy on follow-up studies.

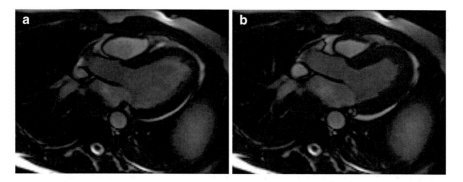

Fig. 24.20 Long-axis cine images in 3 chamber orientation. There is mild impairment of global LV function (EF 47 %) with pronounced wall motion abnormalities. There is a small pericardial effusion (max. 4 mm). A large retrocardiac mass (lymphnodes) is visible adjacent to the left atrium. (**a**) 3-chamber view end-diastole and (**b**) 3-chamber view end-systole

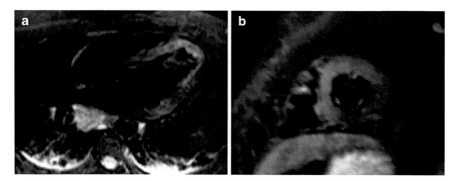

Fig. 24.21 STIR images revealing myocardial oedema (hyperintensity) of the apical anterior and septal wall. (**a**) 3-chamber view and (**b**) apical short axis

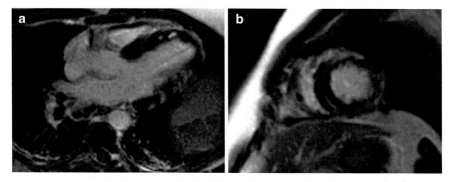

Fig. 24.22 LGE images showing multiple intramyocardial, almost transmural myocardial lesions (hyperenhancement). (**a**) 3-chamber view and (**b**) apical short axis

CMR Report in Sarcoidosis
1. Mediastinal or hilar abnormalities (lymphadenopathy)
2. Myocardial lesions on LGE
3. LV/RV function

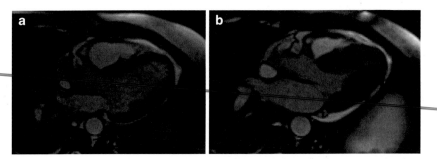

Fig. 24.23 At follow-up following Prednisolone therapy, Cines show full recovery of LV function. The mediastinal mass is no longer detectable. (**a**) Diastole and (**b**) systole

Fig. 24.24 At follow-up apical short-axis STIR image without new signs of myocardial oedema

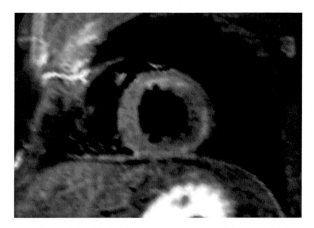

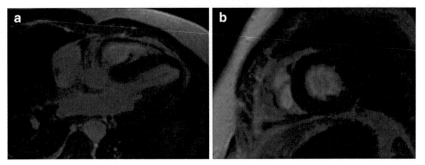

Fig. 24.25 Follow up LGE images: The myocardial lesions are still detectable but are significantly smaller and appear less hyper-intense. (**a**) 4cv and (**b**) apical short axis

Inflammatory Diseases: Vasculitis (Churg-Strauss Syndrome)

CMR Protocol in Churg-Strauss Syndrome
1. Anatomy module
2. LV function module
3. Oedema module
4. T1 mapping/ECV module
5. Late gadolinium enhancement module

Introduction

Churg-Strauss Syndrome is an autoimmune disease affecting small and medium size vessels, including the microcirculation of the myocardium in the later stages of disease.

The Role of CMR in Churg-Strauss Syndrome
1. Accurately assess cardiac function
2. Confirm cardiac involvement

Findings on CMR
- Circular subendocardial hyper-enhancement on late gadolinium enhancement images

Differential Diagnosis
- Multiple myocardial infarctions

Tips and Tricks
1. Hyper-enhancement in Churg-Strauss Syndrome rarely affects more than 50 % of the wall thickness

Key points CMR in Churg-Strauss Syndrome:

- Late gadolinium enhancement images reveal circular subendocardial hyper-enhancement

References:
Petersen et al. (2005b)

Case Example
A 70 year male was hospitalized for dyspnoea at rest (NYHA IV). A CXR showed pulmonary oedema and large bilateral pleural effusions. Blood tests yielded elevated creatine and eosinophilia. p-ANCA was negative.

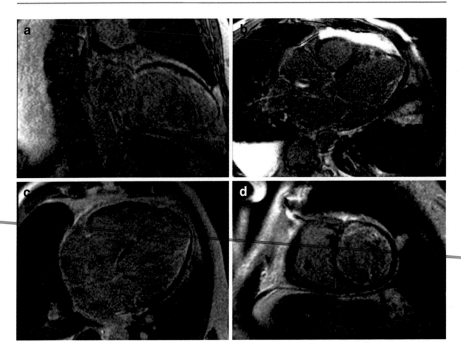

Fig. 24.26 LGE images. There is subendocardial hyper-enhancement that is not confined to a typical coronary territory. There is a persistent large right-sided pleural effusion. (**a**) 2-chamber view, (**b**) 3-chamber view, (**c**) 4-chamber view, and (**d**) short axis

Echocardiography revealed moderate LV dilatation and severely impaired global LV function (EF 22 %). CMR was performed after drainage of the left pleural effusion (Fig. 24.26).

Because of the atypical distribution of hyper-enhancement (subendocardial location not typical for DCM; non-regional distribution and severely impaired LV function despite non-transmural lesions not typical for CAD), cardiac involvement of vasculitis was suspected and a CT scan of the chest was performed which showed multiple small pulmonary infiltrations. Lung biopsy confirmed Churg-Strauss Syndrome.

CMR Report in Churg-Strauss Syndrome
1. LV/RV function
2. Presence and extent of scar on LGE

Infiltrative/Storage Diseases: Amyloidosis

CMR Protocol in Amyloidosis
1. Anatomy module
2. LV function module
3. Oedema module
4. T1 mapping/ECV module
5. Late gadolinium enhancement module

Introduction

Amyloidosis is a systemic disorder where abnormal proteins are produced and deposited in different tissues causing multi-organ damage. While some forms progress slowly, cardiac involvement implies a worse prognosis, with a median survival time of 6 months after diagnosis.

The Role of CMR in Amyloidosis
1. Accurately assess cardiac function
2. Confirm cardiac involvement
3. Assess pericardial effusion

Findings on CMR
- (Very) high global native myocardial T1 values
- High ECV
- Blurry, inhomogeneous suppression of myocardial signal and dark blood on late gadolinium enhancement images
- Restrictive configuration of the heart: small ventricles, large atria, reduced longitudinal shortening of the LV
- Concentric LV hypertrophy
- Pericardial effusion
- Pleural effusions
- Hypertrophy of the inter-atrial septum

Differential Diagnosis
- Other conditions causing LV hypertrophy: arterial hypertension, hypertrophic cardiomyopathy, aortic stenosis: diagnosis based on pattern of LGE. In addition, the amyloid heart tends to have impaired global and longitudinal contraction patterns and the LA and RA are typically enlarged.

- Other conditions causing restrictive pattern: other storage disease: These differential diagnoses cannot usually be made by CMR as the findings are non-specific.

Tips and Tricks
1. In patients where late gadolinium enhancement "doesn't seem to work" despite proper technical procedures, amyloidosis should be considered.
2. If amyloidosis is suspected, a first set of late gadolinium enhancement images should be acquired early (i.e. 3–5 min) after the application of contrast agent, which might demonstrate an epicardial – endocardial signal gradient.
3. Cardiac involvement without hyper-enhancement is possible but rare.
4. Cardiac involvement is usually accompanied by pericardial and pleural effusions.
5. Hypertrophy of the atrial septum is only present in ~20 % of cases.
6. If available, T1 mapping techniques can support the diagnosis by detecting high native myocardial T1 (and high ECV), or to make the differential diagnosis of storage disease (Anderson Fabry's, Siderosis; both leading to low native myocardial T1 and ECV).

Key points of CMR in amyloidosis

- CMR is able to detect cardiac amyloidosis with high sensitivity and specificity
- Myocardial behaviour on late gadolinium enhancement images in amyloidosis is different from any other pathology. It is however not specific and other infiltrative diseases need to be considered.
- Native T1 mapping can make the diagnosis and is helpful to detect other uncommon causes of LVH
- Biopsies in amyloidosis can be negative, so if CMR findings are highly suggestive of infiltration, repeat biopsies, using CMR as a guide to areas worst affected.

References:
Maceira et al. (2005)

Case Example
A 71 year old female was hospitalised for decompensated biventricular heart failure and renal insufficiency. Echo revealed severely impaired LV function and aortic stenosis. She was referred to CMR for evaluation of the aortic valve (Figs. 24.27, 24.28, 24.29, and 24.30).

Fig. 24.27 Localiser and subsequent images show bilateral pleural effusions and mild pericardial effusion (image quality is reduced due to tachyarrhythmia)

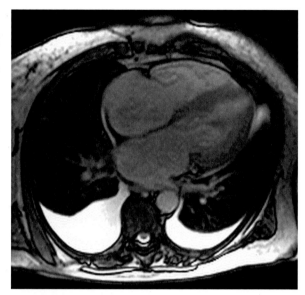

Fig. 24.28 Systolic cine 4-chamber view showing restrictive configuration of heart chambers (small ventricles, large atria), LV hypertrophy, pericardial effusion, and tricuspid insufficiency

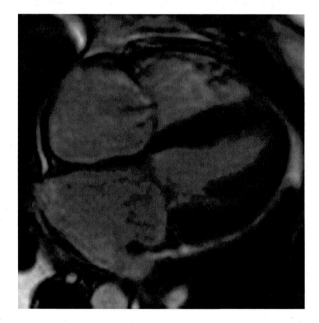

The CMR study excluded severe aortic stenosis and raised the suspicion of cardiac involvement by amyloidosis. Subsequently, blood tests and rectal biopsy revealed AL amyloidosis. Eight weeks later, the patient was re-admitted to hospital after resuscitation from cardiac arrest.

Fig. 24.29 Planimetry of the opening area of the aortic valve revealed mild aortic valve stenosis (1.6 cm^2)

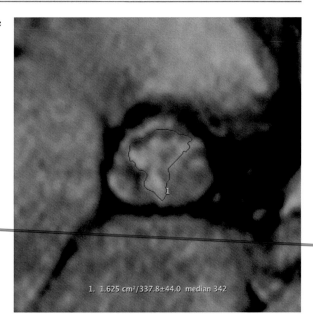

1. 1.625 cm²/337.8±44.0 median 342

Fig. 24.30 Late gadolinium enhancement 4-chamber view with inhomogeneous suppression of myocardium and dark blood

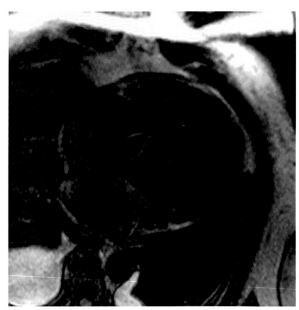

CMR Report in Amyloidosis
1. Global and regional LV/RV function
2. Comment on longitudinal shortening

3. Size of left/right atrium
4. Thickness of interatrial septum
5. Valve regurgitation
6. Enhancement pattern on LGE
7. Myocardial T1, ECV
8. Extracardiac findings (pericardial/pleural effusion)
9. Consider assessment of diastolic function

Infiltrative/Storage Diseases: Siderotic Cardiomyopathy

CMR Protocol in Siderotic Cardiomyopathy
1. Anatomy module
2. LV function module
3. T2* imaging

Introduction

Chronic iron overload, e.g. caused by repetitive blood transfusions for haematological disorders such as thalassemia major, can lead to siderotic cardiomyopathy, characterised by myocardial iron deposition. Cardiac involvement can cause congestive heart failure and arrhythmia, and indicates poor prognosis.

CMR Versus Other Imaging Modalities

CMR has a unique role in the management of iron loading disease. CMR has been shown to reproducibly quantify myocardial iron content and the degree of iron loading directly correlates with outcome. Similar information cannot be provided by other imaging modalities. For this reason CMR is becoming an irreplaceable tool for management of siderotic cardiomyopathy.

The Role of CMR in Siderotic Cardiomyopathy
1. Confirm and quantify cardiac involvement
2. Risk stratification
3. Accurately assess cardiac function
4. Follow-up of iron loading during chelation therapy

Findings on CMR
- Reduced T2* values (<20 ms) in septal myocardium
- Reduced T2* values (<20 ms) in liver tissue
- Reduced LV function
- LV hypertrophy

Differential Diagnosis
- Cardiac amyloidosis
- Other storage disease

Tips and Tricks

1. If other myocardial diseases are considered, a LGE module should be added to the protocol
2. T2* should be assessed in the septal wall since this is the region where susceptibility artefacts are rare (in contrast to the inferolateral wall where they are common due to the proximity to the great cardiac vein)
3. While T2* measurements are currently the method of choice for the assessment of siderosis due to the availability of thorough and extensive validation studies, it has been shown that the presence of iron in the myocardium also leads to shortening of myocardial T1, which can be detected using T1 mapping (Feng et al. 2013). Thus, T1 mapping might present an alternative to T2* measurements if the latter are not available.
4. Patients can have myocardial iron overload without hepatic iron overload and vice versa.

Key points CMR in Siderotic Cardiomyopathy

- T2* mapping can be used to detect and quantify iron overload of the heart and liver

References:
Anderson et al. (2001)

Case Example

A 68 year old female presented with progressive dyspnea on exertion. Since the patient had received multiple blood transfusions in the past 40 years for haemolytic anaemia due to pyruvate kinase deficiency, iron overload of the heart was suspected and the patient was sent for CMR (Figs. 24.31, 24.32, 24.33, and 24.34).

CMR confirmed moderate cardiac and liver iron overload.

Fig. 24.31 Coronal scout image shows large hypo-intense liver

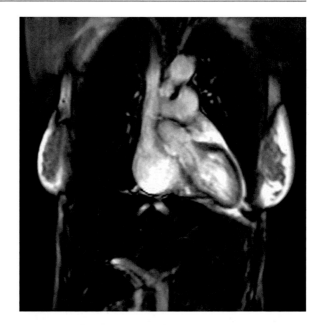

Fig. 24.32 Systolic cine 4-chamber view with dilated atria (image quality is sub-optimal due to atrial fibrillation and poor breath-hold capacity of the patient). LV function was mildly reduced (EF 46 %) with global hypokinesia

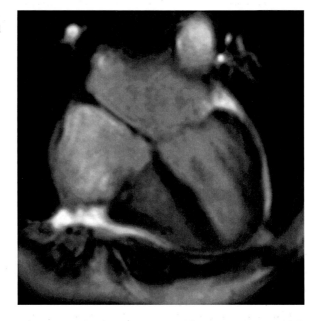

CMR Report in Siderotic Cardiomyopathy
1. LV/RV function and mass
2. T2* values of heart and liver

Fig. 24.33 Mid-cavity short-axis T2* map of the heart. Mean T2* in septal myocardium was 10 ms (normal: >20 ms). *arrows* and *lines* indicate measurement region

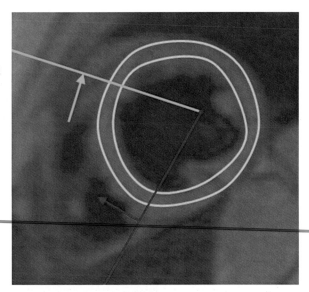

Fig. 24.34 Axial T2* map of the liver (scale: 0–50 ms). Mean hepatic T2* was 2 ms

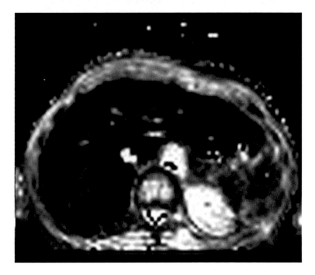

Tako-Tsubo Cardiomyopathy

CMR Protocol in Tako-Tsubo Cardiomyopathy
1. Anatomy module
2. LV function module
3. Oedema module
4. T1 mapping/ECV module
5. Late gadolinium enhancement module

Introduction

In Tako-Tsubo cardiomyopathy, an episode of severe emotional or physical stress to the patient leads to an acute condition mimicking acute coronary syndrome, while coronary arteries are typically normal/unobstructed in these patients. In its typical form, function of the apical and mid-cavity portions of the LV are initially severely impaired ("apical ballooning"), resembling the shape of a traditional Japanese vessel used to catch octopus ("Tako-Tsubo"), although many other patterns of wall motion abnormality have now been described in this condition. It is believed that this acute disease is a 'toxic' reaction to excessive levels of catecholamines.

CMR Versus Other Imaging Modalities

The suspicion of Tako-Tsubo cardiomyopathy usually arises in the cardiac catheter laboratory at the time of primary angioplasty or on an early 'post-infarct' echocardiogram. The main imaging features of this syndrome are characteristic and do not require CMR imaging. However, CMR adds to the diagnosis in uncertain cases, and can on occasions identify unexpected myocardial infarction despite angiographically normal coronary arteries.

The Role of CMR in Tako-Tsubo Cardiomyopathy
1. Confirm diagnosis
2. Rule out myocardial infarction
3. Rule out myocarditis
4. Follow-up functional recovery
5. Detect complications

Findings on CMR
- Typical pattern of functional impairment: apical ballooning or inverted pattern (mid-ventricular ballooning with basal and apical hyperkinesias).
- Quick restoration of LV function: significant amelioration within 5 days, full recovery within 10–14 days after onset.
- Myocardial oedema in the area of wall motion abnormality
- Lack of hyper-enhancement on late gadolinium enhancement images
- LVOT obstruction due to bulging of the basal septum caused by impaired contraction pattern of the LV; reversible with recovery of LV function
- Complications similar to those in acute myocardial infarction: rupture of the LV or papillary muscles

Differential Diagnosis
- thromboembolic or vasospastic myocardial infarction: these will show subendocardial or transmural hyper-enhancement attributable to a coronary artery territory; no immediate recovery of LV function.
- acute myocarditis: may show subepicardial or intramural hyper-enhancement; usually more gradual recovery of LV function.

Tips and Tricks

1. While typical cases do not exhibit any hyper-enhancement on LGE images, there have been reports of cases of histologically proven Tako Tsubo cardiomyopathy that did show infarct-like hyper-enhancement. Given the disastrous histo-pathological damage that has been documented in a large series of "classic" cases, these findings are not surprising and it rather seems remarkable that there are not more of them. If hyper-enhancement is present, the differentiation of Tako-Tsubo from thromboembolic infarction relies on the distribution pattern of the myocardial injury (confined to a coronary territory) and might even be impossible in some cases.

Key points CMR in Tako-Tsubo cardiomyopathy:

- CMR is the best imaging technique to differentiate Tako-Tsubo from thromboembolic myocardial infarction and acute myocarditis.

References:
Wittstein et al. (2005)

Case Example
Six hours after the funeral of her husband, an 83 years female was admitted with acute chest pain, ST elevation in anterior leads, and elevated troponin T. X ray coronary angiography found only minor CAD without a culprit lesion. CMR was performed the next day (Figs. 24.35, 24.36, and 24.37).

Follow-up on echocardiography 1 week later confirmed LV function had returned to normal.

Diagnosis: Apical ballooning syndrome or Tako Tsubo cardiomyopathy.

CMR Report in Tako Tsubo Cardiomyopathy
1. LV/RV volumes and function
2. Presence and pattern of regional wall motion abnormalities, oedema and LGE

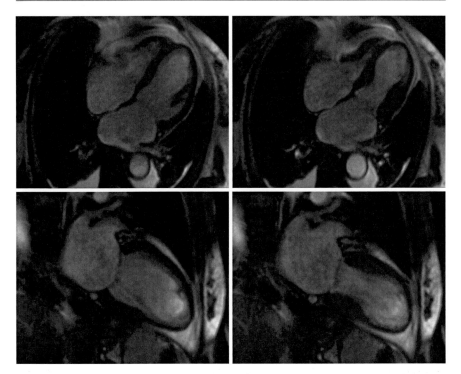

Fig. 24.35 Cine images showing apical ballooning (systolic and diastolic images shown). Ejection fraction is 41 %. There are bilateral pleural effusions indicating acute heart failure

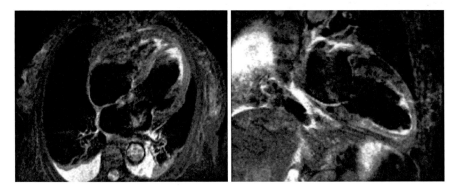

Fig. 24.36 STIR images in 2 chamber (*left*) and 4 chamber views (*right*). There is mild apical hyperintensity of the myocardium (in addition to intra-cavity hyperintensity given by normal slow-flow phenomena)

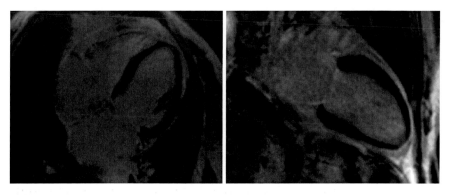

Fig. 24.37 LGE images without signs of myocardial necrosis or scarring

References

Anderson LJ, et al. Cardiovascular T2-star (T2*) magnetic resonance for the early diagnosis of myocardial iron overload. Eur Heart J. 2001;22(23):2171–9.

Assomull RG, et al. Cardiovascular magnetic resonance, fibrosis, and prognosis in dilated cardio-myopathy. J Am Coll Cardiol. 2006;48(10):1977–85.

Authors/Task Force members, Elliott PM, Anastasakis A, Borger MA, Borggrefe M, Cecchi F, Charron P, Hagege AA, Lafont A, Limongelli G, Mahrholdt H, McKenna WJ, Mogensen J, Nihoyannopoulos P, Nistri S, Pieper PG, Pieske B, Rapezzi C, Rutten FH, Tillmanns C, Watkins H. 2014 ESC Guidelines on diagnosis and management of hypertrophic cardiomyopa-thy: the Task Force for the Diagnosis and Management of Hypertrophic Cardiomyopathy of the European Society of Cardiology (ESC). Eur Heart J. 2014;35(39):2733–79. doi:10.1093/eurheartj/ehu284. Epub 29 Aug 2014.

Feng Y, He T, Carpenter JP, Jabbour A, Alam MH, Gatehouse PD, Greiser A, Messroghli D, Firmin DN, Pennell DJ. In vivo comparison of myocardial T1 with T2 and T2* in thalassaemia major. J Magn Reson Imaging. 2013;38(3):588–93.

Ferreira VM, Piechnik SK, Dall'Armellina E, Karamitsos TD, Francis JM, Ntusi N, Holloway C, Choudhury RP, Kardos A, Robson MD, Friedrich MG, Neubauer S. T(1) mapping for the diagnosis of acute myocarditis using CMR: comparison to T2-weighted and late gadolinium enhanced imaging. JACC Cardiovasc Imaging. 2013;6(10):1048–58.

Germans T, Wilde AA, Dijkmans PA, Chai W, Kamp O, Pinto YM, van Rossum AC. Structural abnormalities of the inferoseptal left ventricular wall detected by cardiac magnetic reso-nance imaging in carriers of hypertrophic cardiomyopathy mutations. J Am Coll Cardiol. 2006;48(12):2518–23. Epub 28 Nov 2006.

Kawel N, Nacif M, Arai AE, Gomes AS, Hundley WG, Johnson WC, Prince MR, Stacey RB, Lima JA, Bluemke DA. Trabeculated (noncompacted) and compact myocardium in adults: the multi-ethnic study of atherosclerosis. Circ Cardiovasc Imaging. 2012;5(3):357–66.

Leyva F, Foley PW, Chalil S, Ratib K, Smith RE, Prinzen F, Auricchio A. Cardiac resynchroni-zation therapy guided by late gadolinium-enhancement cardiovascular magnetic resonance. J Cardiovasc Magn Reson. 2011;13:29. doi:10.1186/1532-429X-13-29.

Maceira AM, et al. Cardiovascular magnetic resonance in cardiac amyloidosis. Circulation. 2005;111(2):186–93.

Mahrholdt H, et al. Cardiovascular magnetic resonance assessment of human myocarditis: a com-parison to histology and molecular pathology. Circulation. 2004;109(10):1250–8.

Marcus FI, McKenna WJ, Sherrill D, Basso C, Bauce B, Bluemke DA, Calkins H, Corrado D, Cox MG, Daubert JP, Fontaine G, Gear K, Hauer R, Nava A, Picard MH, Protonotarios N, Saffitz JE, Sanborn DM, Steinberg JS, Tandri H, Thiene G, Towbin JA, Tsatsopoulou A, Wichter T, Zareba W. Diagnosis of arrhythmogenic right ventricular cardiomyopathy/dysplasia: proposed modification of the Task Force Criteria. Eur Heart J. 2010;31(7):806–14. doi:10.1093/eurheartj/ehq025. Epub 19 Feb 2010.

Maron BJ, et al. Contemporary definitions and classification of the cardiomyopathies: an American Heart Association Scientific Statement from the Council on Clinical Cardiology, Heart Failure and Transplantation Committee; Quality of Care and Outcomes Research and Functional Genomics and Translational Biology Interdisciplinary Working Groups; and Council on Epidemiology and Prevention. Circulation. 2006;113(14):1807–16.

McCrohon JA, Moon JC, Prasad SK, McKenna WJ, Lorenz CH, Coats AJ, Pennell DJ. Differentiation of heart failure related to dilated cardiomyopathy and coronary artery disease using gadolinium-enhanced cardiovascular magnetic resonance. Circulation. 2003;108(1): 54–9. Epub 23 Jun 2003.

McKenna WJ, et al. Diagnosis of arrhythmogenic right ventricular dysplasia/cardiomyopathy. Task Force of the Working Group Myocardial and Pericardial Disease of the European Society of Cardiology and of the Scientific Council on Cardiomyopathies of the International Society and Federation of Cardiology. Br Heart J. 1994;71(3):215–8.

Moon JC, et al. The histologic basis of late gadolinium enhancement cardiovascular magnetic resonance in hypertrophic cardiomyopathy. J Am Coll Cardiol. 2004;43(12):2260–4.

Petersen SE, et al. Left ventricular non-compaction: insights from cardiovascular magnetic resonance imaging. J Am Coll Cardiol. 2005a;46(1):101–5.

Petersen SE, Kardos A, Neubauer S. Subendocardial and papillary muscle involvement in a patient with Churg-Strauss syndrome, detected by contrast enhanced cardiovascular magnetic resonance. Heart. 2005b;91(1):e9.

Smedema J-P, et al. Evaluation of the accuracy of gadolinium-enhanced cardiovascular magnetic resonance in the diagnosis of cardiac sarcoidosis. J Am Coll Cardiol. 2005;45(10):1683–90.

Tandri H, et al. MRI of arrhythmogenic right ventricular cardiomyopathy/dysplasia. J Cardiovasc Magn Reson. 2004;6(2):557–63.

Thavendiranathan P, Walls M, Giri S, Verhaert D, Rajagopalan S, Moore S, Simonetti OP, Raman SV. Improved detection of myocardial involvement in acute inflammatory cardiomyopathies using T2 mapping. Circ Cardiovasc Imaging. 2012;5(1):102–10.

Wittstein IS, et al. Neurohumoral features of myocardial stunning due to sudden emotional stress. N Engl J Med. 2005;352(6):539–48.

Wong TC, Piehler K, Meier CG, Testa SM, Klock AM, Aneizi AA, Shakesprere J, Kellman P, Shroff SG, Schwartzman DS, Mulukutla SR, Simon MA, Schelbert EB. Association between extracellular matrix expansion quantified by cardiovascular magnetic resonance and short-term mortality. Circulation. 2012;126(10):1206–16. doi:10.1161/CIRCULATIONAHA.111.089409. Epub 31 Jul 2012.

Cardiac Transplantation

25

Christopher A. Miller and Matthias Schmitt

Abstract

This chapter describes the role of CMR in the assessment of patients following heart transplantation. The transplanted heart presents unique anatomical, physiological, pathological and practical considerations. Post-transplant anatomy is described and typical CMR appearances in the early and chronic phases post-transplantation are explained. The common conditions affecting the transplanted heart, and the role of CMR in their detection, are described. A heart transplantation CMR protocol is provided, and tips and tricks for scanning heart transplant recipients are given.

Keywords

Heart transplant • Acute rejection • Primary graft dysfunction • Cardiac allograft vasculopathy • Chronic graft failure • Imaging • Cardiovascular magnetic resonance • Tissue characterisation • Late gadolinium enhancement

C.A. Miller, BSc(Hons),MBChB(Hons),MRCP,PhD (✉)
Cardiac MRI Unit, University Hospitals of South Manchester NHS Foundation Trust,
North West Heart Centre, Southmoor Road, Wythenshawe, Manchester M23 9LT, UK
e-mail: chrismiller@doctors.org.uk

M. Schmitt, MD, PhD
Cross-Sectional Cardiac Imaging Unit, Cardiovascular Division,
University Hospital of South Manchester, Southmoor Road, Wythenshawe,
Manchester M23 9LT, UK
e-mail: mattschmitt@doctors.org.uk

© Springer International Publishing 2015
S. Plein et al. (eds.), *Cardiovascular MR Manual*,
DOI 10.1007/978-3-319-20940-1_25

Heart Transplantation CMR Protocol
1. Anatomy module
2. LV function module
3. Special views – SSFP imaging of the aorta (sagittal oblique ("candy cane view")) and right ventricular outflow tract/main pulmonary artery
4. Oedema perfusion aortic modules as appropriate
5. LGE module

Introduction

Heart transplantation is an established treatment for end-stage heart failure. It is estimated that approximately 6000 heart transplants are carried out worldwide per year at present. Median survival of transplant recipients is 11 years, although in those surviving up to 1 year post-transplant it is 13 years (Lund et al. 2013).

The transplanted heart presents unique anatomical, physiological, pathological and practical considerations. Due to the nature of conditions that affect the transplanted heart, and its denervation, allograft disease often remains asymptomatic until an advanced stage, or presents non-specifically. As such, there is a low threshold for performing cardiac imaging in this population.

CMR Versus Other Imaging Modalities

Echocardiography remains the first line imaging modality for transplant recipients presenting with cardiovascular symptoms. In addition, for the reasons stated in the introduction, patients undergo regular screening echocardiography with the aim of detecting allograft dysfunction at an earlier stage. However, factors such as the non-standard position of the transplanted heart and immunosuppression-related raised body mass index, mean accurate echocardiographic assessment is often challenging. With its independence of acoustic windows, high inherent tissue contrast, ability to image the vascular anastomoses and being free from ionising radiation (important given the frequency that transplant recipients undergo investigations and their high risk of malignancy), CMR is an ideal second line tool. Furthermore, CMR provides unique additional information regarding the state of the graft myocardium (tissue characterisation).

Role of CMR in Heart Transplant Disease
1. To investigate the aetiology of graft dysfunction
2. To assess graft function when echo windows are poor (common), particularly in patients presenting with non-specific symptoms (common).
3. To detect otherwise unrecognised myocardial infarction
4. To assess for vascular complications

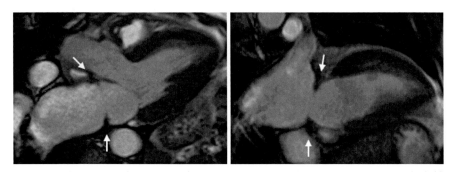

Fig. 25.1 LVOT and VLA cine images showing the left atrial anastomosis (anastomosis indicated by *arrows*)

Heart Transplant Anatomy

Heterotopic heart transplantation, where the recipient's heart is left in situ and the donor heart is connected in parallel fashion, is performed very rarely. Orthotopic transplantation, where the majority of the recipient's heart is removed, is the standard technique. The posterior aspect of the recipient's left atrium is typically left in place in order to preserve pulmonary venous connections. The donor left atrium is sutured to the recipient's left atrium, which can result in a 'double' left atrial appearance (Fig. 25.1). Increasingly, the most common method of anastomosis for the base of the right heart is the bi-caval technique, where the recipient's right atrium is almost completely resected, leaving an atrial cuff at the juncture of the superior and inferior venae cavae, and the donor superior and inferior venae cavae are sutured to the recipient atrial cuffs (Fig. 25.2). Whilst more complex than the standard right atrial anastomosis, where the posterior aspect of the recipient's right atrium is left in place and the donor right atrium is sutured to it, the bi-caval technique aims to preserve right atrial function, and appears to be associated with a lower incidence of tricuspid regurgitation, sinoatrial node dysfunction and atrial arrhythmias. Aortic anastomosis is performed in the ascending aorta at a variable position between the ST junction and the origin of the brachiocephalic artery (Fig. 25.3). The pulmonic anastomosis is in the main pulmonary artery (Fig. 25.4). The great vessel suture lines are usually apparent and a donor-recipient size mismatch is not uncommonly observed. The transplanted heart often does not sit in the standard position in the chest, typically being laterally displaced (Fig. 25.5).

The Early Post Operative Period (Up to 1 Year)

Typical CMR Appearances

Ventricular contraction often appears 'stiff' in the early post operative period. Long-axis function is often reduced but radial contraction is typically preserved and ejection fraction is usually normal or near normal. Pericardial effusion is common (two-thirds of patients at 3 months). Global myocardial oedema may be evident in the first few

Fig. 25.2 Cine images show
the Bi-caval anastomosis.
Arrows superior vena cava
anastomosis, *triangles*
inferior vena cava
anastomosis

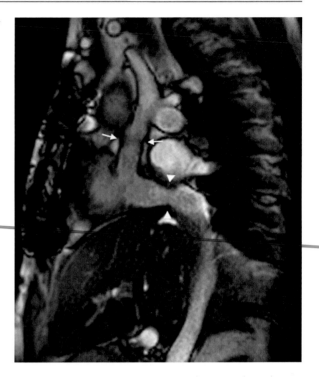

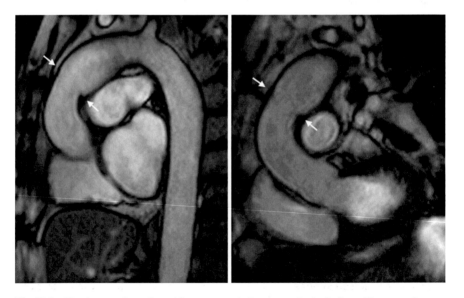

Fig. 25.3 Cine images show the aortic anastomosis (anastomosis site indicated by *arrows*)

Fig. 25.4 Cine images of the RVOT show the pulmonic anastomosis (*arrows*)

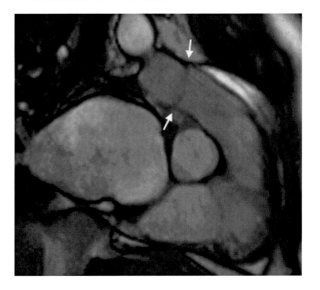

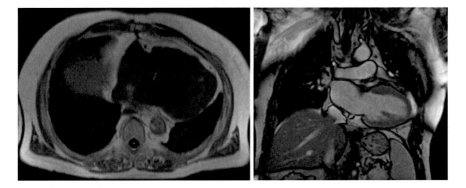

Fig. 25.5 Abnormal lateral and horizontal position of the transplanted heart

months, likely reflecting the considerable insults to which the donor heart is subjected in the peri-transplant period (e.g. brain death and its sequelae, ischemia and reperfusion).

Complications

The most common conditions affecting the transplanted heart in the early phase are primary graft dysfunction, myocardial infarction and acute rejection.

Primary Graft Dysfunction/Failure

Primary graft dysfunction (PGD) is a clinical syndrome manifesting as severe ventricular dysfunction that develops within hours to days after transplantation, with requirements for high-dose inotropic and/or mechanical circulatory support. It represents the most common cause of death in the first 30 days post-transplant (Lund et al. 2013). It is usually diagnosed clinically and with echocardiography. CMR appearances include global severe LV dysfunction. There may be evidence of diffuse oedema (global high T1 and T2). Typically there is no late gadolinium enhancement (LGE). In surviving patients, EF usually improves over the first 6–12 months, but generally remains moderate-severely reduced.

Myocardial Infarction

Myocardial infarction (MI) can occur peri-operatively, or may have been unrecognised in the donor heart. CMR appearances include regional wall motion abnormalities, with LGE extending from the endocardium outwards.

Acute Rejection

Acute rejection affects approximately 20 % of patients in the first year post-transplantation, and represents a leading cause of death during this period (Lund et al. 2013). Clinical features are unreliable and therefore patients undergo routine screening via histological analysis of right ventricular myocardial tissue obtained at endomyocardial biopsy.

Left ventricular (LV) wall thickness, mass, EF, and pericardial effusion, are insensitive markers of rejection. Nevertheless, an acute global reduction in LV EF should prompt further investigation, and in this regard the higher reproducibility of CMR may be advantageous over echocardiography for serial follow-up. LGE is usually not evident during acute rejection. Single-centre studies of selected patients have reported that acute rejection is associated with high myocardial T2 and high signal on early gadolinium enhancement (Marie et al. 2001; Usman et al. 2012). However, there is currently no data from unselected populations, particularly in the period when rejection is most relevant clinically (first 6–12 months), although work is underway. Furthermore, as described, CMR markers of oedema may be routinely elevated in the early period post-transplant and are raised in PGD. As such, despite the recognized limitations of endomyocardial biopsy, at present, there is no good evidence to support the routine use of CMR for diagnosing acute rejection.

The Chronic Phase Post-transplant (Beyond 1 Year)

Typical CMR Appearances

Hypertension is almost ubiquitous by 5 years post-transplant, primarily due to calcineurin inhibitor immunosuppression, and concentric left ventricular hypertrophy (LVH) is common. Ventricular ejection fraction is usually normal or near normal in the absence of complications, although contraction often remains 'stiff' beyond the early post-operative period, particularly in the presence of LVH. Repeated bioptome passage across the tricuspid valve (for endomyocardial sampling) leads to a high

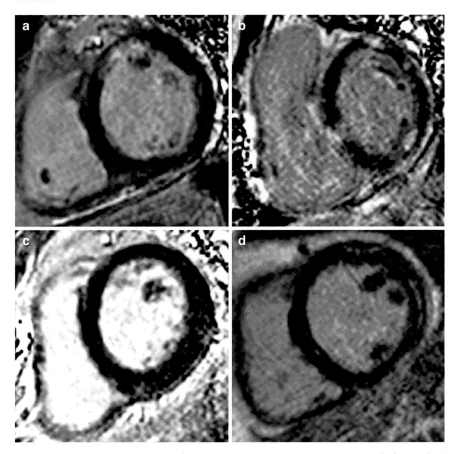

Fig. 25.6 Late gadolinium enhancement (LGE) patterns seen chronically post-transplant. (**a**) Infarct-typical LGE (anteriorly) and infarct-atypical inferior septal insertion point LGE; (**b–d**) infarct-atypical LGE, specifically (**b**) multiple 'punched-out' LGE lesions; (**c**) inferolateral epicardial LGE; (**d**) mid-wall LGE

prevalence of tricuspid regurgitation, which is moderate to severe in up to a third of patients, and can lead to right ventricular dilatation. Infarct-atypical LGE is seen in approximately half of patients by 3 years post-transplant, with a variety of patterns observed, including septal insertion point, mid-wall, epicardial and 'punched-out' lesions (Fig. 25.6) (Steen et al. 2008; Miller et al. 2014). Pericardial LGE is also described. It has been proposed that the atypical LGE may relate to cumulative previous rejection episodes. Of note, it does not appear to relate to allograft vasculopathy.

Complications

The most common conditions affecting the transplanted heart in the chronic phase are allograft vasculopathy, acute rejection and chronic graft failure. CMR is useful for investigating the aetiology of LV dysfunction detected on echocardiography, and

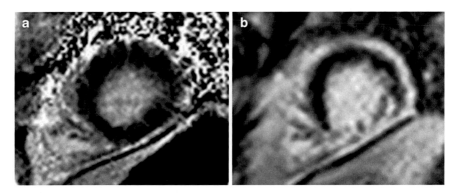

Fig. 25.7 LGE images from the same patient 4 months (**a**) and 4 years (**b**) post-transplant, demonstrating a new apical inferior wall infarct. The patient was entirely asymptomatic and echocardiography was reported as normal

for further assessment of graft structure and function in the presence of (often non-specific) symptoms and unremarkable echocardiographic findings. Vascular complications also occur and extracardiac findings are common.

Cardiac Allograft Vasculopathy (CAV)

CAV affects approximately 50 % of patients by 5 years post transplant and is responsible for approximately 15 % of deaths annually, although it represents a major pathophysiological factor in chronic graft failure (section "Chronic graft failure"), and as such its impact is likely to be much wider (Lund et al. 2013). It is characterized by diffuse and concentric intima-media proliferation. Due to denervation of the transplanted heart, symptoms of angina are rare and therefore, despite its limited sensitivity, regular angiographic screening is performed.

The prevalence and extent of infarct LGE on CMR correlates with the degree of CAV seen at angiography. However, more importantly, CMR LGE frequently detects MIs that are otherwise (clinically, echocardiography, angiographically) unrecognized (Fig. 25.7) (Steen et al. 2008). Indeed, a quarter of patients with only apparently mild disease at angiography display infarct on CMR LGE. MI in transplant recipients is associated with a poor prognosis and as such, CMR has an important role. Due to the diffuse nature of the disease, affecting both epicardial and microvascular coronary compartments, qualitative assessment of all functional imaging modalities, including perfusion CMR, have limited sensitivity for detecting CAV. Quantitative perfusion CMR appears to be advantageous, and contrast-enhanced MRI of the coronary vessel wall also appears to hold promise (Miller et al. 2014; Hussain et al. 2013).

Acute Rejection

The role of rejection screening beyond the first year post-transplant is unclear and many centres stop routine biopsies at 1 or 2 years. A deterioration in LV function

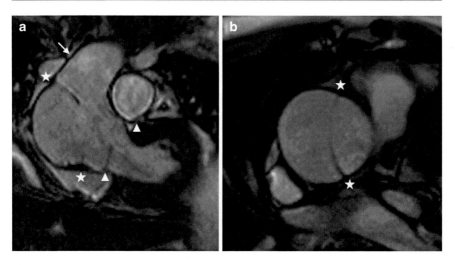

Fig. 25.8 Dilatation and dissection of the donor ascending aorta. (**a**) coronal and (**b**) axial views. *Arrow* anastomosis, *stars* dissection flap, *triangle* aortic valve (with aortic regurgitation visible)

detected on CMR, particularly in the absence of infarct, should prompt consideration of endomyocardial biopsy.

Chronic Graft Failure

Chronic deterioration in graft function is common, leads to a clinical syndrome analogous to native chronic heart failure, and is responsible for 15–25 % of deaths beyond the first year post-transplant (Lund et al. 2013). Its pathophysiology includes chronic myocardial ischaemic injury secondary to CAV, exaggerated activation of the renin-angiotensin-aldosterone, and sympathetic nervous, systems, immunological factors and standard cardiovascular risk factors. CMR appearances include global ventricular dysfunction, often with additional regional wall abnormalities secondary to CAV-related MIs. Infarct typical and infarct-atypical LGE are common. The initial detection of ventricular dysfunction, in the absence of infarction, should prompt consideration of biopsy to assess for rejection (section "Acute rejection").

Vascular

CMR is ideal for assessing the integrity of donor aortic and pulmonic tissue and the anastomosis sites, and for identifying and following-up vascular complications such as dilatation of the donor ascending aorta (Fig. 25.8).

Extracardiac Findings

Malignancy is the leading cause of death beyond the first year post-transplant. Cutaneous malignancies are the most common, but there is a high incidence of lymphomas and solid tumours (lung and breast cancer being among the most common)

(Lund et al. 2013). CMR scans should be carefully inspected for extracardiac findings.

Key Points of CMR Following Heart Transplant

1. Heart transplant patients present non-specifically; have a low threshold for imaging.
2. Recognise the normal findings; LVH and infarct-atypical LGE are common.
3. Myocardial oedema is not specific for acute rejection, particularly in the first 6 months post-transplant.
4. CMR frequently detects infarct that is otherwise unrecognised.
5. An acute deterioration in ventricular function in the absence of infarction warrants further investigation for rejection.
6. Look out for extracardiac abnormalities; malignancy is common.

Tips and Tricks

1. **Retained pacing/ICD wires** – Prior to undergoing transplantation, patients frequently have CRT ± ICD devices in situ. The device and wires are usually removed during the transplant procedure, but occasionally wires that are heavily fibrosed within the venous system cannot be completely removed. It is therefore important to review a chest x-ray to exclude retained wires prior to CMR.
2. **Renal function** – renal dysfunction is common after transplantation. Ensure renal function is checked prior to giving gadolinium contrast agents.
3. **ECG** – due to the abnormal (often lateral) position of the transplanted heart it can be difficult to get a good ECG trace. This can usually be overcome by obtaining an initial localiser to identify the location of the heart and then adjusting the position of the ECG pads accordingly.
4. **High resting heart rate** – vagal denervation of the transplanted heart means resting heart rate is often higher than in the non-transplant population. Appropriate methods to speed up image acquisition are usually required.
5. **Adenosine sensitivity** – The denervated sinus and atrioventricular nodes can have enhanced sensitivity to adenosine which can lead to bradyarrhythmias during adenosine infusion. Close monitoring is required (ECG, pulse oximeter, blood pressure).
6. **Delayed tachycardic response to adenosine** – The loss of sympathetic innervation means that heart rate response to adenosine is dependent on plasma catecholamine stimulation. As a result, heart rate response is often delayed, submaximal and can continue to rise after termination of adenosine.

References

Hussain T, Fenton M, Peel SA, et al. Detection and grading of coronary allograft vasculopathy in children with contrast-enhanced magnetic resonance imaging of the coronary vessel wall. Circ Cardiovasc Imaging. 2013;6(1):91–8.

Lund LH, Edwards LB, Kucheryavaya AY, et al. The Registry of the International Society for heart and lung transplantation: thirtieth official adult heart transplant report–2013; focus theme: age. J Heart Lung Transplant. 2013;32(10):951–64.

Marie PY, Angioi M, Carteaux JP, et al. Detection and prediction of acute heart transplant rejection with the myocardial T2 determination provided by a black-blood magnetic resonance imaging sequence. J Am Coll Cardiol. 2001;37(3):825–31.

Miller CA, Sarma J, Naish JH, et al. Multiparametric cardiovascular magnetic resonance assessment of cardiac allograft vasculopathy. J Am Coll Cardiol. 2014;63(8):799–808.

Steen H, Merten C, Refle S, et al. Prevalence of different gadolinium enhancement patterns in patients after heart transplantation. J Am Coll Cardiol. 2008;52(14):1160–7.

Usman AA, Taimen K, Wasielewski M, et al. Cardiac magnetic resonance T2 mapping in the monitoring and follow-up of acute cardiac transplant rejection: a pilot study. Circ Cardiovasc Imaging. 2012;5(6):782–90.

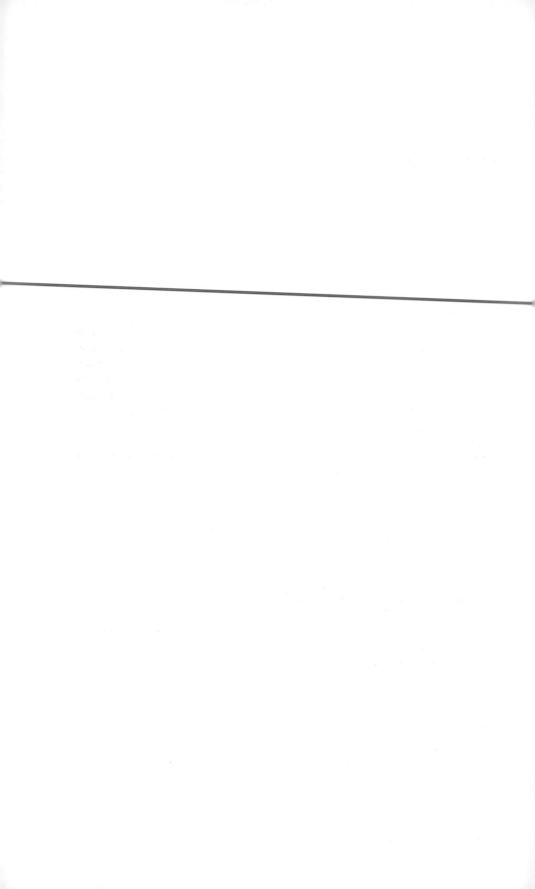

Pericardial Disease

Charles Peebles

Abstract

The investigation and management of pericardial disease remains difficult due to the limitations of echocardiography in visualising the entire pericardium. This chapter explores the role for CMR in pericardial disease, covering pericardial effusion, constrictive pericarditis, congenital pericardial abnormalities, and pericardial tumours. The ability of CMR to identify pericardial anatomy as well the the functional consequences of pericardial pathology is emphasised.

Keywords

Pericardial constriction • Ventricular coupling • Pericardial effusion • Pericardial defect • Pericardial tumour • Pericardial cyst • Pericarditis

Pericardial Effusion

CMR Protocol in Pericardial Effusion
1. Anatomy module including T1 & T2 weighting
2. LV function module
3. Targeted sequences depending on findings e.g. tumour protocol, valve imaging, real-time dynamic respiratory cine.
4. Late Gadolinium Enhancement module

C. Peebles, MBBS, MRCP, FRCR (✉)
Department of Cardiothoracic Radiology, University Hospital Southampton,
E level, North wing, Tremona Rd, Southampton Hampshire SO16 6YD, UK
e-mail: charles.peebles@uhs.nhs.uk

© Springer International Publishing 2015
S. Plein et al. (eds.), *Cardiovascular MR Manual*,
DOI 10.1007/978-3-319-20940-1_26

Introduction

The aetiology of pericardial effusions is varied and can be broadly divided into transudates, exudates, haemorrhage and chyle. A full review of the causes of pericardial fluid is beyond the scope of this text. The role of imaging is to identify the effusion, assess its physiological significance and, if possible, diagnose the cause. Exudative processes tend to be associated with more complex effusions and greater pericardial inflammation, transudates conversely are generally simpler. Cross-sectional imaging has a specific role in assessing the extracardiac structures to identify malignancy and other systemic diseases.

CMR Versus Other Imaging Modalities

Echocardiography remains the primary investigation for diagnosis of pericardial effusions but is susceptible to both false negative and positive results due to the presence of loculated fluid, poor acoustic windows or adjacent pleural fluid. CMR demonstrates the whole of the pericardium, as well as the surrounding structures, making it an ideal tool for secondary imaging.

The functional significance of a pericardial effusion is also primarily assessed by clinical and echocardiographic examination. CMR provides similar information to echo regarding compromise to RV and RA filling but is advantageous if acoustic windows are poor or difficult to interpret.

Findings on CMR

The pericardial space normally contains a trace of pericardial fluid (<30 ml) which may be observed on CMR. There are no absolute CMR criteria for differentiating a physiological effusion from a pathological one but as a guideline a pericardial width of >4 mm is considered abnormal. An effusion measuring >5 mm anterior to the RV is likely to be a moderate volume (100–500 ml). Most effusions show a gravitational distribution being deepest posterolateral to the left ventricle.

Black Blood Images (Spin Echo Sequence)

It is important to initially scan the whole thorax when imaging a pericardial effusion. This will usually be performed with a fast black blood sequence and the intention is to identify extra-cardiac pathology such as lung tumours, lymph nodes, pleural effusions etc. Echocardiography provides little or no information about the extra-cardiac structures and this is a major advantage for CMR. Computed tomography (CT) fulfils a similar role but provides more detail relating to the lungs as well

Table 26.1 Findings on CMR in pericardial effusion of different aetiology

	T1 signal (SE)	Cine appearances and signal intensity (b-SSFP)
Transudate	↓	Simple ↑
Exudates	↓↑	Complex ↓↑
Haemorrhage	↓↑	Complex ↓↑
Chylous	↑↑	Simple ↑

as the abdomen. CT and MRI are thus complementary and may well both be indicated (In practice CT is generally used if there is a strong suspicion of underlying malignancy whilst MRI is favoured if functional information is required)

In principle T1 characteristics of the fluid can give an indication of the nature of the effusion (see Table 26.1). In practice the signal return from the fluid is more influenced by flow voids and loculation than by pure T1 effects. A more useful finding is the complexity of the effusion and degree of pericardial thickening and enhancement – transudates tend to be simple with little pericardial inflammation while exudates and haemorrhage are complex with greater pericardial thickening.

CINE Imaging (b-SSFP)

Pericardial fluid generally appears as high signal on b-SSFP techniques, comparable to pleural effusions (if these should be present). Loculation and soft tissue stranding is well visualised as areas of mixed or reduced signal within the fluid effusion.

As with echocardiography the size of the effusion has a limited relationship with the physiological consequences, being more related to the duration and rate of accumulation of fluid. CMR criteria for functionally important effusion are similar to echocardiography; diastolic compression of the RV free wall, early systolic collapse of the RA, distortion of the LV and RV morphology and potentially paradoxical interventricular septal motion during inspiration (ventricular coupling – more commonly seen in constrictive pericarditis).

Targeted Sequences

Depending on the initial findings further sequences may be indicated:

1. Pericardial inflammation – linear high signal with T1 weighted gadolinium enhanced images.
2. Tumour – first pass perfusion, T1 weighted post-gadolinium images, myocardial delayed enhancement, myocardial tagging.
3. Myocardial disease – additional tissue characterisation sequences (T1/T2/STIR/ T1 & 2 mapping), myocardial delayed enhancement

The Role of CMR in Pericardial Effusion
1. CMR is useful in confirming the presence and size of a pericardial effusion if doubt exists on Echo (particularly if loculated).
2. CMR may identify the cause of a pericardial effusion or give indications as to the aetiology.
3. CMR provides functional information about the haemodynamic consequences of the effusion.
4. CMR is complementary to other imaging modalities.

Case Example

A 65 years old lady presented with increasing breathlessness on exertion and swollen ankles. She had a long history of Rheumatoid arthritis. An Echo suggested a pericardial effusion but this was not well visualised so that CMR was requested.

Following pericardial drainage the effusion was found to be an exudate and was rheumatoid factor positive. She was diagnosed with constrictive-effusive pericarditis and required a surgical pericardial window followed by pericardectomy (Figs. 26.1, 26.2, and 26.3).

Tips and Tricks
1. Cine images usually show pericardial effusions as high signal, if a pleural effusion is present the signal will often be similar on cine images but differ on TSE sequences.

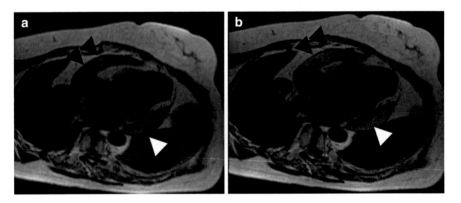

Fig. 26.1 (**a**) T1 TSE image in a 3-chamber view shows an intermediate signal pericardial effusion (*arrow heads*). (**b**) T2 weighted image in the same position again showing an intermediate signal (*arrow heads*). The signal intensity suggests a proteinaceous effusion/exudate rather than a simple transudate which should be lower signal on T1 images

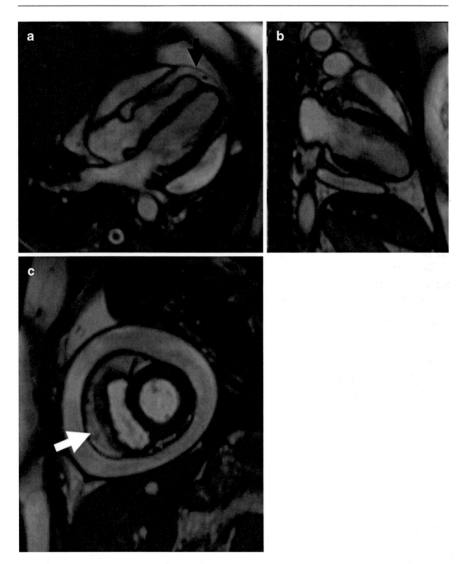

Fig. 26.2 (a) 4-Chamber cine image showing a loculated pericardial effusion anterior to the RV and posterior to the LV. The RV chamber is distorted and compressed suggesting that the effusion is haemodynamically significant. Normal pericardium is seen over the apex (*arrow*). (b) 2-Chamber cine image. The loculated effusion has a similar distribution to Fig. 26.3a. (c) Short axis cine. The effusion is circumferential and has a typical high signal on SSFP images. Epicardial fat (*arrow*) is easily visualised

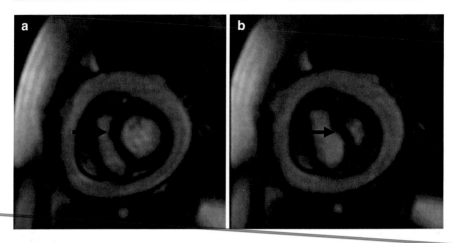

Fig. 26.3 (**a**) Real-time short axis cine image taken during expiration shows a normal interventricular septal position (*arrow*). (**b**) Real-time short axis cine image taken from the same cine loop during early inspiration. There is clear septal displacement to the left side (*arrows*) confirming a constrictive physiology

CMR Report in Pericardial Effusion

Morphology (descriptive)

1. Pericardial Thickness: describe as local or circumferential and list thickness measurements
2. Pericardial effusion : presence and extent

Ventricular parameters

1. LV volumes
2. Ventricular wall motion:
   Systolic wall motion
   Septal motion during normal respiration and breath holding.
3. Presence or absence of atrial inversion

Late Gadolinium Enhancement in RV, LV and pericardium

Key Points CMR in Pericardial Effusion

1. Useful adjunct to Echo
2. Gives functional and anatomical information
3. May identify or indicate the cause

Constrictive Pericarditis

CMR Protocol in Constrictive Pericarditis
1. Anatomy module including T1 & T2 weighting
2. LV function module
3. Targeted sequences depending on findings e.g. real-time dynamic respiratory cine, tagging, mitral valve flow.

Introduction

Constrictive pericardial disease is the end result of a number of inflammatory, infective, or malignant processes involving the pericardium causing a constrictive physiology. Usually this is associated with macroscopic thickening of the visceral and/or parietal pericardium which may become adherent to the myocardium and regularly calcifies (particularly if tuberculous in origin). Constrictive pericarditis may however be associated with a pericardial effusion (effusive-constrictive pericarditis) or a normal thickness pericardium. Generally it is a progressive and chronic condition but may be acute or rarely transient.

The physiological consequence of pericardial constriction is reduced ventricular diastolic filling. Ventricular filling pressures therefore increase in a similar way to restrictive cardiomyopathy, the main differential diagnosis. In constrictive pericarditis, however, the pericardial volume becomes fixed creating competition for diastolic filling between the ventricles – ventricular coupling or interdependence. The end result is preferential RV filling during inspiration (when negative intrathoracic pressure encourages systemic venous return), and preferential LV filling during expiration (when positive intrathoracic pressure encourages pulmonary venous return). The CMR sequelae of this is paradoxical displacement of the interventricular septum to the left side during early inspiration and normalisation during expiration. Ventricular coupling is not seen in restrictive cardiomyopathy.

The Role of CMR in Constrictive Pericarditis

The primary role of cross-sectional imaging in patients with signs and symptoms suggestive of constrictive pericarditis or restrictive cardiomyopathy is to identify pericardial thickening. The presence of thickened pericardium in the appropriate clinical context effectively differentiates constrictive pericarditis from restrictive cardiomyopathy and allows planning of pericardial stripping. Echocardiography is relatively poor at visualising the pericardium and hence cross-sectional imaging is superior. CT demonstrates the pericardium well and has the advantage of being very sensitive to pericardial calcification. CMR, as well as showing the pericardium, has a much greater ability to provide functional information to support the diagnosis of constriction. CT and CMR are therefore often complementary particularly in the difficult diagnostic case.

Findings on CMR

Pericardial Thickening
The normal pericardium is seen over the RV free wall and the atrioventricular and interventricular grooves where there is abundant surrounding fat. The pericardium is usually pencil thin except over the diaphragmatic reflections. A thickness of >4 mm on spin-echo sequences is generally considered to be pathological. Pericardial thickening is often patchy and may in some cases be absent.

Cine images readily differentiate pericardial effusion from thickening but tend to overestimate the thickness.

Indirect Signs of Constrictive Physiology
1. Distortion of RV and LV shape. The RV in particular may be flattened and tubular. This is best demonstrated with cine imaging.
2. Atrial dilatation (in the absence of ventricular dilatation).
3. IVC and SVC dilatation (reflecting elevated filling pressures).
4. Pericardial adhesions between the thickened pericardium and the epicardial surface of the myocardium. This may be highlighted by tagged cine imaging demonstrating loss of the normal slippage of the pericardium over the myocardium.
5. Ventricular coupling. Paradoxical diastolic interventricular septal motion during early inspiration. This is best seen with a real-time cine sequence during deep breathing.

Tips and Tricks
1. Use real-time dynamic respiratory sequence in several short axis views and a 4-chamber view.
2. The 4-chamber view demonstrates the whole length of the interventricular septum, the paradoxical septal motion often being limited to one part of the septum.
3. The short axis views show the diaphragmatic position clearly, allowing assessment of the respiratory phase.
4. Obtaining several short axis views samples the septum at a number of levels.

The Role of CMR in Constrictive Pericarditis
1. CMR identifies pericardial thickening.
2. CMR provides functional information that may support or indicate constrictive physiology.
3. CMR helps exclude restrictive cardiomyopathy.
4. CMR is complementary to other imaging modalities.

Case

This 80 year old man presented with a history of increasing exertional breathlessness and upper abdominal pain. An Echocardiogram suggested reduced RV function and diastolic dysfunction. He was referred for a CMR scan which diagnosed constrictive pericarditis. He subsequently underwent pericardiectomy and has made a full recovery (Figs. 26.4, 26.5, 26.6, 26.7, and 26.8).

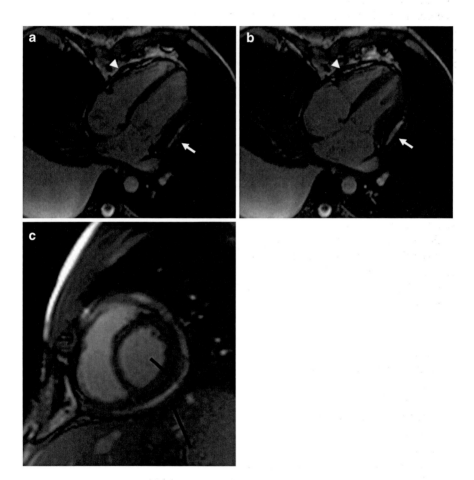

Fig. 26.4 (a–c) 4 chamber cine image in diastole (**a**) and systole (**b**). There is pericardial thickening over the lateral wall with a trace of pericardial fluid (*white arrow*). There is further pericardial thickening anterior to the RV (*arrow head*). There is subtle distortion of the LV free wall during diastole and bi-atrial dilatation – features suggesting a constrictive physiology. Note the substantial right pleural effusion. (**c**) Short axis cine image showing thickened parietal (*long black arrow*) and visceral (*short black arrow*) pericardium separated by a thin pericardial effusion

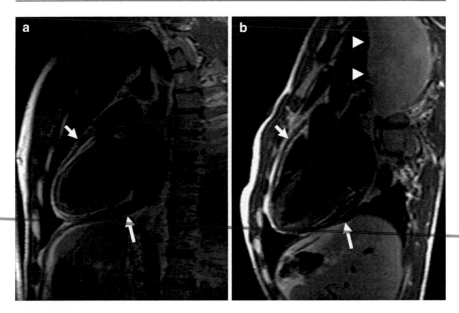

Fig. 26.5 (**a, b**) T1 weighted TSE image in a 2-chamber plane (**a**) and T2 weighted image in the 3-chamber plane (**b**) showing diffuse pericardial thickening (*arrows*) sparing the apex. This measures up to 1 cm in thickness. Note is made of the pleural effusion (*arrowhead*)

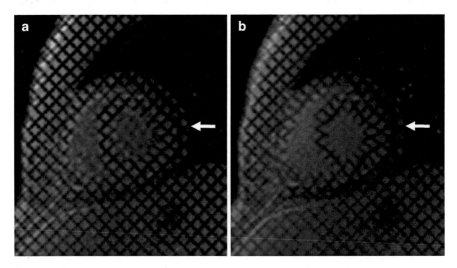

Fig. 26.6 (**a, b**) Myocardial tagged image in the short axis plane at end-diastole (**a**) and end-systole (**b**). There are adhesions between the pericardium and the myocardium over the lateral wall demonstrated on the images as failure of 'slippage' of the tag lines between the myocardium and pericardium during the cardiac cycle (in the region of the *arrows*)

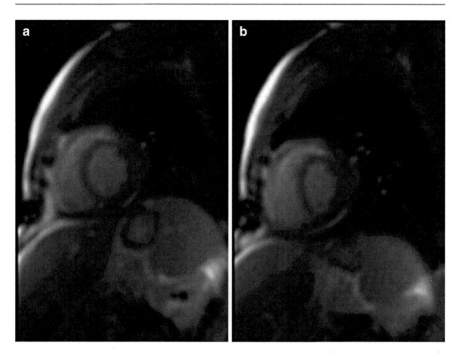

Fig. 26.7 (**a**, **b**) Two diastolic images taken from a real-time dynamic respiratory sequence. During expiration (**a**) the interventricular septal contour is normal, during inspiration there is subtle flattening of the septum indicating abnormal ventricular coupling. This finding is useful for differentiation between restrictive cardiomyopathy and constrictive pericarditis (although in this case is not marked)

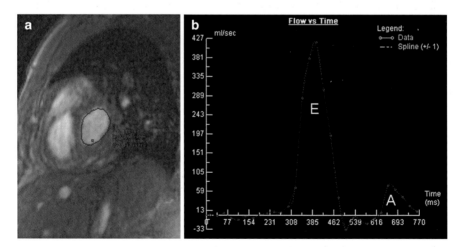

Fig. 26.8 (**a**, **b**) Phase contrast flow mapping of the mitral in-flow shows a pronounced E wave with rapid deceleration time and a small A wave. This indicates a restrictive or constrictive physiology. Respiratory variation would be seen in constriction but CMR does not have the ability to demonstrate this due to the need for breath-hold acquisition or respiratory averaged images

Case 2

This patient demonstrates transient pericardial constriction. The initial CMR clearly demonstrates pericardial thickening and constrictive physiology which resolves on a follow-up scan 3 months later (Figs. 26.9 and 26.10).

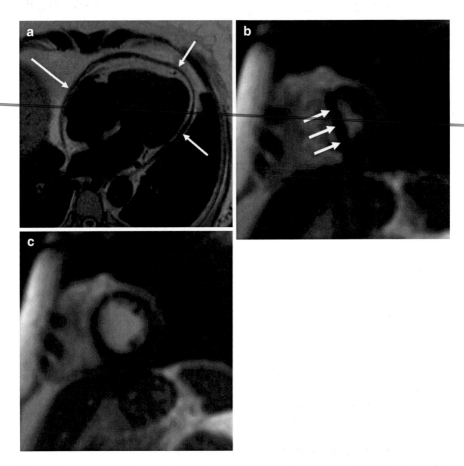

Fig. 26.9 (a–c) Axial T1 weighted TSE image (**a**) demonstrating pericardial thickening (*white arrows*). Real-time dynamic respiratory sequence shows a diastolic image during inspiration (**b**) and expiration (**c**). The inversion of the interventricular septum during inspiration (*white arrows*) indicates pathological ventricular coupling and a constrictive physiology

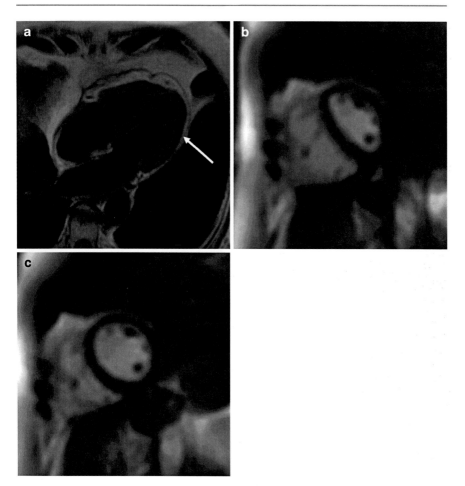

Fig. 26.10 (**a–c**) Axial T1 weighted TSE image (**a**) 3 months later shows partial resolution of the pericardial thickening, particularly over the LV (*white arrow*). Real-time dynamic respiratory images (**b, c**) now show a normal interventricular septal position confirming physiological recovery

CMR Report in Pericardial Constriction
Morphology (descriptive)
1. Pericardial Thickness: describe as local or circumferential and list thickness measurements
2. Pericardial effusion : presence and extent

Ventricular parameters
1. LV volumes
2. Ventricular wall motion:
   Systolic wall motion
   Septal motion during normal respiration and breath holding.
3. Presence or absence of atrial inversion

Late Gadolinium Enhancement in RV, LV and pericardium

Key Points CMR in Constrictive Pericarditis
1. Identification of thickened pericardium in the appropriate clinical context is diagnostic of constriction
2. CMR gives indirect physiological information that may support the diagnosis
3. Pericardial constriction may be present with a normal pericardial thickness or patchy thickening
4. CMR is complementary to CT, Echo and cardiac catheterisation

Pericardial Tumours

CMR Protocol in Pericardial Tumours
1. Anatomy module including T1 & T2 weighting. Images should cover the whole thorax.
2. LV function module.
3. Myocardial Tagging.
4. First pass perfusion imaging.
5. T1 weighted post contrast images.
6. Late Gadolinium Enhancement module.

Introduction

Pericardial tumours are divided into primary and secondary lesions. The commonest are secondaries with breast cancer, lung cancer or haematological tumours.

Primary pericardial tumours are rare, the commonest being mesothelioma (not associated with asbestos exposure) followed by sarcomas and intrapericardial teratomas. Pericardial tumours tend to cause complex pericardial effusions but may encase the pericardium and result in constrictive physiology. The volume of tumour in pericardial metastasis may be small and not macroscopically visible.

Tumours in the lung and mediastinum may directly invade the pericardium and CMR has a useful role in identifying such invasion and staging thoracic malignancies.

CMR Versus Other Imaging Modalities

Echocardiography remains the initial investigation for most patients with pericardial tumours as the presentation is often that of pericardial effusion. If there is a suspicion of tumour clinically or on other imaging modalities a CMR is likely to be the next imaging modality. Its excellent soft tissue differentiation and large field of view make it an ideal tool to identify pericardial tumour and delineate its origin and extent. CT has a complementary role although is less versatile at dynamic imaging or multiplanar imaging. CT is, however, more robust in identifying other thoracic lesions including lung primaries, pulmonary metastases and mediastinal nodes, all of which may be instrumental in making a definitive diagnosis.

Having identified a pericardial tumour attention turns to delineating its extent and the presence of local invasion. CMR is ideal for this and using the full range of imaging sequences can also provide useful information about the nature of the lesion and its physiological consequences. Coronary angiography may be needed if surgical resection is needed to identify distortion/invasion of the coronaries although CT and CMR will provide adequate information in most cases.

Findings on CMR

The whole of the thorax should be imaged in patients with suspected pericardial tumours to identify primary lesions, other secondaries and mediastinal nodes.

CINE Imaging (b-SSFP)

Standard cine images will identify a pericardial effusion if present and also show areas of thickened pericardium. This alone may be enough to confirm a pericardial mass or pericardial deposits as well as extra-pericardial tumours invading the pericardium.

Most pericardial tumours will show similar signal to the myocardium but greater heterogeneity of the tumour and slight increase in signal will usually allow differentiation. Tethering and/or invasion of the adjacent myocardium or great vessels are generally easily identified and are an indicator of malignancy. Well defined or encapsulated lesions are more likely to be benign.

Cine images provide additional direct or indirect information about the physiological consequences of the tumour (see the sections on "Pericardial effusion" and "Constrictive pericarditis").

Myocardial Tagging

Tagging may help to differentiate tumour (which is non-contractile) from myocardium and subsequently indicate the extent of myocardial invasion.

Black Blood Images (TSE)
Characterisation of tumours is difficult although differentiation of benign and malignant lesions can be indicated by well defined/encapsulated margins versus soft tissue invasion respectively. Lipomas can be positively identified by their fat content on T1/T2 weighted TSE images and fat suppressed sequences. Most soft tissue tumours will have similar signal characteristics to myocardium although increased tissue oedema may be manifest by slight increase in signal on T2 weighting.

First-Pass Perfusion Imaging
Both primary and secondary pericardial tumours will show some degree of enhancement on first pass perfusion imaging. Enhancement on first pass perfusion imaging helps to confirm the presence and extent of the tumour and differentiate it from haematoma or complex effusion.

Post Contrast T1 TSE and Delayed Enhanced Images
As indicated above most soft tissue tumours will display some contrast enhancement and delayed contrast wash-out. T1 TSE images early following contrast may show heterogenous enhancement in the tumour as will delayed inversion recovery sequences. These findings help confirm the presence and extent of tumour but give little information regarding the pathological diagnosis.

> **The Role of CMR in Pericardial Tumours**
> 1. CMR identifies and delineates focal pericardial masses.
> 2. CMR demonstrates extracardiac tumours invading the pericardium and is useful in staging mediastinal and thoracic tumours.
> 3. Excellent soft tissue differentiation allows accurate assessment of extent of pericardial tumours and invasion of adjacent structures.
> 4. CMR may provide useful tissue characterisation e.g. lipoma.
> 5. CMR provides additional functional information.

Case Example
A 61-year-old man presented with a 3 week history of shortness of breath, dry cough, chest tightness, and orthopnoea. Having been previously fit he was now breathless on climbing one flight of stairs. Examination primarily showed evidence of right-sided failure with raised JVP and swollen legs. Echocardiogram showed a large pericardial effusion and on pericardiocentesis two litres of blood stained fluid was drained.

The patient was transferred to our institution with the drain in-situ and a repeat echocardiogram suggested a pericardial clot. CMR imaging helped to clarify the anatomical findings. The patient underwent surgical resection of the lesion which on histology was a synovial sarcoma (Figs. 26.11, 26.12, 26.13, 26.14, and 26.15).

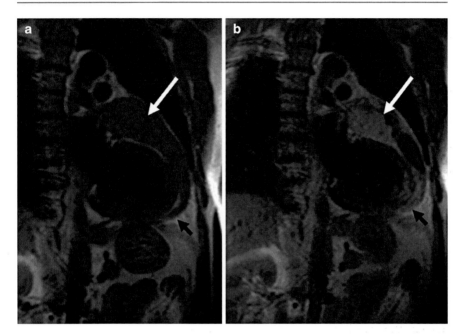

Fig. 26.11 (**a, b**) T1 weighted TSE pre and post gadolinium in a 2 chamber view. Pre-contrast (**a**) there is 4×6 cm soft tissue mass (*white arrow*) arising from the pericardium with more diffuse pericardial thickening elsewhere (*black arrow*). The mass appears not to involve the myocardium with preservation of the epicardial fat. Post-contrast (**b**) the mass enhances (*white arrow*) and becomes differentiated from the adjacent pericardial thickening

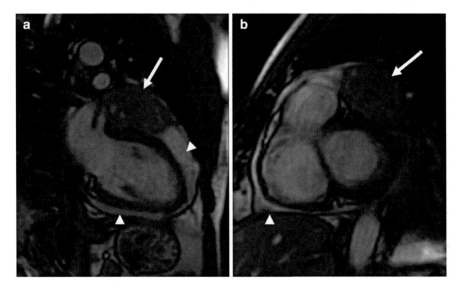

Fig. 26.12 (**a, b**) Cine SSFP 2 chamber and short axis views. The soft tissue mass (*white arrows*) seems to arise from the pericardium with normal myocardial signal and motion. The fat around the interventricular groove and LAD is preserved. The pericardial effusion has homogeneous high signal (*arrow heads*)

Fig. 26.13 1st pass perfusion study. An arterial phase image from a first-pass perfusion study shows heterogenous enhancement of the mass (*arrow*). This effectively precludes a pericardial haematoma and makes a soft tissue tumour the most likely diagnosis

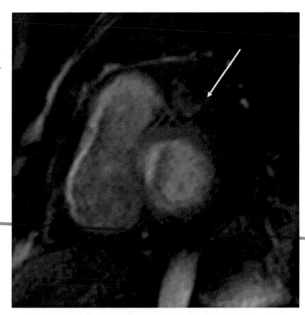

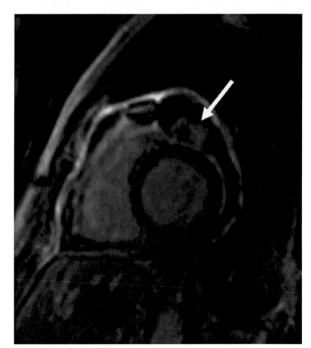

Fig. 26.14 TSE inversion recovery late gadolinium enhanced image. There is patchy high signal within the lesion. The myocardium remains of normal low signal. This is a non-specific finding but again helps to exclude an haematoma

Fig. 26.15 Angiogram. The coronary angiogram shows normal coronaries with capillary filling of the soft tissue lesion (*arrows*)

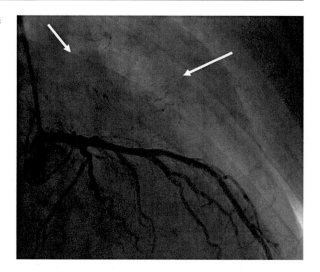

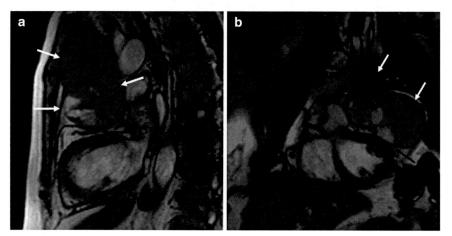

Fig. 26.16 (**a**) Coronal Cine image. The large heterogenous anterior mediastinal mass is well demonstrated (*white arrows*) and appears to invade the pericardium (*black arrows*). Although the epicardial fat is effaced the myocardium is not obviously involved. (**b**) Sagittal Cine image. In this plane the tumour abuts the pericardium and distorts the Left anterior descending coronary artery although does not clearly invade it. There is again no tumour invasion of the myocardium

Case 2

A 35 year old man presented with a large anterior mediastinal mass closely applied to the pericardium. CMR was used to assess myocardial invasion. The tumour was a thymic carcinoma and was resected. As the CMR demonstrates the tumour invaded the pericardium but could be removed from the myocardium and coronary arteries. CMR is a powerful tool for staging mediastinal tumours prior to surgery (Fig. 26.16).

CMR Report in Pericardial Tumours
1. Location (pericardial, myocardial, valve relationship, chamber relationship)
2. Size (cross-sectional dimensions)
3. T1 signal intensity (homogeneous, heterogeneous, hyper, iso or hypo intense to myocardium/or chest wall (specify reference tissue))
4. T1 fat sat images signal intensity (if performed) (homogeneous, heterogeneous, hyper, iso or hypo intense to myocardium/or chest wall (specify reference tissue))
5. T2 signal intensity (homogeneous, heterogeneous, hyper, iso or hypo intense to myocardium/or chest wall (specify reference tissue))
6. STIR signal intensity
7. Perfusion pattern (if perfusion performed)
8. Late gadolinium enhancement pattern on static/delayed images (if gadolinium administered)
9. Relationship to myocardium/pericardium, mediastinum
10. Margins (e.g., smooth, irregular, infiltrating, pediculated)
11. Cine CMR appearance (pedunculated, motion with myocardium/pericardium)
12. Myocardial function (if performed, qualitative or quantitative as appropriate)
13. Pericardial abnormalities if present (pericardial thickness should be reported along with determination of the presence or absence of a pericardial effusion)

Key Points CMR in Pericardial Tumours
1. Useful for identifying primary and secondary pericardial tumours
2. Useful for assessing pericardial involvement from other mediastinal or lung tumours
3. Accurate tumour characterisation is usually not possible and requires histological confirmation

Congenital Abnormalities of the Pericardium

CMR Protocol in Congenital Abnormalities of the Pericardium
1. Anatomy module including T1 & T2 weighting (page X)
2. LV function module (page X)
3. Targeted sequences depending on findings e.g. first pass perfusion, tagging,

Pericardial Cysts and Pericardial Defects

Introduction

Pericardial cysts are caused by embryonic remnants of pericardium which become fluid filled. They generally lie adjacent to the pericardium but may rarely be intrapericardial. If they communicate with the pericardium they are termed diverticulae but usually they are separate. Approximately 70 % are located in the right cardiophrenic angle and 20 % on the left. The majority of patients are asymptomatic and present coincidentally following a chest X-ray with a right paracardiac mass. Occasionally patients present with symptoms from complications such as pressure effects or secondary infection.

Pericardial defects or agenesis are congenital abnormalities that often pass unnoticed. Part of or all of the pericardium fails to develop, possibly as a result of vascular insufficiency during pericardial embryogenesis. One third of cases are associated with other cardiac malformations and the condition is more common in males. Complete agenesis is rare (9 %) and is considered benign as symptoms are uncommon. Partial defects are more common and are generally over the left heart (70 %). They may result in herniation of cardiac structures through the defect with potential strangulation or compromise of the herniated structure e.g. the left atrial appendage. Cases of coronary compromise have been described. Repair of partial pericardial defects has therefore been recommended.

The Role of CMR in Congenital Pericardial Abnormalities

CMR is used to confirm the position and nature of cystic lesions around the heart which have been identified by CXR or Echocardiography. Likewise pericardial defects can be demonstrated on CMR if there is a radiological or clinical suspicion, but are more commonly incidental findings.

Additional physiological information can be gained if there is compression or distortion of an adjacent cardiac chamber or vessel.

Findings on CMR

Pericardial cysts are fluid filled thin walled lesions usually abutting the pericardium. The fluid is a transudate and as such appears simple on MRI with low T1 signal, high T2 signal and high signal on SSFP sequences. Occasionally the cyst will contain proteinaceous fluid and show higher T1 signal. They are generally round and well defined but may conform to surrounding structures as they are under low pressure, indeed they may change shape during respiration. Occasionally they become tense and distort or compress the adjacent intrapericardial structures with significant haemodynamic consequences particularly if the cyst itself is intrapericardial. The main differential is from other paracardiac masses and this is usually straight forward given the simple cystic nature of the lesion and the location.

Pericardial defects are identified by absence of the normal pericardium and a subsequent change in the normal cardiac contour. The heart may shift leftward or specific chambers may herniated through the defect. Likewise paracardiac structures that are normally separated from the heart may lie in direct contact with heart and create abnormal contours, such as the lung extending into the aorto-pulmonary window. In clinical practice these defects are rarely seen.

The Role of CMR in Congenital Abnormalities of the Pericardium
1. CMR identifies the normal pericardium and pericardial defects.
2. CMR demonstrates and characterises cystic lesions relating to the pericardium.
3. CMR is complementary to other imaging modalities.

Case Example
This patient presented following an abnormal CXR as part of a health screening assessment. He has no symptoms of cardiac disease (Figs. 26.17, 26.18, and 26.19).

Case Example 2
This patient presented following a CT scan of the chest for atypical chest discomfort, the CT showed an unusual cardiac orientation. He had a long history of intermittent breathlessness and chest discomfort that was positional (Figs. 26.20 and 26.21).

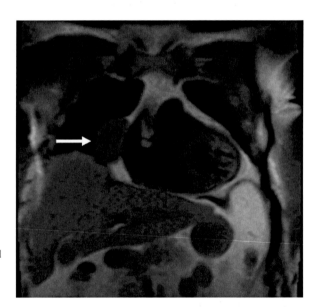

Fig. 26.17 Coronal HASTE image. A pericardial cyst is demonstrated in the typical position (*white arrow*)

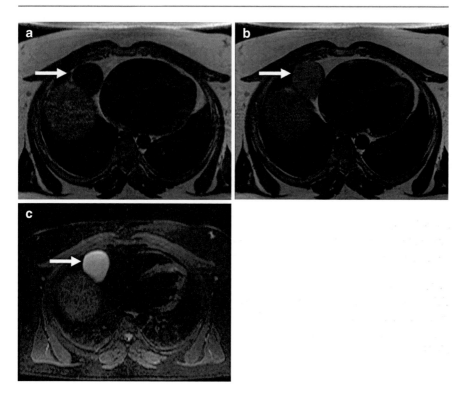

Fig. 26.18 (**a–c**) TSE images in an axial plane with T1, T2 and Fat suppressed weighting respectively. The cyst (*white arrow*) is well defined and abuts the pericardium. It is low signal on T1 weighted images, intermediate signal on T2 weighting and high signal on T2 weighted fat suppressed images consistent with a simple transudate

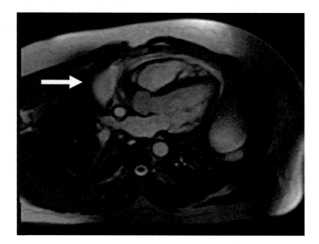

Fig. 26.19 3-chamber cine image (SSFP). The pericardial cyst (*arrow*) shows high signal without septations. There is no distortion of the adjacent cardiac structures

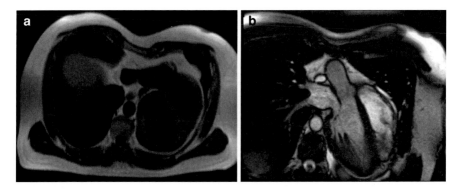

Fig. 26.20 (**a**, **b**) Axial HASTE image and axial cine (SSFP) image respectively. There is complete absence of the pericardium allowing the heart to lie in a dependent position in the left hemithorax with the apex against the posterior chest wall and the left ventricle adjacent to the spine

Fig. 26.21 Axial cine image in a prone position. The heart now lies anteriorly against the chest wall demonstrating abnormal mobility within the thorax

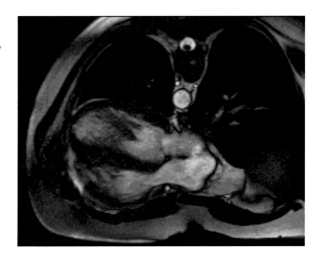

Tips and Tricks
1. Imaging with the patient in supine and prone positions may help highlight absence of the pericardium.

CMR Report in Congenital Pericardial Abnormalities
1. Morphology of the abnormality
2. Appearance on different CMR image types
3. Associated pathologies

Key Points: CMR in Congenital Pericardial Abnormalities
1. Used to confirm the typical cystic nature and location of pericardial cysts.
2. Excludes other causes of paracardiac mass lesions.
3. Identifies congenital pericardial absence or pericardial defect.
4. Demonstrates any functional consequence of pericardial abnormality.

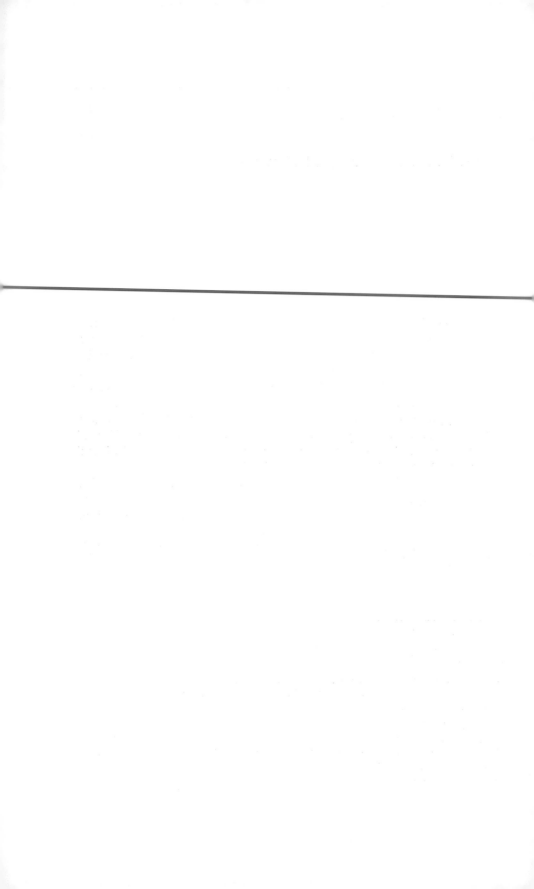

Cardiac Masses

27

John P. Greenwood and Manish Motwani

Abstract

Tumours of the heart are generally uncommon and can be either primary or secondary, the former of which can be either benign or malignant. CMR is an important imaging modality for the assessment of any suspected cardiac or paracardiac mass, as it can determine tumour size, location, relationship to other cardiac structures, invasion into the pericardium or extra-cardiac spread (e.g. invasion into the great vessels), which is vital for any proposed surgical planning. It is typically performed after a transthoracic echocardiogram has identified an abnormality and further characterisation is required. Increasingly, cardiac CT is used as it can provide high spatial resolution anatomical imaging, but CMR is still important due to its ability to provide additional functional information.

This chapter will highlight a standard approach to imaging suspected cardiac tumours using a multi-parametric MR imaging protocol. Each of the most common referral indications for investigation of a suspected cardiac mass will be discussed in turn, highlighting their clinical features, frequency and MR imaging/tissue characteristics; and each will be illustrated by a typical case example highlighting the imaging features.

J.P. Greenwood, MBChB, PhD, FRCP (✉)
Department of Cardiology, Leeds General Infirmary,
Great George Street, Leeds LS1 3EX, UK

Leeds Institute for Cardiovascular and Metabolic Medicine & Multidisciplinary
Cardiovascular Research Centre, University of Leeds, Leeds LS2 9JT, UK
e-mail: j.greenwood@leeds.ac.uk

M. Motwani, MB ChB
Division of Cardiovascular and Diabetes Research, Leeds Institute of Cardiovascular and
Metabolic Medicine, Multidisciplinary Cardiovascular Research Centre, University of Leeds,
Leeds LS2 9JT, UK
e-mail: M.Motwani@leeds.ac.uk

© Springer International Publishing 2015
S. Plein et al. (eds.), *Cardiovascular MR Manual*,
DOI 10.1007/978-3-319-20940-1_27

Keywords

Myxoma • Lipoma • Papillary Fibroelastoma • Fibroma • Rhabdomyoma • Haemangioma • Sarcoma • Lymphoma • Metastatic tumours • Thrombus • Pericardial cyst • Pseudo-tumours

The Role of CMR in the Diagnosis of a Potential Cardiac Mass Is
1. To confirm or refute the presence of a mass identified on CXR or Echo
2. To establish the tumours location, size and relationship to surrounding cardiac structures (including extra-cardiac involvement)
3. To assist with tissue characterization and vascularity
4. To guide potential surgical intervention

CMR Protocol for Cardiac Masses (see Chap. 20: components of CMR protocols)
1. High resolution trans-axial BB T1-weigthed stack, diaphragm to aortic arch
2. Cine imaging in all standard planes and additional targeted planes
3. In two optimised orthogonal planes:
   (a) BB T1w with/without fat suppression and pre/post contrast
   (b) T2w
   (c) 1st pass myocardial perfusion imaging
   (d) Early and Late Gadolinium Enhancement imaging

Introduction

Cardiovascular magnetic resonance (CMR) imaging is an important technique for the evaluation of a suspected cardiac mass. CMR imaging offers a larger field of view, multi-planar imaging and superior tissue contrast compared to echocardiography. With recent improvements in MR pulse-sequence technology, tissue characterization is possible by comparing the T1 and T2 values of the mass to a reference tissue (Table 27.1). Thus CMR is an important imaging modality for the assessment of any suspected cardiac or paracardiac mass as it can determine tumour size, location, relationship to other cardiac structures, invasion into the pericardium or extra-cardiac spread (e.g. invasion into the great vessels), which is vital for any proposed surgical planning. Serial CMR studies can also be performed for monitoring tumour regression after surgical resection or chemotherapy.

Tumours of the heart can be either primary or secondary, the former of which can be either benign or malignant (Table 27.2). Primary cardiac tumours are very rare with a quoted prevalence of between 0.001 and 0.3 % in autopsy series. Approximately 75 % of primary cardiac tumours are benign. Secondary cardiac tumours occur with a frequency of 30–50 times that of primary malignant cardiac tumours. Benign primary cardiac tumours tend to be well circumscribed,

Table 27.1 CMR tissue characteristics of common cardiac masses

Cardiac mass	T1-w imaging[a]	T2-w imaging[a]	Post-contrast (LGE)
Pseudotumours			
Thrombus	Low (high if recent)	Low (high if recent)	No uptake[b]
Pericardial cyst	Low	High	No uptake
Benign			
Myxoma	Isointense	High	Heterogeneous
Lipoma	High[c]	High[c]	No uptake
Fibroma	Isointense	Low	Hyperenhancement[d]
Rhabdomyoma	Isointense	Isointense/high	No/minimal uptake
Malignant			
Angiosarcoma	Heterogenous	Heterogenous	Heterogeneous
Rhabdomyosarcoma	Isointense	Hyperintense	Homogeneous
Undifferentiated sarcoma	Isointense	Hyperintense	Heterogeneous/Variable
Lymphoma	Isointense	Isointense	No/minimal uptake
Metastasis[e]	Low	High	Heterogeneous

Reproduced with permission from (Motwani et al. 2013)
Note – typical characteristics are presented in table, but all tumours can have atypical appearances due to altered tissue composition
T1-w T1-weighted, *T2-w* T2-weighted, *LGE* late gadolinium enhancement
[a]T1-w and T2-w imaging signal is given relative to myocardium
[b]Best seen on early gadolinium enhancement imaging (no uptake) 2 min after contrast (Fig. 27.5)
[c]Similar to surrounding fat signal and characterized by marked suppression with fat-saturation pre-pulse
[d]However, fibromas are non-enhancing on perfusion-imaging due to avascularity
[e]The exception is metastatic melanoma which has a high T1-w and a low T2-w signal

Table 27.2 Primary cardiac tumours in adults

Benign (~70 %)		Malignant (~30 %)	
Myxoma	30 %	Angiosarcoma	9 %
Lipoma	10 %	Rhabdomyosarcoma	5 %
Papillary fibroelastoma	10 %	Mesothelioma	4 %
Fibroma	4 %	Fibrosarcoma	3 %
Rhabdomyoma	7 %	Lymphoma	2 %
Haemangioma	3 %		

homogeneous, do not invade local structures and tend not to be associated with pleural or pericardial effusions. The most common primary malignant cardiac tumours are the various sarcomas and lymphomas. Unfortunately due to the small numbers studied and their variable presentation reliable tissue differentiation by CMR is still not possible.

A CMR scan is usually performed after a transthoracic echocardiogram has identified an abnormality and further characterisation is required. For example, CMR can provide detailed information on extra-cardiac involvement, lesion vascularity and tissue characterisation (Table 27.3). With the advent of cardiac CT, comparable anatomical information can be obtained from this modality, but CMR is still important due to its ability to provide additional functional information.

Benign Cardiac Tumours

Myxoma

This is the most common primary cardiac tumour accounting for ~30 % of all cardiac masses and half of all benign tumours. Myxomas typically present between the third and sixth decades of life, more commonly in women and whilst 20 % may be asymptomatic, the classic triad of symptoms relate to obstruction, constitutional symptoms and the effects of embolisation.

Typically, myxomas are solitary and located in the left atrium (75 %) with a predilection for the inter-atrial septum. Internally they are heterogeneous tumours containing cystic areas, haemorrhage, necrosis and calcification. On CMR imaging, they appear spherical and often the pedunculated point of attachment to the endocardial surface can be identified on cine imaging. Cine imaging is also particularly useful as myxomas are highly mobile and may be seen prolapsing through the mitral valve causing obstruction. With SSFP cine techniques, myxomas appear hyperintense relative to the myocardium but hypointense relative to the blood pool. On T1-weighted imaging, myxomas are characterized by an isointense (similar to myocardium), but often heterogeneous signal intensity due to their complex architecture. On T2-weighted imaging myxomas may show marked increased signal intensity due to the high extracellular water content. After contrast, there may be moderately high contrast enhancement mixed with non-enhancing areas which are cystic or necrotic giving a typical heterogeneous pattern on LGE imaging (Fig. 27.1). Many myxomas also have a surface layer thrombus, with peripheral low signal on LGE images.

Lipoma

This is the second most common benign cardiac tumour. Typically solitary, encapsulated and well circumscribed. Lipomas can arise subepicardially (25 %), subendocardially (50 %) or from the myocardium and arise most commonly from the right atrium or left ventricle. On CMR, lipomas are characterized by high signal intensity on T1-weighted imaging, slightly less signal on T2-weighted imaging, and a marked reduction in signal intensity on T1-weighted imaging when a fat saturation prepulse is used (compare appearance to that of subcutaneous fat). They do not enhance following the administration of contrast (Fig. 27.2).

Lipomatous hypertrophy is a non-encapsulated fatty infiltration, typically seen in the inter-atrial septum and is usually contiguous with the epicardial fat. It can usually be distinguished from a true encapsulated lipoma by its morphological

Table 27.3 Typical CMR scanning protocol for a suspected cardiac mass

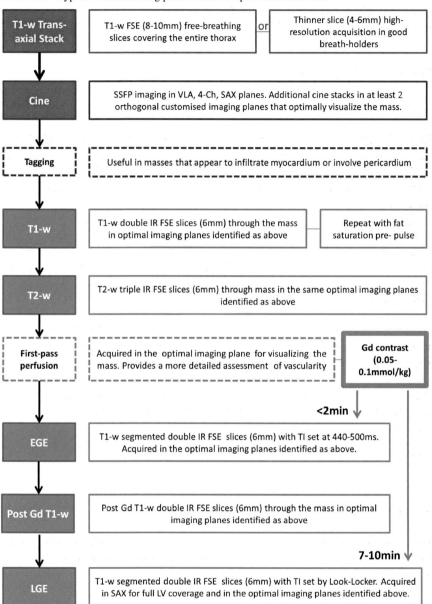

Sequences in *red* are used for 'localisation' of the mass. Sequences in *blue* are used for 'tissue characterization'. Tagging and first-pass perfusion sequences are optional sequences that can supplement the core dataset. The second bolus of gadolinium (Gd) contrast is given with the first-pass perfusion sequence if performed – or alternatively as a 'top-up dose' prior to EGE imaging

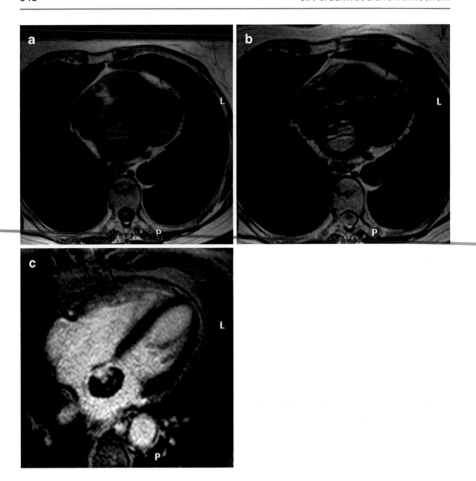

Fig. 27.1 Eighty four year female presenting with syncope and embolic phenomena. CMR characteristics of a left atrial myxoma: (**a**) T1-weighted black blood image in axial orientation showing an oval mass in the left atrium. (**b**) T2-weighted imaging using the same geometry. (**c**) LGE image confirming the heterogeneous nature of the lesion

features – the fatty mass in lipomatous hypertrophy is by definition greater than 2 cm in transverse diameter and classically involves the limbus of the fossa ovalis, sparing the fossa ovalis membrane, giving rise to a bilobed dumbbell shape

Papillary Fibroelastoma

These represent the third most common benign cardiac tumour, typically occurring on the valves (90 %) as a frond like structure. They are generally not visualized well by CMR due to their small size (usually <1.5 cm) and high mobility.

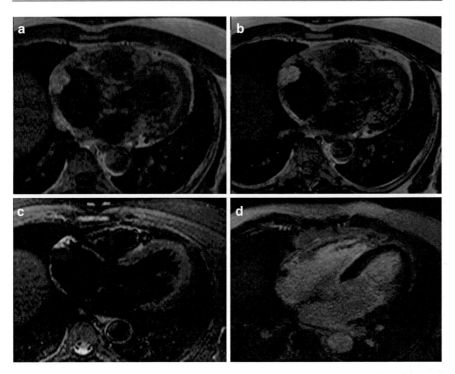

Fig. 27.2 Forty five year female presenting with palpitations. CMR features of a right atrial lipoma demonstrated by: (**a**) T1-weighted black blood image in transaxial plane. (**b**) T2-weighted black blood imaging. (**c**) T1-STIR (fat suppression pre-pulse). (**d**) LGE image confirming no contrast uptake into the lesion (Images courtesy of G. McCann, Leicester)

Fibroma

These are congenital tumours that typically first present in young adult life. Fibromas are usually solitary and located within the ventricular myocardium (LV more frequently than RV). The tumour typically exerts a local 'mass' effect and are frequently associated with malignant ventricular arrhythmias. On CMR, fibromas appear homogeneous, well-demarcated and solitary. On T1-weighted imaging they appear isointense compared to normal myocardium and skeletal muscle; and on T2-weighted imaging they appear characteristically hypointense (unlike other masses). With gadolinium administration, fibromas generally show non-enhancement during perfusion imaging, due to their avascularity. However, using the LGE technique 10–15 min after contrast, fibromas classically show intense homogeneous hyperenhancement (Fig. 27.3). The explanation of this LGE pattern is that microscopically fibromas are a collection of fibroblasts interspersed with large amounts of collagen and therefore have a very large extracellular space component.

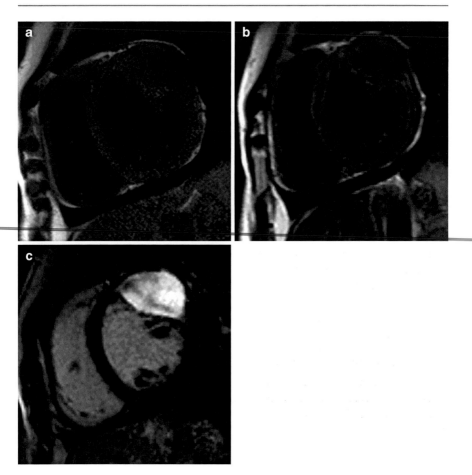

Fig. 27.3 Thirty two year female presenting with palpitations. CMR features of a fibromas demonstrated by: (**a**) T1-weighted black blood image in short axis. (**b**) T2-weighted black blood imaging. (**c**) LGE image confirming hyperenhancement confined to the lesion

Rhabdomyoma

These tumours are the most common primary cardiac tumour in infants and children. They typically present in the first year of life and are often associated with a diagnosis of tuberous sclerosis. They arise in the ventricular myocardium (LV > RV), but unlike fibromas, they are multiple in 90 % of cases. Microscopically they are hamartomas, and macroscopically they are well-circumscribed and vary from a few millimeters to a few centimeters in size. On CMR rhabdomyomas appear homogeneous and isointense on T1-weighted imaging and hyperintense on T2-weighted imaging compared to normal myocardium. They typically show minimal or no enhancement with gadolinium consistent with their hamartomatous composition.

Haemangioma

Arteriovenous haemangioma are rare accounting for 5–10 % of benign cardiac tumours. They are typically solitary, non homogeneous and found in the LV or RV. With CMR, haemangiomas are typically heterogenous and hyperintense on T1- and T2-weighted imaging due to slow blood flow. During and after contrast administration they intensely hyperenhance due to their vascular content – but there may be areas of inhomogeneity due to calcification or fibrous septa

Malignant Cardiac Tumours

Sarcomas

This group of tumours occurs mainly in adulthood, usually between the third and fifth decades, and carries an extremely poor prognosis. They account for approximately 95 % of primary malignant cardiac tumours and include angiosarcomas, leiomyosarcomas, fibrosarcomas, liposarcomas and osteosarcomas. Angiosarcomas are the most common of this group and typically arise in the RA, and are irregular or nodular. They often infiltrate into the cardiac chambers or extend along the pericardium. Due to their associated haemorrhage and necrosis, on CMR they appear heterogeneous with areas of increased signal intensity on T1- and T2- weighted images. After contrast they continue to appear heterogeneous on LGE imaging due to peripheral fibrosis (surface hyperenhancement) and focal hypoenhancement due to central necrosis (Fig. 27.4). Other sarcomas are rare and beyond the scope of this text.

Lymphoma

Primary cardiac lymphomas are very rare, and cardiac metastases from extra-cardiac forms of lymphoma are far more common (~25 % of patients with lymphoma have cardiac involvement on post-mortem studies). Nearly all primary cardiac lymphomas are aggressive B-cell lymphomas and they predominantly occur in immunocompromised patients, especially those with HIV infection. They most commonly involve the right side of the heart, particularly the RA, but any chamber can be involved and there are frequently multiple lesions. Unlike other malignant tumours such as sarcomas, lymphomas generally lack areas of central necrosis and hemorrhage. As a result, lymphomas are typically homogenous and isointense on T1 and T2 weighted imaging, which can be a useful discriminating feature. Similarly, unlike other malignant tumors, there is generally minimal contrast uptake on LGE imaging. The transaxial anatomy stacks should be carefully examined for mediastinal lymph nodes to identify extra-cardiac involvement and for the purpose of biopsy targets.

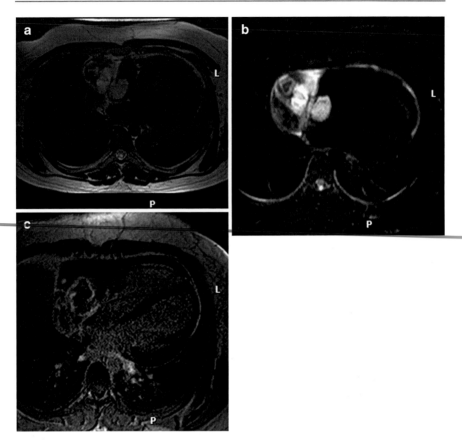

Fig. 27.4 Twenty five year male presenting with clinical features of tamponade. CMR imaging features included: (**a**) T1-weighted black blood imaging transaxially showing large heterogeneous mass compressing the right atrium and invading through the wall into the right atrial cavity. (**b**) T2-weighted images and (**c**) LGE images confirmed the heterogeneous nature of the tumour

Metastatic Tumours

Metastatic spread to the heart is most commonly associated with lung cancer, breast cancer, lymphoma, and melanoma. Spread to the heart may be by direct invasion, and by haematological or lymphatic spread. Transvenous spread can also occur for example, via the IVC in the case of hepatic or renal tumours. The commonest site of involvement is the pericardium (usually from direct invasion or lymphatic spread) and malignant pericardial effusions are the commonest consequence of cardiac metastasis. Usually, haemorrhagic and exudative pericardial effusions have a high signal on T1-weighted imaging, whereas benign transudates have a low signal. Typically metastases tend to have low signal intensity on T1-weighted images, appear brighter on T2-weighted images and enhance after contrast. Melanoma is the exception which appears bright on T1 weighted imaging due to the paramagnetic metals bound by melanin.

Others Masses & Tumours

Thrombus

This is one of the most common causes of an intra-cardiac mass and is typically found in the LA in association with chronic AF or mitral valve disease, or in the LV in association with myocardial infarction. The CMR appearances are variable depending on age of the thrombus; fresh thrombus appears bright on T1 and T2-weighted imaging, older thrombi typically have lower signal intensity on T2-weighed images. After contrast administration, intra-cavity thrombus appears very dark on both the early and late gadolinium enhancement images (Fig. 27.5).

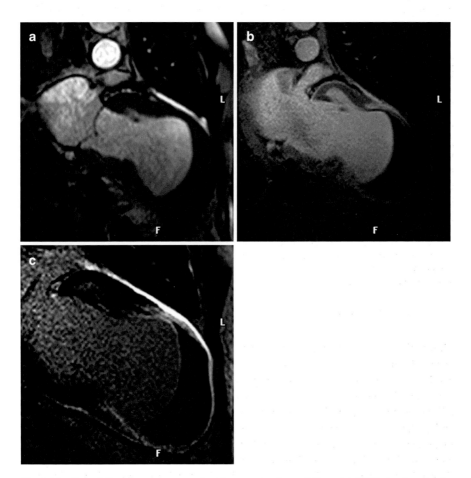

Fig. 27.5 Sixty five year male presented with worsening heart failure. (**a**) SSFP cine imaging in the VLA orientation showed a large antero-apical aneurysm which appeared to be lined with thrombus. (**b**) Early gadolinium enhancement and (**c**) LGE images in the VLA orientation confirmed the presence of thrombus (very dark area at the apex)

Cysts

Pericardial cysts are usually located in the right pericardiophrenic angle and are often discovered incidentally on CXR or by echocardiography. Usually the patient is asymptomatic unless the cyst exerts a local compressive effect. The cyst is usually filled with clear fluid and on CMR they characteristically appear very bright on T2-weighted imaging (Fig. 27.6).

Pseudo-Tumours

Not infrequently normal intra-cardiac structures or remnants can be mistaken for a tumour e.g. Crista terminalis, Thebesian valve, Eustachian valve, or a Coumadin ridge. Other structures outside the heart can also give 'cause for concern' such as

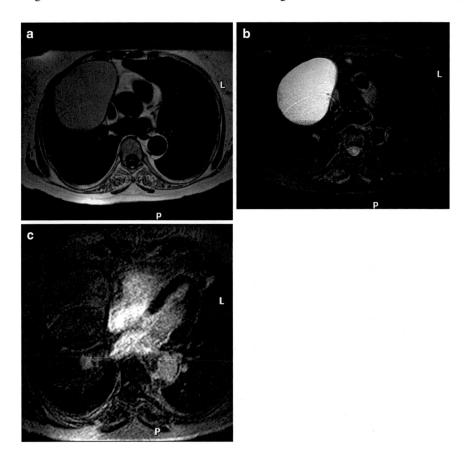

Fig. 27.6 Seventy one year female presented with shortness of breath and a large mass lesion seen on the CXR and echocardiogram. CMR features included: (**a**) T1-weighted black blood imaging showing large well demarcated lesion exerting local compression of the right hilum, RA and SVC. (**b**) T2-weighted imaging showing very high signal intensity from the fluid filled cyst. (**c**) LGE image shows no contrast uptake

prominent coronary sinus, AV malformations, and left sided SVC. With its large field of view and high spatial resolution CMR can rapidly characterise these structures.

Tips and Tricks
1. Identify the lesion on multi-slice, multi-phase cine imaging in at least two orthogonal planes.
2. For tissue characterisation always perform multiple pulse sequence acquisitions (e.g. BB T1-weighted sequences with and without a fat saturation prepulse, BB T2-weighted imaging and late gadolinium enhancement imaging) using the same planning geometry.
3. 1st pass myocardial perfusion imaging can be extremely helpful in the determination of vascularity.

Key Points: CMR in Diagnosis of Cardiac Masses
1. CMR is the principle modality for the diagnosis and follow-up intra-cardiac tumours.
2. CMR allows detailed assessment of tumour location and its involvement of other cardiac/extra-cardiac structures, to assist with surgical planning.
3. Very small, highly mobile masses (e.g. valvular vegetations) may be best visualised by echocardiography.
4. Whilst CMR can provide information on tissue characterisation, it cannot give a histological diagnosis and thus further assessment (e.g. biopsy) may be required.

Standard CMR Report for Cardiac Masses
1. Location (pericardial, myocardial, valve relationship, chamber relationship)
2. Size (in three cross-sectional dimensions)
3. Signal intensity on T1, T1 fat, T2 and STIR images (homogeneous, heterogeneous, hyper-, iso- or hypo-intense to myocardium/or chest wall (specify reference tissue))
4. Relationship to myocardium/pericardium, mediastinum
5. Margins (e.g., smooth, irregular, infiltrating)
6. Cine CMR appearance (pedunculated, motion with myocardium/pericardium)
     Optional (if performed)
7. Perfusion pattern
8. Late gadolinium enhancement pattern

Additional Reading

Chiles C, Woodard PK, Gutierrez FR, Link KM. Metastatic involvement of the heart and pericardium: CT and MR imaging. Radiographics. 2001;21:439–49.

Hoffmann U, Globits S, Frank H. Cardiac and paracardiac masses. Eur Heart J. 1998;19:553–63.

Motwani M, Kidambi A, Herzog BA, Uddin A, Greenwood JP, Plein S. MR imaging of cardiac tumors and masses: a review of methods and clinical applications. Radiology. 2013;268:26–43.

Valvular Heart Disease

28

Amedeo Chiribiri and Timothy Fairbairn

Abstract

Echocardiography remains the principal investigation for valvular heart disease (VHD). Cardiovascular MR provides accurate and reproducible information about the valves (flow, velocities, pressure gradient, volumes, regurgitant fraction), the left ventricle (volumes, mass, function, ischaemia and fibrosis) and the aorta (root measurements and coarctation). This detailed yet diverse information can be appropriately used in complex VHD/congenital cases to further grade disease severity and risk stratify the patient.

Keywords

Stenosis • Regurgitation • Phase-contrast • Through-plane • In-plane • Continuity equation • Planimetry • Prosthetic • TAVI

CMR Protocol in Valvular Heart Disease

1. LV structure and function module
2. Cine images specific to individual valves :
   - Aortic valve : LVOT views, coronal view and in-plane view of valve
   - Mitral valve : LVOT view, VLA view and in-plane view of valve
   - Pulmonary valve : RVOT views and in-plane view of valve
   - Tricuspid valve : RV long axis view and in-plane view of valve

A. Chiribiri, MBBS, CCST in Cardiology, PhD (✉)
Department of Cardiovascular Imaging, King's College London/St Thomas's Hospital,
4th Floor Lambeth Wing, London SE1 7EH, UK
e-mail: amedeo.chiribiri@kcl.ac.uk

T. Fairbairn, MBChB, PhD
Department of Cardiology, Liverpool Heart and Chest Hospital,
Thomas Drive, Liverpool L14 3PE, UK
e-mail: timothy.fairbairn@lhch.nhs.uk

© Springer International Publishing 2015
S. Plein et al. (eds.), *Cardiovascular MR Manual*,
DOI 10.1007/978-3-319-20940-1_28

3. Flow measurement perpendicular to the vessel and distal from the edge of valve leaflets
4. Contiguous stack of 5 mm cines aligned with the direction of inflow and transecting the principal line of coaptation to assess valve morphology.
5. Gradient echo/EPI rather than SSFP cine to visualize regurgitant jets

Introduction

Echocardiography remains the first and most important imaging modality for the evaluation of valvular heart disease. However, increasingly CMR is used in cases of inadequate echocardiographic examination and in order to provide additional information on regurgitant volumes and cardiac chamber size. Phase-sensitive sequences provide accurate measurements of flow (Fig. 28.1). The CMR evaluation of valvular heart disease should include the quantification of lesion severity (quantification of the regurgitation or stenosis), the measurement of the consequences of the valvular defect on the cardiac chambers (volume, mass, and function), and the assessment of valve morphology.

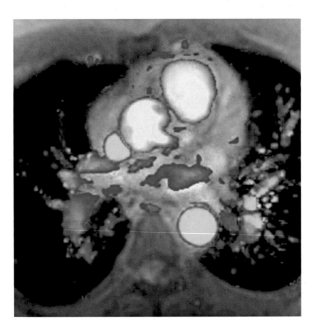

Fig. 28.1 Phase-sensitive flow sequence with colour-encoded reconstruction, showing a systolic frame acquired at the level of the pulmonary artery and of the ascending aorta. Blood flow pulling away from the reader is represented in *yellow-red*; blood flow crossing the image plane towards the reader is represented in *cyan-blue*

CMR Versus Other Imaging Modalities

Echocardiography is the principle imaging modality for the assessment of heart valve disease. CMR may be useful in specific clinical scenarios, for example when image quality by echocardiography is poor. CMR is also an excellent and more reproducible test for the measurement of chamber volumes and can accurately quantify regurgitant fractions, although the clinical relevance of such CMR derived measurements remains to be established. Since the publication of the 2004 appropriateness criteria for CMR [1], new methodology such as multi-dimensional flow, and clinical studies have been published that are expected to enhance the role of CMR in valvular heart disease in the future (Table 28.1).

CMR may also be useful in assessing valvular masses (tumors, vegetations or thrombi). In congenital heart disease, assessment of valvular morphology is a routine component of CMR protocols.

Furthermore, in selected cases CMR can assess the presence of turbulence and the direction of jets, and can provide essential information on concomitant vascular abnormalities (aortic dilatation or coarctation and dilatation of the pulmonary artery).

> **Role of CMR in Valvular Heart Disease**
> 1. Provides accurate measurements of ventricular function and mass (Class I indication)
> 2. Provides accurate measurements of regurgitant blood volume (Class I indication)
> 3. Useful for valve morphology description, particularly to identify bicuspid aortic valve (Class II indication)

Congenital

Bicuspid aortic valve is a frequent congenital abnormality. Cine SSFP or cine turbo gradient echo sequences allow a direct visualization of the shape of the valvular orifice and of the number of cusps. The evaluation is usually possible also in severely calcified valves, using a flow sequence and evaluating the shape of the forward flow (Fig. 28.2).

Table 28.1 Clinical indications for CMR in valvular heart disease

Indication	Class
1. Valve morphology	II
Bicuspid aortic valve	III
Other valves	Inv
Vegetations	
2. Cardiac chamber anatomy and function	I
3. Quantification of regurgitation	I
4. Quantification of stenosis	III
5. Dewtection of paravalvular abscesses	Inv
6. Assessment of prosthetic valves	Inv

Adapted from: Clinical indications for CMR: consensus panel report [1]

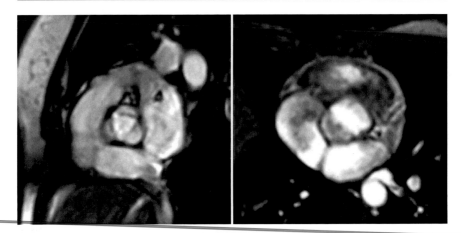

Fig. 28.2 Tricuspid (*left*) and Bicuspid (*right*) aortic valve

CMR also allows a complete evaluation of the abnormalities that are usually associated with a bicuspid aortic valve, such as aortic regurgitation, dilatation of the ascending aorta or aortic coarctation, and is very useful to obtain repeated measurements during the follow-up of the patient (Fig. 28.3).

In patients with Ebstein's anomaly, CMR provides a complete assessment of tricuspid valve displacement, valve morphologic abnormalities, volume and function of the residual RV, and presence and size of an associated interatrial defect (Fig. 28.4).

Where mitral valve masses are suspected, CMR can often provide unique diagnostic information that help to characterise the lesion (see also Chap. 27, Cardiac Masses). (Fig. 28.5).

CMR allows the visualization of the left ventricular outflow tract and a precise differential diagnosis between different types of sub-aortic stenosis. In patients with hypertrophic cardiomyopathy, systolic anterior movement of the anterior leaflet of the mitral valve can confirm the diagnosis of obstruction of the left ventricular outflow tract. CMR is also a valuable tool to identify other causes of obstruction, such as a subvalvular fibrous ridge (Fig. 28.6).

Regurgitation

CMR can accurately quantify valvular regurgitation. Clinical indications vary depending on the valve concerned. CMR is the modality of choice for the evaluation of pulmonary valve regurgitation. Due to the through-plane motion of the pulmonary artery (PA) during the cardiac cycle, care must be taken to avoid the appearance of the right ventricle outflow tract (RVOT) or the right and left branches of the PA in the imaging plane (though-plane) of the flow sequence used to measure the regurgitant fraction. CMR also offers a complete evaluation of the size and function of the right ventricle (RV), of the RVOT, and of the PA.

Patients with known or suspected aortic regurgitation can be fully evaluated with CMR. Flow measurements at the level of the aortic valve allow a reliable

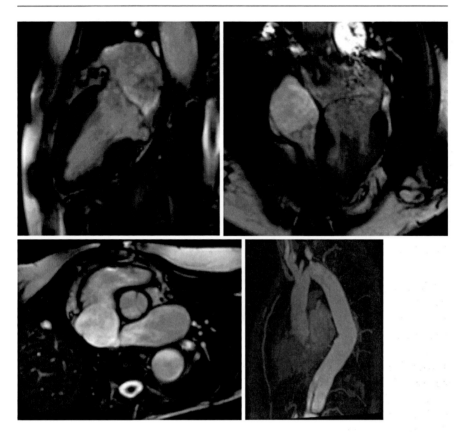

Fig. 28.3 Evaluation of a patient with Marfan's syndrome and previous valve-sparing aortic root replacement and aortic repair for Stanford type B aortic dyssection. 2-chamber and 4-chamber SSFP cine (end systolic frame) demonstrating prolapse of the mitral and tricuspid valves (*top images*). Native tricuspid aortic valve (*bottom left*) and aortic angiography demonstrating residual distal aortic dissection (MPR image, *bottom right*)

measurement of regurgitant fraction (Fig. 28.7). CMR can also provide an accurate measurement of left ventricular (LV) function and mass, and can diagnose associated abnormalities such as bicuspid aortic valve, dilatation of the ascending aorta, or aortic coarctation. In a study of 113 patients with echocardiographic moderate or severe aortic regurgitation a CMR derived aortic regurgitant fraction of more than 33 % was strongly associated with the development of typical symptoms and referral for aortic valve surgery [2].

Due to the movement of the atrio-ventricular valves during the cardiac cycle, a reliable evaluation of the transvalvular blood flow is precluded with bi-dimensional flow sequences (Fig. 28.8). Mitral regurgitant volume can be indirectly quantified as the difference between LV stroke volume and aortic forward flow or as the difference between LV stroke volume and RV stroke volume in case of normal function of the tricuspid and pulmonary valve. Cine long-axis views (particularly with turbo gradient echo sequences) allow the visualization of the regurgitant jet in the atrial cavities.

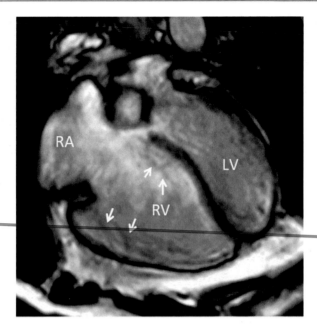

Fig. 28.4 SSFP-Image of an atrialised RV in Ebstein's anomaly. The dilated right atrium (*RA*) is connected to the *RV* by a dysplastic tricuspid valve that is displaced towards the apex of the heart (*arrows*)

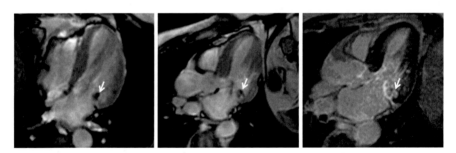

Fig. 28.5 SSFP-cine and late gadolinium enhancement images in a case of mitral annulus calcification (calcified mass indicated by the *arrows* on the posterior leaflet of the mitral valve). Cine images in diastole and systole identify the mass. Late gadolinium enhanced images (*right*) show the mass to have a fibrous component. Additional CMR images may be acquired to further characterise the lesion

New approaches using a moving slice for flow measurement were proposed but are not implemented for clinical use in the majority of the CMR scanners [3].

In mitral or tricuspid regurgitation, a contiguous stack of thin (5 mm) cine images in the inflow direction and transecting the valve's coaptation line or a stack of cines oriented radially along the long axis of the LV or RV enables assessment of tethering, prolapse, or regurgitation through the different scallops of the valve leaflets.

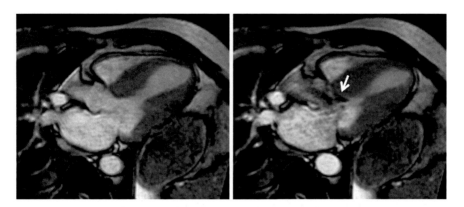

Fig. 28.6 SSFP-cine images in end diastolic (*left*) and end-systolic phase (*right*), showing the systolic anterior motion (SAM) of the anterior leaflet of the mitral valve in a patient with hypertrophic cardiomyopathy. The dynamic obstruction in the left ventricular outflow tract causes significant turbulence of the blood in systole, seen as a signal void originating from the outflow track and extending above the aortic valve (*arrow*)

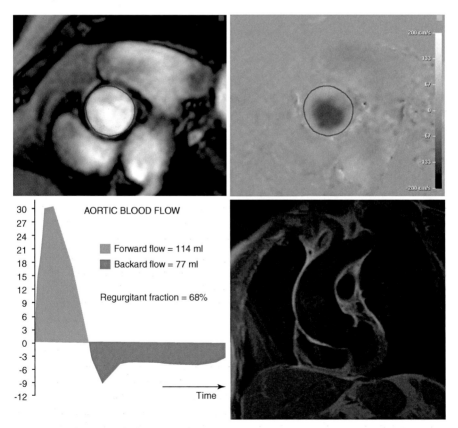

Fig. 28.7 Aortic regurgitation. Modulus and phase images are reconstructed from a gradient-echo flow sequence (*top*, *left* and *right* respectively). Post-processing of the data (*left bottom*) allows an accurate measurement of forward and backward flow across the valve

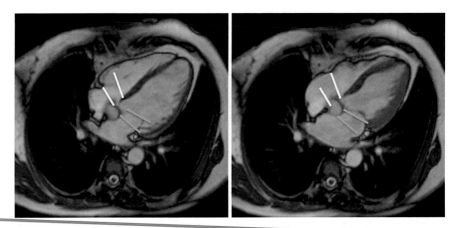

Fig. 28.8 4-chamber view showing the end-diastolic (*left*) and the end-systolic frame (*right*). The atrio-ventricular valves have a marked movement throughout the cardiac cycle (tricuspid valve: *white lines*; mitral valve: *green lines*). For this reason the evaluation of transvalvular blood flow is not reliable using a bidimensional flow sequence

Stenosis

Semi-lunar valve stenosis: CMR can provide useful data for the evaluation of patients with aortic or pulmonary stenosis. Short axis slices of the aortic valve may better identify valve morphology (bicuspid vs tricuspid), and determine the severity of stenosis compared to echo (Fig. 28.9) [4]. Thin slices (5 mm) with no gap should be performed to allow planimetry of the valve at the tip of the leaflets during maximal systolic opening. Planimetry should be performed on the cross section that delineates the orifice or flow jet most clearly. Alternatively, aortic valve area can be measured by the continuity equation as (Velocity time integral LVOT/Velocity time integral aorta)×Area LVOT. Phase contrast (PC) imaging (VENC 400) planned at the STJ in line with the stenotic jet, will provide additional functional information about the peak velocity through the AV, mean and peak pressure gradients.

Atrioventricular valve stenosis: CMR represents a second line investigation in patients with known mitral stenosis. It allows a precise determination of the atrial size, and of the number and location of the pulmonary veins in those patients undergoing ablation of atrial fibrillation. CMR can also provide an estimate of the planimetric opening area of the mitral valve but it is likely to underestimate the severity of mitral stenosis due to the translational motion of the heart. As in mitral or tricuspid regurgitation, a contiguous stack of thin (5 mm) cine enables detailed assessment of the morphology of the valve substructures.

Prosthetic Valves

With the exception of some older ball and cage prosthetic valves, implanted metallic heart valves are not a contraindication to CMR. Metal parts of the prosthesis create a local artifact that affects the interpretation of the image (Fig. 28.10).

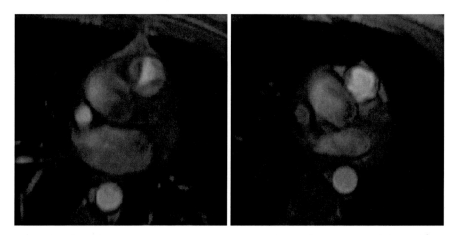

Fig. 28.9 Pulmonary valve (PV) stenosis. Turbo-gradient echo cine images acquired in short axis at the level of the PV (end-systolic frame). In case of PV stenosis, the opening of the valve is usually incomplete. In this case the shape is triangular (*left*), different from the almost circular shape of a normal PV (*right*)

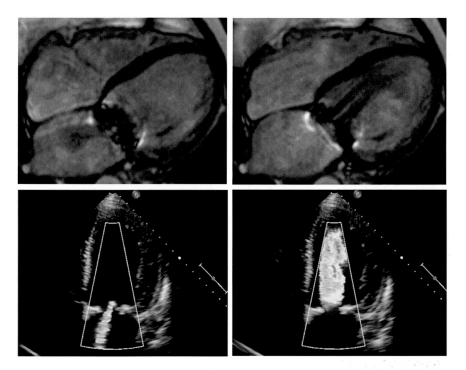

Fig. 28.10 Example of a dysfunctioning bio-prosthetic valve in mitral position in a patient referred for dyspnoea. CMR cine images identified the regurgitant jet in the left atrium (*left image*) and a turbulent diastolic flow towards the left ventricle (*right*). These findings were confirmed with colour-Doppler echocardiography. The diagnosis of the prosthetic dysfunction was made despite the artifact from the metallic components of the prosthesis

Transcatheter Aortic Valve Implantation

Transcatheter Aortic Valve Implantation (TAVI) is recommended for symptomatic severe aortic stenosis (AS) patients who are at a high operative risk. Cardiac imaging plays an integral role in assisting the multidisciplinary 'heart team' make an informed decision regarding patient selection, operative risk versus benefit and guiding the procedure (Table 28.2). Cardiovascular MRI can provide detailed and accurate pre-operative information to assess a patients' anatomical suitability for the procedure and determine the likelihood of clinical benefit. It remains an underutilized imaging strategy due to perceived difficulties in patient tolerability, however several studies have now demonstrated its feasibility and usefulness [5, 6].

Patient Selection

Aortic Valve Assessment
PC imaging of peak velocity and regurgitant fraction (pre and post TAVI [paravalvular]) is simple and reproducible when compared to the difficulties of 2D and 3D echocardiography [7]. AR severity provides additional prognostic information post TAVI [8].

Left Ventricle
The accurate EF and stroke volume (SV) quantification afforded by CMR can identify individuals with previously unrecognised reduced systolic function or SV; Low-flow low gradient AS (LF LG AS: EF< 40 %, mean pressure gradient <40 mmHg) and paradoxical low flow-low gradient AS (Paradoxical LF LG AS: EF>40 %, mean pressure gradient <40 mmHg, SV <35 ml/m^2) These patients form the two groups of AS patients who are either misdiagnosed or refused SAVR and yet have the poorest outcomes without intervention.

Table 28.2 Imaging assessment for TAVI

Assessment	TTE/TOE	MDCT	CMR
AV stenosis/regurgitation	+++	+	++
LV function	+++	+	+++
LV wall thickness (septal)	+++	++	+++
Concomitant valve disease	+++	+	+++
AV morphology	++	++	++
AV calcification	++	+++	–
AV annulus	++	+++	+++
AV root	++	+++	+++
Annulus to coronary distance	+	+++	+++
Coronary artery disease	–	++	+
Peripheral artery disease	–	+++	++
Myocardial fibrosis/viability	–	–	+++

AV aortic stenosis, LV left ventricle
Diagnostic accuracy and appropriate use criteria:
+++ high, ++ moderate, + poor, – unsuitable

Coronary Artery Disease

Half of all TAVI patients will have significant CAD and 25 % will have had a previous myocardial infarct. CMR cannot assess CAD anatomical severity with the same detail as MDCT or coronary angiography. However, it does provide additional information concerning myocardial ischaemia and viability [8]. Significant myocardial ischaemia may help guide the need for pre-TAVI revascularisation. LGE scar burden has been shown to predict reverse remodelling post TAVI [5]. In comparison, in low EF patients stress echocardiography only predicts operative mortality not likely benefit.

Myocardial Fibrosis

Myocardial fibrosis (MF) is prevalent is AS (30–50 %). This can be detected as either diffuse interstitial fibrosis (increase in extracellular volume) by T1 mapping, or as focal replacement fibrosis by late gadolinium enhancement. The presence and burden of fibrosis is a poor prognostic marker and may influence the timing of any intervention and patient selection (Fig. 28.11).

Anatomical Suitability

CMR imaging can help determine anatomical suitability, the type of device used and the best operative route (Transfemoral, subclavian, transaortic or transapical).

Aortic Root and LVOT

Annular measurements are essential in the accurate sizing of the TAVI device. The aortic annulus is actually ovoid in shape, requiring 3D assessment for accurate measurement of the diameter (d). MDCT is the modality conventionally used, however MDCT, 3D TEE and CMR have similar levels of reproducibility and accuracy [6]. CMR is of particular use in the individuals with chronic kidney disease and the need to avoid contrast. Sagittal and coronal cine imaging of the LVOT can be used to measure LVOT, annulus (Eq. 28.1) and sinus diameters (Fig. 28.12).

$$\text{mean annular diameter} \left(\text{Mean d} = \left(\text{LVOT Min d} + \text{Coronal max} \right) / 2 \right)$$

A short axis cine stack can be used to calculate the annular perimeter or area, which are believed to be more reproducible and predict AR with greater accuracy. Multiplanar cine imaging can measure the distance between the aortic annulus (hinge) and coronary arteries. A minimum height of 8–10 mm is recommended to prevent coronary obstruction during device expansion,

Ascending Aorta and Peripheral Vasculature

A sagittal-oblique cine stack of the aorta and contrast enhanced MR angiography (CE-MRA) or non-contrast 3D SSFP sequence provides accurate and reproducible measurements of the ascending aorta and peripheral vasculature as well as MDCT, but cannot assess the degree of calcification. Measurements of the ascending aorta and sinus of valsalva are important as an ascending aortic diameter of >43 mm is considered a contraindication to implantation. A transfemoral approach is the preferred route of TAVI access yet bulky delivery sheaths can result in major vascular complications and increased 30 day mortality. A minimum artery diameter of 6 mm is recommended to reduce complications.

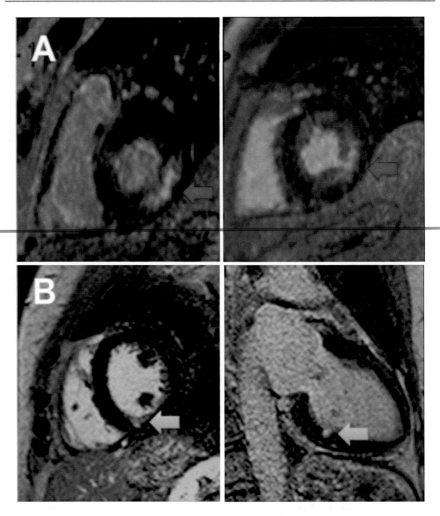

Fig. 28.11 Late gadolinium enhanced imaging: Mid-wall pattern Myocardial Fibrosis, (**a**, *red arrow*) and Myocardial scar (**b**, *blue arrow*)

Vegetations

CMR is less effective than echocardiography in the detection of mobile vegetations of the valvular leaflets. Nevertheless, infective endocarditis is not a contraindication itself to the CMR examination.

Paravalvular Abscesses

Just a few cases are described in the literature of paravalvular abscesses identified with CMR. When a paravalvular abscess is suspected, echocardiography is the method of choice to confirm the diagnosis. In patients with prosthetic valves (particularly for

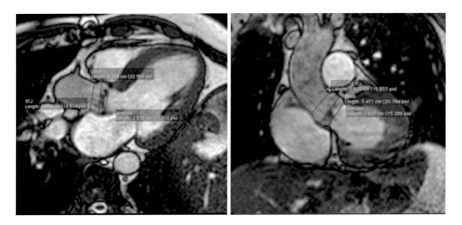

Fig. 28.12 Aortic root measurements

mechanical valves), artifacts and signal loss due to the metallic valve components usually preclude the evaluation of the area surrounding the prosthesis.

Key Points CMR in Valvular Heart Disease
1. CMR is the method of choice for assessment of ventricular function.
2. Patients with prosthetic valves can safely undergo CMR at 1.5 and 3 T, except patients with the old ball and cage Starr-Edwards prosthesis
3. Determine left and right ventricular stroke volume from cine stacks to measure single valve regurgitation.
4. Mitral regurgitation can be measured by subtracting aortic flow from LV stroke volume.
5. Multiple valve lesions can be assessed from comparison of the aortic and pulmonary diastolic regurgitant flow and the LV and RV stroke volumes.
6. Measure aortic valve area by direct planimetry or continuity equation.
7. Calculate peak mitral valve gradient from peak mitral valve flow
8. CMR provides a wealth of functional and anatomical information in the assessment of a TAVI patient

Tips and Tricks
1. During flow measurements, adapt velocity encoding (VENC) to the actual velocity (the lowest value without aliasing) and use the shortest possible TE.
2. The best value for velocity encoding can be estimated from previous echocardiographic evaluations where available or with an iterative approach, increasing the value at each acquisition until an image without aliasing is obtained.
3. The software for flow measurement is usually available on the scanner. A quick evaluation of the results of flow sequences to exclude the aliasing artifact is advisable before discharging the patient.

4. Arrhythmias can lead to the acquisition of low quality images and obscure the diagnostic evaluation of the patient. If cardioversion is indicated and feasible, the CMR examination should be postponed until the patient is in sinus rhythm.

CMR Report in Valvular Heart Disease
1. LV and RV dimensions and volumes.
2. Morphology of each component of the valve complex (e.g. leaflets, annulus, chordae)
3. Presence of any insufficiency or reduced valvular excursion
4. If indicated mitral regurgitant
5. Peak velocity (single value when recorded across semilunar valves or a vessel in cross-section, both early (E) and late (A) peak velocities for atrioventricular valves)
6. Forward stroke volume and peak and mean transvalvular gradients;
7. Regurgitant volume and fraction
8. Valve area (mention the method of determination);

References

1. Pennell DJ, Sechtem UP, Higgins CB, Manning WJ, Pohost GM, Rademakers FE, van Rossum AC, Shaw LJ, Kent Yucel E. Clinical indications for cardiovascular magnetic resonance (CMR): consensus panel report. Eur Heart J. 2004;25:1940–95.
2. Myerson SG, d'Arcy J, Mohiaddin R, Greenwood JP, Karamitsos TD, Francis JM, Banning AP, Christiansen JP, Neubauer S. Aortic regurgitation quantification using cardiovascular magnetic resonance. Association with clinical outcome. Circulation. 2012;126:1452–60.
3. Kozerke S, Schwitter J, Pedersen EM, Boesiger P. Aortic and mitral regurgitation: quantification using moving slice velocity mapping. J Magn Reson Imaging. 2001;14:106–12.
4. Garcia J, Marrufo OR, Rodriguez AO, Eric L, Philippe P, Lyes K. Cardiovascular magnetic resonance evaluation of aortic stenosis severity using single plane measurement of effective orifice area. J Cardiovasc Magn Reson. 2012;14:23.
5. Fairbairn TA, Steadman CD, Mather AN, Motwani M, Blackman DJ, Plein S, McCann GP, Greenwood JP. Assessment of valve haemodynamics, reverse ventricular remodelling and myocardial fibrosis following transcatheter aortic valve implantation compared to surgical aortic valve replacement: a cardiovascular magnetic resonance study. Heart. 2013;99(16):1185–91.
6. Zamorano JL, Gonçalves A, Lang R. Imaging to select and guide transcatheter aortic valve implantation. Eur Heart J. 2014;35(24):1578–87.
7. Cawley PJ, Hamilton-Craig C, Owens DS, Krieger EV, Strugnell WE, Mitsumori L, D'Jang CL, Schwaegler RG, Nguyen KQ, Nguyen B, Maki JH, Otto CM. Prospective comparison of valve regurgitation quantitation by cardiac magnetic resonance imaging and transthoracic echocardiography. Circ Cardiovasc Imaging. 2013;6(1):48–57.
8. Abdel-Wahab M, Zahn R, Gerckens U, Linke A, Sievert H, Schäfer U, Kahlert P, Hambrecht R, Sack S, Hoffmann E, Senges J, Schneider S, Richardt G. Predictors of 1-year mortality in patients with aortic regurgitation after transcatheter aortic valve implantation: an analysis from the multicentre German TAVI registry. Heart. 2014;100(16):1250–6.

Ischemic Heart Disease

29

Adam N. Mather, Neil Maredia, and Sven Plein

Abstract

CMR is increasingly used to investigate patients with suspected ischaemic heart disease, and to guide the management of those with established coronary artery disease. Vasodilatory stress first pass myocardial perfusion imaging and dobutamine stress CMR have been shown to be highly accurate in diagnosing significant coronary disease and are now recommended in major society guidelines. STIR imaging may be used to identify oedema, a marker of recent myocardial injury. Microvascular obstruction represents an important prognostic marker in the acute infarct setting. Late gadolinium enhancement imaging permits the detection of myocardial infarct scar, assessment of myocardial viability by scar thickness and identification of alternative pathologies that may mimic an acute coronary syndrome.

Keywords

Ischaemia • Perfusion • Ischaemic heart disease • Viability • Oedema • Late Gadolinium Enhancement • Microvascular obstruction • Myocardial infarction • Adenosine • Dobutamine • Regadenoson

A.N. Mather, MBBS, MD, MRCP
Department of Cardiology, Castle Hill Hospital, Hull and East Yorkshire
Hospitals NHS Trust, Hull, East Yorkshire, UK
e-mail: adam.mather@hey.nhs.uk; a.n.mather@doctors.org.uk

N. Maredia, MB ChB, MRCP (UK), MD
Department of Cardiology, James Cook University Hospital, Middlesbrough, UK
e-mail: neil.maredia@stees.nhs.uk

S. Plein, MD, PhD (✉)
Division of Biomedical Imaging, Leeds Institute of Cardiovascular and
Metabolic Medicine, University of Leeds & Leeds Teaching Hospitals,
Clarendon Way, Leeds LS1 9JT, UK
e-mail: s.plein@leeds.ac.uk

© Springer International Publishing 2015
S. Plein et al. (eds.), *Cardiovascular MR Manual*,
DOI 10.1007/978-3-319-20940-1_29

Introduction

Cardiovascular magnetic resonance offers a wide-ranging assessment of ischaemic heart disease (IHD), including:

- Accurate measurement of global and regional myocardial contractile function.
- Detection of myocardial ischaemia with either myocardial perfusion imaging during vasodilator stress (akin to nuclear scintigraphy) or wall motion assessment during inotropic stress (akin to stress echocardiography).
- Accurate delineation of the extent of myocardial infarction and residual viability with LGE to inform revascularisation decisions.
- Assessment of contractile reserve during low dose inotropic stimulation.
- In acute coronary syndromes, identification of myocardium at risk with T2-weighted imaging as well as delineation of infarcted myocardium and infarct characteristics such as microvascular obstruction with LGE.
- Direct visualisation of coronary anomalies and stenoses with coronary MR angiography.

CMR is thus a highly versatile imaging modality for the diagnosis and management of patients with known or suspected IHD. In addition to its unparalleled versatility, CMR offers several conceptual advantages over other current imaging modalities. Compared with nuclear scintigraphy, specific advantages of CMR are its higher spatial resolution, lack of ionising radiation and more accurate assessment of LV function and viability. Compared with echocardiography, image quality by CMR is more consistent and viability assessment by LGE is a unique feature. Compared with cardiac CT, CMR does not expose patients to ionising radiation and it is more versatile, although coronary CT is superior to coronary CMR for the visualisation of coronary stenoses.

Although CMR remains less available and used than nuclear perfusion imaging or stress echocardiography, in many centres CMR has become an invaluable addition to the available diagnostic tools for the assessment of IHD. In some centres CMR has replaced these investigations as a first-line test for the detection of IHD and CMR has been included in all recent IHD guidelines. Importantly, the evidence base for using CMR in IHD has steadily increased and studies have demonstrated the diagnostic accuracy and prognostic relevance of a normal or abnormal CMR study.

Stress Myocardial Perfusion Imaging for the Detection of Myocardial Ischaemia

CMR Protocol for Stress Perfusion CMR
1. Anatomy module
2. LV function module
3. Myocardial perfusion module "dummy" scan
4. Myocardial Perfusion module during vasodilator stress
5. Myocardial Perfusion module at rest (optional)
6. LGE module

CMR first pass myocardial perfusion imaging is used to analyse the flow of blood through the myocardial capillary bed. Because of autoregulation, which keeps resting myocardial blood flow constant until epicardial coronary stenosis becomes critical, it is necessary to acquire perfusion data during physiological or pharmacological stress in order to reveal myocardial ischaemia. In the ischaemic cascade, a perfusion defect is the first manifestation of ischaemia, which subsequently leads to wall motion abnormalities, symptoms and ECG changes. In principle, perfusion assessment is therefore the most sensitive test for ischaemia.

Practically, CMR perfusion imaging is most commonly performed during vasodilator stress, induced by adenosine, dipyridamole or regadenoson. It is important to emphasize that these agents do not usually induce ischaemia, but induce maximal vasodilation and thus delineate myocardial perfusion reserve. A "perfusion defect" by first pass perfusion CMR is therefore identified as an area that has reduced perfusion reserve because of epicardial coronary stenosis or microvascular pathology. In specific pathophysiological states such as two-vessel coronary stenosis, myocardial ischaemia may occur during vasodilator stress because of coronary steal, but this phenomenon is relatively rare.

CMR provides sufficiently high spatial resolution to delineate subendocardial perfusion, which is much more sensitive to ischaemia than the subepicardial layer. The analysis of CMR myocardial perfusion data in clinical practice is usually visual, by comparing contrast uptake patterns in different parts of the heart, but methods for objective quantitative measurement of myocardial blood flow are available.

Myocardial Perfusion CMR Versus Other Imaging Modalities

The most commonly used method for assessment of myocardial perfusion is nuclear scintigraphy with single photon emission computed tomography (SPECT) or positron emission tomography (PET). Although based on similar principles, i.e., the measurement of myocardial blood flow at rest and during stress, the acquisition and analysis of nuclear scintigraphy and CMR myocardial perfusion imaging are different in many key areas:

Contrast agents: Contrast agents used for nuclear myocardial perfusion imaging are either potassium analogues that are taken up in perfused myocardium or labelled perfusion molecules such as water. CMR uses gadolinium based and mostly extracellular contrast agents, which readily diffuse into the extracellular space.

Data acquisition: In SPECT, data are acquired some time after the administration of the tracer and over several minutes. This makes the test susceptible to movement artefacts. In addition, attenuation of signal can lead to diagnostic errors. Myocardial perfusion CMR assesses the first myocardial passage of the contrast agent. This requires very rapid data acquisition with the associated technical challenges. It also means that unlike SPECT or PET, myocardial perfusion CMR does not usually cover the entire heart.

Spatial resolution: The in-plane spatial resolution in PET is around 6 mm, in SPECT around 10 mm and in CMR less than 3 mm. The higher spatial resolution of CMR may improve the detection of subendocardial ischaemia and multi-vessel disease, when balanced ischaemia can pose a diagnostic challenge in SPECT analysis.

Contractile function and scar assessment: With cine and late gadolinium enhanced imaging, the reference tests for assessment of contractile function and presence of scar are routinely acquired as part of a stress perfusion CMR study, further enhancing its diagnostic value.

Ionising radiation: Both PET and SPECT expose patients to considerable doses of ionising radiation, in the order of 10 mSv (with a wide variation depending on the isotope used, patient size and other variables), while CMR uses no ionising radiation.

In particular because of its higher spatial resolution and lack of ionising radiation, CMR may be a more accurate test for myocardial perfusion assessment than nuclear perfusion imaging. Several studies have suggested better diagnostic performance of CMR compared with SPECT. The single-centre CE-MARC trial is the largest trial to date comparing CMR and SPECT for the diagnosis of significant coronary artery disease (Greenwood et al. 2012). In a population of 752 patients with a 39 % prevalence of significant coronary disease, multiparametric CMR assessment was found to have a significantly higher sensitivity (87 %) vs SPECT (67 %) but similar specificity (both 83 %). Similar results were found irrespective of angiographic cutoff applied and in single and multi-vessel disease subgroups (Greenwood et al. 2012) (Fig. 29.1).

Myocardial perfusion can also be assessed with contrast echocardiography, but to date there has been no comparison between CMR and perfusion echocardiography. A 2012 meta-analysis of SPECT, CMR and PET imaging for the detection of obstructive coronary disease demonstrated pooled sensitivity of 88 % for SPECT, 89 % for CMR and 84 % for PET (Jaarsma et al. 2012). Specificities were 61, 76 and 81 % respectively. However, this analysis only included studies published up to 2010, and CMR was consequently under-represented (37 CMR studies vs 114 SPECT studies).

Reflecting the growing evidence base for stress perfusion CMR, recent guidelines rate stress perfusion CMR as equivalent to SPECT, PET and stress echocardiography with a Class 1a indication for patients at intermediate risk of CAD (Windecker et al. 2014).

Prognostic Performance

In a 2013 meta-analysis of stress CMR, vasodilator stress CMR myocardial perfusion imaging was found to be a reliable method of estimating prognostic risk (Lipinski et al. 2013). The annualised event rate was 0.8 % in patients with negative results and 4.9 % in those with a positive result..

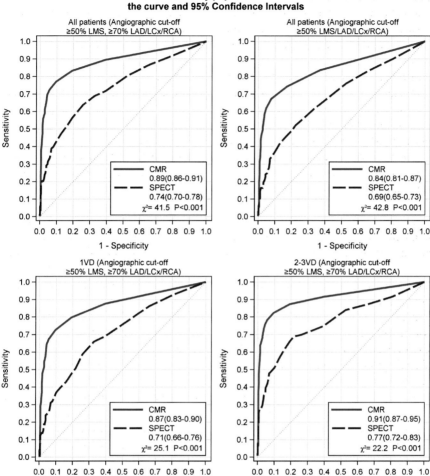

Fig. 29.1 Comparison of diagnostic accuracy of multiparametric CMR assessment against SPECT showed significantly higher sensitivity for CMR in patients with single and multivessel coronary artery disease, and irrespective of whether a 50 or 70% angiographic definition of significant luminal stenosis was applied (Reproduced from Greenwood et al. 2012)

The Role of Myocardial Perfusion CMR in IHD
1. Detect reduced myocardial perfusion reserve as a marker of ischaemia.
2. Combine perfusion assessment with LV function and viability assessment.
3. Indications:
    (a) Detect IHD in patients with intermediate likelihood of IHD
    (b) Identification of culprit lesions to guide revascularisation

How to Perform a CMR Myocardial Perfusion Study

Important: Instruct patients in the invitation letter to refrain from caffeine (coffee, tee, caffeinated beverages or foods e.g., chocolate, caffeinated medications), theophylline and dipyridamole for 24 h prior to the examination. Caffeine is a competitive analogue of adenosine and can thus reduce the response to vasodilator stress. Some centres also ask patients to refrain from smoking and beta-blockers prior to vasodilator stress testing.

Protocol:

- Scout imaging to plan a true short axis view of the left ventricle
- Plan perfusion imaging
  - Use the '3 of 5' method to plan position of 3 slices in the SAX orientation. On a systolic VLA and HLA image, position 5 slices to cover the heart from the mitral valve plane to the apex. Then remove the outer slices. This leaves three slices in accurate and reproducible positions.
  - Before starting adenosine, run a "dummy" perfusion sequence (**without** contrast), assessing for:
    (a) Presence of artefact. Move/increase FOV if necessary
    (b) Satisfactory VCG triggering. Change lead position if needed.
    (c) Patient compliance with breathing commands. We ask patients to hold their breath in end-expiration during the first pass of contrast, taking shallow breaths after that should they be unable to hold their breath for the entire scan duration.
- Consider removing patient from magnet bore to improve monitoring.
  - If using adenosine, commence intravenous infusion at 140 mcg/kg/min and scan after 3–4 min of the infusion have elapsed (but with the infusion continuing).
  - If the patient shows no haemodynamic response and has no symptoms after 3–4 min, some centres increase the adenosine dose to 210 mcg/kg/min.
  - If using regadenoson give bolus dose and scan during subsequent 60–90 sec
  - Monitoring (irrespective of stressor):
    (a) VCG for arrhythmia.
    (b) Patient for symptoms. Reassure as necessary.
    (c) Blood pressure.
- First pass perfusion imaging. A power injector is used to deliver an intravenous bolus of contrast agent (typical infusion rate 3–7 ml/s) and a subsequent saline flush (typically 15–30 ml at the same rate). The patient is instructed to hold their breath in expiration from the moment contrast enters the right ventricle. Imaging should continue for 40–50 cardiac cycles, to ensure that the entire first pass of contrast is observed. The dose of contrast to be delivered may be between 0.05 and 0.1 mmol/kg, according to local protocols.
- Rest perfusion may be performed a minimum of 15 min after the stress perfusion study, using identical slice geometry and scan settings as the stress perfusion sequence.

Note: Quantitative CMR myocardial perfusion assessment has shown that the vasodilatory effect of regadenoson extends beyond 15 min (even when aminophylline is used to counter its effect), making rest perfusion imaging at this time point potentially unreliable (Bhave et al. 2012). This has led to some centres removing rest perfusion imaging from their regadenoson stress CMR protocol. In these modified protocols, stress perfusion images are compared against LGE images to determine whether there is reversible or "fixed" (infarct-related) hypoperfusion.

Vasodilator Stress Agents
Adenosine
1. Most widely used agent for stress perfusion imaging
2. Produces coronary artery vasodilatation – preferentially dilating non-stenosed vessels
3. Very short half-life (<10 s)
4. Adverse events easily reversed by cessation of infusion
5. Can demonstrate perfusion abnormalities (reduced perfusion reserve) without inducing myocardial ischaemia

Side-Effects
Severe side-effects are extremely rare and adenosine is therefore a very suitable agent for pharmacological stress in the MR environment. Side effects include:
1. Dyspnoea
2. Wheezing
3. Chest heaviness
4. Facial flushing
5. AV nodal block (usually self-limiting)

Contra-Indications (Kramer et al. 2008)
1. Known hypersensitivity to adenosine
2. Second or third degree AV nodal block
3. Reversible airways disease
4. Sinus bradycardia (HR <45 bpm)
5. Systemic arterial hypotension (<90 mmHg)

Dipyridamole
1. Longer half-life
2. More frequently requires aminophylline administration in event of adverse effects
3. Mechanism of action, side effects and contraindications similar to adenosine

Regadenoson
1. Selective A_2 adenosine receptor agonist
2. Similar vasodilatory action to adenosine
3. Single bolus dose
4. Lower side effect profile than adenosine

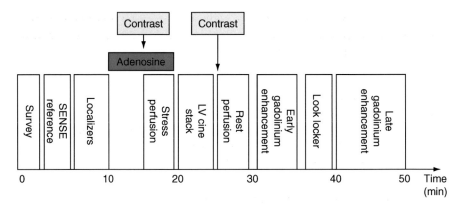

Fig. 29.2 A comprehensive IHD protocol, which can be performed in less than 50 min in most patients. Depending on the dose of contrast used for stress and rest perfusion studies, an additional "top-up" of contrast may be delivered after rest perfusion imaging in order to achieve a total dose of 0.15–0.2 mmol/kg prior to late gadolinium enhancement imaging

In most instances, the above protocol will be performed as part of a larger comprehensive ischaemic heart disease study as outlined in Fig. 29.2. The comprehensive protocol has superior overall accuracy than any of its individual components for the detection of ischaemic heart disease (Plein et al. 2004). Importantly, it was also shown that omission of (potentially time-consuming) coronary artery imaging did not reduce the diagnostic accuracy obtained by a combination of the remaining three components.

Safety Considerations

The administration of any form of stress in the MR environment requires particular consideration for patient and staff safety. ECG monitoring is limited because of magneto-hydrodynamic effects. ST segment changes as occur during myocardial ischaemia can therefore not be reliably detected. Heart rhythm monitoring is possible, but p-waves cannot be detected reliably, so that lower grade AV conduction block may not be recognised and higher grade AV block is only evident because of changes in ventricular rate. It is therefore essential to monitor patients' symptoms very closely and respond to symptoms quickly. Furthermore, resuscitation within the magnetic field is limited and it is usually impractical for the hospital's resuscitation team to enter the magnet room. An efficient evacuation procedure to a safe and suitable resuscitation environment close to the magnet room has to be in place and must be regularly practiced. Finally, staff involved in stress testing must be trained in basic and advanced life support.

Safety Considerations
1. A physician should always be present to supervise stress CMR studies
2. A resuscitation protocol must be in place **and practised regularly**
3. Contraindications to specific stress agents should be identified and an appropriate agent chosen accordingly

<u>**Additional Equipment**</u>
1. Sphygmomanometer for blood pressure monitoring
2. Intravenous infusion pump for administration of pharmacological stressor.
3. If not MR compatible, devices must be located outside the scan room and connected to the patient via waveguide tunnels through the wall
4. Heart rhythm monitoring (Vectorcardiograph).
5. Resuscitation equipment:
   (a) Defibrillator (to be kept <u>outside</u> the scan room!)
   (b) Medications for cardiac arrest scenarios and management of arrhythmia
6. Other Medications
   (a) Iv aminophylline for reversal of vasodilator (particularly if using dipyridamole)
   (b) Salbutamol inhaler
   (c) Beta-blocker (esmolol or metoprolol)
   (d) GTN spray
7. MR compatible rapid infusion pump for delivery of contrast bolus (most general MRI Units will already have one of these)

Analysis of CMR Perfusion Images

In clinical practice, myocardial perfusion CMR data are usually analysed visually by scrolling through the series of dynamic images. Where there is a physiologically significant obstruction to myocardial blood flow, the entry of contrast agent will be impaired, with later contrast arrival, a slower uptake and lower amplitude. This manifests as a darker area, "a perfusion defect", in the poorly perfused myocardium.

Table 29.1 Analysis of perfusion/LGE CMR studies

Stress	Rest	LGE	Diagnosis
Positive	Negative	Negative	Inducible ischaemia
Positive	Positive	Positive	Infarction
Positive	Positive	Negative	Likely Artefact

A true perfusion defect has the following characteristics:

- most prominent in the subendocardium
- occurs in segments that anatomically correlate to a particular coronary artery distribution
- persists for several RR intervals.

As outlined in Chap. 20 (p219), endocardial dark rim artefacts can affect CMR perfusion images. Often comparison is made with rest perfusion images and if available also late gadolinium enhanced images that delineate scar. By using information these data, artefacts can usually be identified:(Thomson et al. 2007) (Table 29.1).

Perfusion should be assessed and recorded in accordance with the 17-segment American Heart Association model (Fig. 29.3) (Cerqueira et al. 2002). However, a three short axis slice acquisition strategy will not provide views of segment

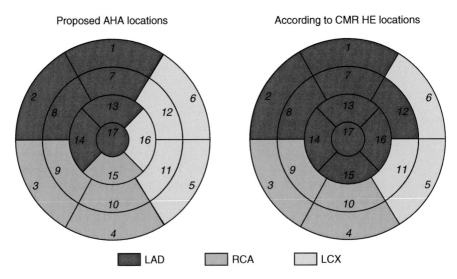

Fig. 29.3 Distribution of coronary artery supply to the myocardium. The left bulls-eye plot represents the official segmentation proposed by the American Heart Association in 2002 (Cerqueira et al. 2002). The right bulls-eye plot is derived from a recent CMR study analysing the pattern of late gadolinium enhancement in patients undergoing primary percutaneous intervention for acute myocardial infarction (Jose et al. 2008)

17 (true apex) so only 16 segments may be reported in this instance. Perfusion defects should be graded according to transmurality. Stress perfusion images should be compared with late gadolinium enhancement (+/− rest perfusion images – see earlier discussion) to identify inducible ischaemia, infarction, artefacts and normal areas of perfusion.

Tips and Tricks
1. Intravenous cannulae should be inserted into both arms for stress perfusion. Adenosine should be administered through a cannula in the opposite arm to that used for contrast administration. This prevents the interruption of adenosine delivery by the inflation of the sphygmomanometer.
2. Patient compliance may be improved by removing them from the magnet bore during the first phase of stress administration.
3. Recent studies have suggested that splenic perfusion is reduced during appropriate adenosine vasodilatation. Present splenic perfusion may be a sign of inadequate adenosine response.
4. Some centres increase the dose of adenosine to 210 mcg/kg/min if the standard dose causes no haemodynamic and symptomatic response.
5. Normal rest perfusion study with presence of a dark rim at stress does not always rule out artefact at stress. Differences in heart rate, haemodynamics and background signal can alter the appearances between stress and rest images.

Key Points Myocardial Perfusion CMR in IHD
1. Higher in plane spatial resolution than SPECT and PET
2. At least similar diagnostic performance as SPECT and PET
3. Included with Class 1a indication in patients with intermediate pretest probability 2014 revascularisation guidelines
4. Usually combined with cine and scar imaging
5. Safety in MR environment requires special consideration

Case Examples

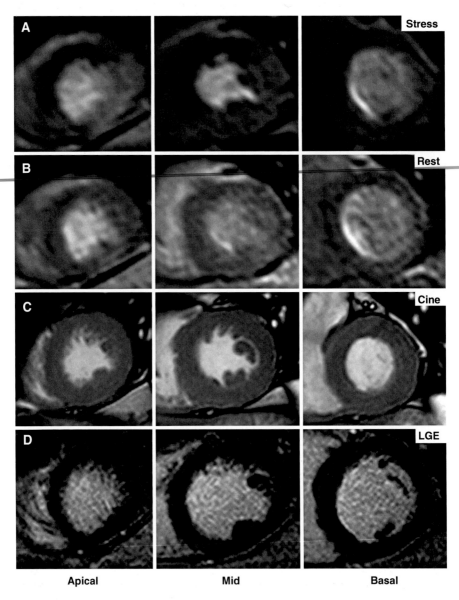

Case 1 A 49 year-old gentleman presented with angina. Three-slice adenosine stress perfusion revealed a transmural perfusion defect in the left anterior descending (LAD) artery territory (*row A*). No defect was seen at rest (*row B*). Left ventricular systolic function was normal (*row C* shows the end-systolic cine images). Late gadolinium enhancement imaging did not reveal any scar (*row D*). Coronary angiography subsequently demonstrated a severe proximal LAD stenosis

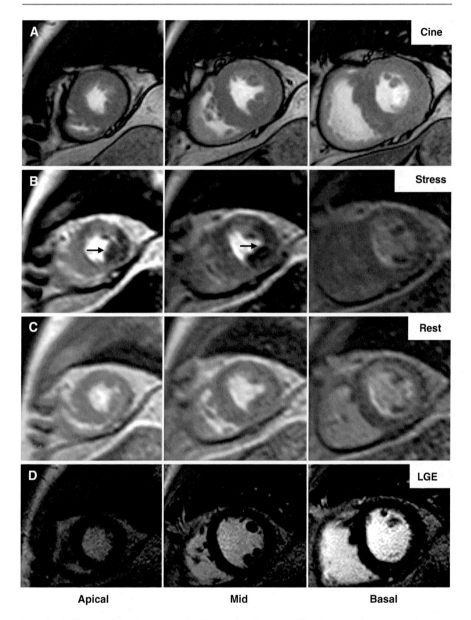

Case 2 A 62 year-old male presented with exertional angina. Cine imaging demonstrated normal left ventricular systolic function (*row A*). Adenosine stress perfusion highlighted a perfusion defect in the lateral wall (*row B*, see *arrows*). There were no perfusion defects at rest (*row C*). Late gadolinium enhancement did not demonstrate any scar (*row D*). Coronary angiography subsequently revealed a significant stenosis in the circumflex artery

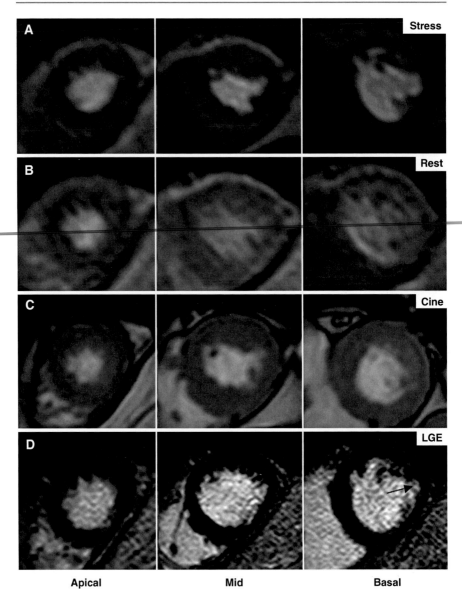

Case 3 A 67 year-old gentleman presented with angina. Perfusion defects were evident in all three coronary artery territories during adenosine stress but absent at rest (*rows A* and *B*). LV systolic function was normal (*row C* shows the end-systolic cine images). Late gadolinium enhancement imaging shows a small focal lateral subendocardial infarction (*row D*, *arrow*). Coronary angiography subsequently confirmed severe three-vessel coronary artery disease

CMR Report for Myocardial Perfusion
1. Report global and LV and RV volumes and function
2. Report regional wall motion abnormalities using the AHA segmentation
3. Describe distribution of scar and its transmural extent using the AHA segmentation
4. Describe perfusion abnormalities using the AHA segmentation. Note transmurality of perfusion defect.
5. Correlate ischaemia and scar
6. In the summary, report on presence and extent of scar and perfusion defect (as No of segments affected or percentage of total LV). If requested, give an overall assessment of suitability for revascularisation based on presence of ischaemia, contractile function and viability of myocardium.

CMR Stress Wall Motion Imaging for the Detection of IHD

Dobutamine Stress CMR Protocol
1. LV function module
2. Rest cine images in at least 3 SAX slices and 2–3 long axis views
3. Start dobutamine and increase at 3 min intervals in increments of 10 mcg/kg/min minute until target heart rate [85 % × (220-age)] reached
4. Consider adding Atropine to increase heart rate response
5. Repeat cine images at each stress level
6. Check blood pressure at each stage of the protocol, and monitor ECG throughout
7. View cine loops online as they are being acquired.
8. Stop test for new wall motion abnormality, serious side effect, or achievement of peak heart rate.

Introduction

The echocardiographic assessment of left ventricular wall motion during stress is now a well-established method of detecting myocardial ischaemia. By applying similar techniques using CMR imaging, it is possible to achieve a comparable level of diagnostic accuracy for the detection of IHD.

Table 29.2 Key differences between dobutamine stress CMR and dobutamine stress Echo

Key differences between dobutamine stress CMR and dobutamine stress Echo	
Favouring CMR	Favouring Echo
Higher spatial resolution	Real time imaging may allow earlier identification of ischaemia
Excellent slice reproducibility	ECG ST segment monitoring is possible (not possible using the VCG in CMR)
No reliance on a good "acoustic window" and more reproducible image quality	Bed-side testing permits better interaction with patient and swifter management of complications

CMR Versus Other Imaging Modalities

Dobutamine stress echocardiography and dobutamine stress CMR are based on the same principle of detecting ischaemia through inducible wall motion abnormalities. However, several notable differences between the two tests need to be considered (Table 29.2).

A direct comparison of dobutamine stress echocardiography and dobutamine stress CMR was performed by Nagel et al. in 1999, showing higher sensitivity and specificity for the CMR technique than its echo equivalent (Nagel et al. 1999). In a subanalysis, the differences in diagnostic accuracy occurred in particular in those studies where image quality by echocardiography was suboptimal. However, it should be noted that with harmonic imaging, echocardiographic contrast agents and other more recent technical improvements, the reliability of DSE is improved through better definition of the endocardial border. No contemporaneous comparison of current state of the art DSE and DSCMR is available.

Diagnostic Performance

Dobutamine stress CMR has proven to be an effective method of diagnosing myocardial ischaemia. In a 2007 meta-analysis, studies using dobutamine or exercise as the stressor were found to have a sensitivity of 0.85 and specificity of 0.86 for the detection of IHD (Nandalur et al. 2007). By comparison, a pooled analysis of 102 DSE studies found a weighted mean sensitivity of 0.81 and specificity of 0.84 (Heijenbrok-Kal et al. 2007).

Prognostic Performance

A 2013 meta-analysis demonstrated that dobutamine stress CMR is also a reliable indicator of prognostic risk (Lipinski et al. 2013). Annualised combined adverse event rates for patients with negative and positive studies were 0.7 and 4.7 % respectively.

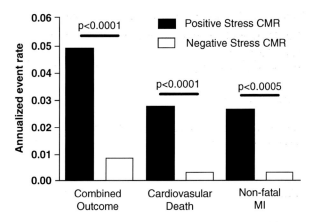

Fig. 29.4 Weighted mean annualised event rates for patients with a positive or negative stress CMR study (either vasodilator or dobutamine stress) (Reproduced from (Lipinski et al. 2013)

The overall ability of stress CMR to stratify prognosis, whether vasodilatory or dobutamine stress, appears good (Fig. 29.4).

The Role of Dobutamine Stress CMR
1. Detect reduced myocardial ischaemia by inducing wall motion abnormalities.
2. Combine with low dose dobutamine stress to assess contractile reserve
3. Indications:
   (a) When perfusion CMR is contraindicated
   (b) Detect IHD in patients with intermediate likelihood of IHD
   (c) Second line test if other investigations have been inconclusive
   (d) Identification of culprit lesions to guide revascularisation

Method

- Resting LV function is assessed using a full LV cine stack.
- Three short axis slices through the left ventricle are planned using the 3 of 5 technique described previously.
- A horizontal long axis, vertical long axis and three short axis cine slices are acquired at rest and at each increment of the dobutamine stress protocol. A 3-chamber view may be added.
- Intravenous dobutamine is commenced at 5 or 10 mcg/kg/min. The dobutamine dose is increased every 3 min, at increments of 10 mcg/kg/min up to a maximum of 40 mcg/kg/min. Blood pressure should be measured at each stage of the protocol, and continuous VCG monitoring occurs throughout.
- Uptitration ceases when 85 % of the patient's maximum predicted heart rate is achieved (200 minus age for women, 220 minus age for men). If this is not

achieved at a dobutamine dose of 40 mcg/kg/min, intravenous atropine may be administered in increments of 0.25 mg up to a maximum dose of 2 mg (Kramer et al. 2008).

- Reasons for stopping the study prematurely include:
  - New regional wall motion abnormality (View cine loops online as they are being acquired!)
  - Arrhythmia
  - Other serious side effects/patient request

Safety Considerations

The administration of intravenous dobutamine is associated with a small but definite risk of inducing ventricular arrhythmias (ventricular tachycardia and ventricular fibrillation) and myocardial infarction. Arrhythmias occur in approximately 3–4/1,000 cases. Even more than for vasodilator stress myocardial perfusion CMR, careful consideration needs to be given to patient safety prior to commencing a dobutamine stress service. As outlined earlier, these include in particular patient evacuation from the magnet room in case of a complication occurring and the rapid and safe transfer to an appropriate resuscitation environment.

Because ECG-monitoring is limited in the magnet room, ischaemia detection should be based on immediate review of acquired cine loops at every stress level. The test should be terminated as soon as an inducible wall motion abnormality is identified or other endpoints reached (as outlined above).

Dobutamine
1. β_1 agonist. Beta-blockers should be omitted for 24 h before the test.
2. Less preferable for perfusion imaging due to its positive chronotropic effect.
3. High heart rates may require compromises in slice coverage or image resolution

Side Effects
1. Nausea
2. Palpitations
3. Dyspnoea
4. Dizziness

Contraindications (Kramer et al. 2008)
1. Severe systemic arterial hypertension ($\geq$220/120 mmHg)
2. Unstable angina pectoris
3. Significant aortic stenosis (Peak valve gradient >50 mmHg or aortic valve area <1 cm^2)

4. Complex cardiac arrhythmias including atrial fibrillation
5. Hypertrophic obstructive cardiomyopathy
6. Myocarditis, endocarditis, pericarditis
7. Uncontrolled congestive heart failure

Atropine
Administered when target heart rate not achieved with maximum dose of dobutamine (see page 386)

Contraindications (Kramer et al. 2008)
1. Narrow-angle glaucoma
2. Myasthenia gravis
3. Obstructive uropathy
4. Obstructive gastrointestinal disorders

Analysis

For each imaging orientation (HLA, VLA and SA), cine images from each dobutamine increment should be viewed side-by-side, allowing the effect of stress to be determined. Wall motion may be assessed qualitatively according to the AHA 17 segment model as follows:

- Normal or Hyperkinetic
- Hypokinetic
- Akinetic
- Dyskinetic

A wall motion score index may be calculated by dividing the sum of the wall motion scores by the number of segments assessed. Quantitative assessment of % wall thickening or strain may also be performed. It should be noted if global LV function does not improve or worsens during stress.

Four typical patterns of wall motion are seen with dobutamine stress:

- Normal – Normal resting myocardial contraction, becoming more vigorous as dobutamine dose increases
- Reversible Ischaemia – Contractile function deteriorates as stress increases
- Biphasic Response – An initial improvement in contractile function is seen with low dose dobutamine (up to 10 mcg/kg/min) but further increases in stressor dose lead to a deterioration in contractile function. This response is typical of ischaemic "hibernating" myocardium.
- No response – Poorly contracting myocardium at rest, which fails to show any improvement with dobutamine. This is characteristic of non-viable myocardium.

The report should conclude with a summary of myocardial viability and any inducible wall motion abnormalities identified.

Tips and Tricks
1. Dobutamine stress images must be analysed as they are acquired so that dobutamine may be stopped promptly in the event of a new regional wall motion abnormality.
2. Adapt the SSFP cine sequence to optimize temporal resolution
3. as needed as the heart rate increases.

Case Example

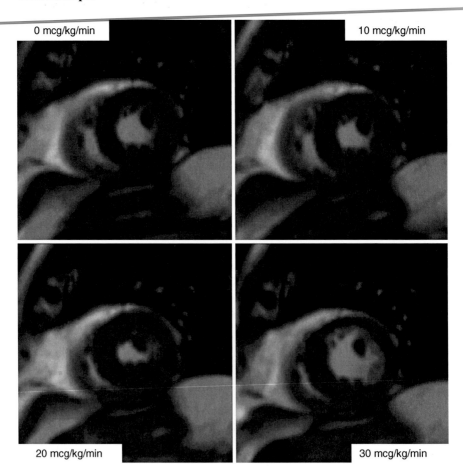

Case 4 End-systolic short axis cine images from a dobutamine stress CMR study. Inducible isch-aemia was identified by the development of new wall motion abnormalities in the anterior and inferolateral walls at 30 mcg/kg/min of dobutamine. The study was terminated at this point (Images courtesy of Charles Peebles, Southampton)

Dobutamine Stress CMR Report
1. Comment on global LV and RV volumes and function
2. Comment on resting regional wall motion abnormalities using the AHA segmentation
3. Comment on improvement of regional wall motion during low dose stress
4. Comment on inducible regional wall motion abnormalities using the AHA segmentation
5. Provide wall motion index.
6. Comment if global LV function fails to improve during stress.
7. Comment if valvular regurgitation occurs or worsens during stress.
8. Summarise resting function, contractile reserve and ischaemia for coronary territories. Provide an estimate of extent of ischaemia (in no of segments affected of percentage of total LV)

Which Pharmacological Stress Agent Should I Choose?

For most patients, either vasodilator or inotropic stress will be applicable, with a similar level of confidence in the result. The decision often comes down to local preference. However, there are certain situations in which one modality may be preferred:

- Absolute contraindications to a specific stressor agent
- Chronic renal impairment of sufficient severity to preclude the use of contrast agent (see Chap. 19 (p189)). In this situation, DSCMR clearly represents the best option.

CMR for Assessment of Viability

CMR Protocol for Viability Assessment
1. LV function cine imaging at rest
2. LGE module
3. Consider low-dose dobutamine cine imaging in particular if LGE shows 25–75 % transmural infarction

Introduction

The delineation of myocardial scar and viability in patients with IHD is of great clinical relevance. Contractile abnormalities of myocardium in IHD can be caused by stunning (if it recovers function spontaneously), hibernation (if it recovers after revascularisation) or scar. Myocardial stunning is commonly seen in patients with early reperfusion after coronary artery occlusion. Patients with hibernating myocardium often present with either multi-vessel coronary artery disease and global left ventricular dysfunction or a history of previous myocardial infarction and infarct scar with associated regional wall motion abnormality. Several studies have shown that revascularisation of hibernating myocardium improves clinical outcomes. CMR with LGE has become the gold standard imaging modality for the delineation of myocardial infarction. LGE-CMR can accurately determine the presence, location and extent of infarcted tissue and assess the likelihood of functional recovery. It is therefore extremely useful in planning coronary arterial revascularization. It is also an important tool in the identification of complications of myocardial infarction.

CMR Versus Other Imaging Modalities

The detection of myocardial infarction by CMR with LGE has been compared with PET and SPECT. In both comparisons, CMR detected myocardial infarction more frequently than nuclear imaging, in particular if the infarcts were small or limited to the subendocardium. The reason for the higher sensitivity of CMR to detect myocardial infarction is its much higher spatial resolution and the direct anatomical correlation. Echocardiography can provide information on myocardial viability through measurements of myocardial thickness, contractile function and contractile reserve. Contrast echocardiography has also been used to assess viability.

CMR Methods for Viability Assessment

Cine Imaging

Myocardial infarction is first suspected by the observation of myocardial thinning with associated akinesia, as seen on initial cine images. However, recent studies suggest that in the absence of scar on LGE, even severely thinned myocardium may recover function after revascularisation, making myocardial thickness alone an unreliable predictor of viability.

Contractile Reserve

Viable myocardium should demonstrate improved contractility in response to a suitable inotropic stimulus. The most widely used method of stimulation is the intravenous infusion of low dose dobutamine, up to 10 mcg/kg/min. Dobutamine is a β_{1-} receptor agonist and, therefore, patients should avoid beta-blockers for 24 h prior to the CMR scan. Regular blood pressure measurements should also be taken. Side effects of dobutamine include nausea, dizziness, dyspnoea, chest pain and palpitations. Cine imaging in the standard planes should be performed in order to assess wall thickness and contractility with stress.

Fig. 29.5 A 65 year old male presented with an acute inferior ST-elevation myocardial infarction. LGE images clearly demonstrated inferior LV infarction with transmural hyperenhancement (*white arrow*) spreading from the endocardial to the epicardial border

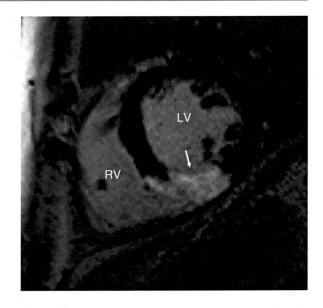

Late Gadolinium Enhancement

Most Gadolinium-based contrast agents in current use are extracellular and extravascular agents that diffuse freely in to the interstitial space. Their distribution volume is therefore increased in both acute myocardial infarction, where cell barriers are destroyed and chronic infarction where myocardial cells are replaced with a fibrotic matrix. In viable myocardium, on the other hand, extracellular space is small and the volume of distribution of gadolinium is lower. Several minutes after contrast administration, a steady state evolves with larger contrast concentrations in infarcted tissue, which can be imaged with an appropriate T1-sensitive imaging method – a technique called late gadolinium enhancement (LGE). LGE due to myocardial infarction occurs in the perfusion territory of the occluded artery. Occlusion of a coronary artery initiates a process of myocyte necrosis, which spreads from the sub-endocardium to the epicardial borders. Therefore, LGE always extends from the endocardium outwards with infarction (Fig. 29.5). Complete sparing of the endocardial border suggests that the cause of LGE is not infarction.

LGE also occurs in areas of fibrosis and therefore the method can be used to identify pathologies such as infiltrative cardiomyopathy and myocarditis. If the presence of LGE appears unusual, images should be re-acquired after changing the phase encode direction of the slice (*phase swapping*) in order to exclude artefact. If the LGE remains in the same position, then one can assume the abnormality to be genuine.

Functional improvement of stunned myocardium can be predicted by LGE. The likelihood of improvement and complete recovery decreases with increasing transmurality of LGE (Fig. 29.6). As can be seen in the Figure, functional recovery is variable in infarction between 25 and 75 % transmurality. In such instances, additional low dose dobutamine imaging may add prognostic information.

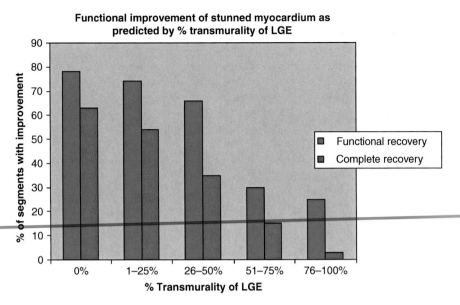

Fig. 29.6 Graph demonstrating % of dysfunctional segments with functional improvement and complete recovery after myocardial infarction according to transmurality of LGE (Beek et al. 2003)

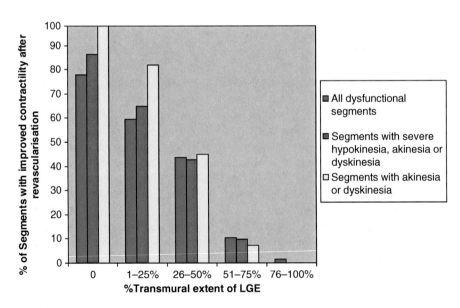

Fig. 29.7 Graph demonstrating the relationship between the transmural extent of LGE before revascularization and the likelihood of increased contractility after revascularization (Kim et al. 2000)

LGE can also identify hibernating myocardium prior to revascularization. The likelihood of improvement in contractility after revascularization also reduces with increasing transmural extent of LGE. Dysfunctional myocardium which demonstrates <50 % transmural extent of LGE has a high likelihood of functional recovery (Fig. 29.7).

Case Examples

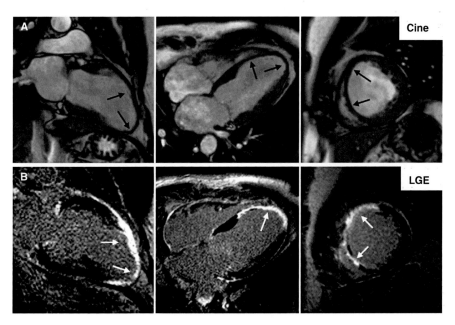

Case 5 A 54 year-old male presented with breathlessness after suffering an anterior myocardial infarction. CMR was requested to look for viable myocardium. Cine imaging demonstrated thinned and akinetic myocardium in the anterior wall and apex (*row A*, see *arrows*). Late gadolinium enhancement showed transmural scar in the anterior wall and apex (*row B*, see *arrows*). It was, therefore, concluded that the anterior wall was non-viable

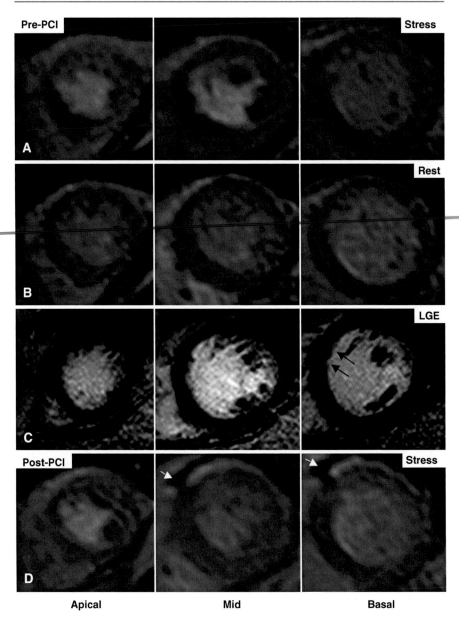

Case 6 73 year-old male with a history of prior myocardial infarction, presented with recurrent angina. CMR was requested to look for reversible ischaemia and viable myocardium. At first presentation, a reversible perfusion defect was noted in the apical and mid septum (*rows A* and *B*). Late gadolinium enhancement imaging demonstrated minimal focal subendocardial scar in the basal septum (*row C, arrows*). Percutaneous coronary intervention (PCI) was performed to an occluded left anterior descending artery. Six months later, stress perfusion imaging revealed no defect (*row D*). Note the prominent artefact arising from the LAD stent (*white arrows*)

CMR Report for Viability
1. Quantitative measurements of left ventricular volumes and function.
2. Describe regional wall motion abnormalities according to the 17 segment model as proposed by the American Heart Association
3. Describe presence and pattern of LGE according to the 17 segment model. If quantified, use at least >2 SD above the average signal intensity of normal myocardium as cut-off for infarction. Describe LGE pattern as subepicardial, intramural, subendocardial, or transmural.
4. Provide transmural extent of the LGE as 0, ≤25 %, 26 % to ≤50 %, 51 % to ≤75 %, and 76–100 %.
5. Report total amount of infarcted tissue (grams or % of LV).
6. Comment on contractile reserve if using low dose dobutamine inotropic stimulation

CMR in Acute Coronary Syndromes

Introduction

CMR has the unique ability to characterize a range of pathophysiological effects of acute myocardial infarction (AMI). Multi-parametric CMR assessment with cine imaging, T2-weighted (T2W) imaging and early or late gadolinium enhanced (EGE and LGE) acquisition, delineates contractile function, myocardial oedema, microvascular obstruction (MVO), intracardiac thrombus and myocardial scar. Many of these parameters have prognostic significance, for example, left ventricular (LV) ejection fraction, extent of scar and presence of MVO. Therefore, CMR can contribute to the risk stratification of patients with AMI and may play an important future role in assessing the efficacy of treatment strategies.

CMR Protocol for Acute Myocardial Infarction
1. Cine imaging for LV function
2. T2-weighted imaging for oedema
3. EGE for MVO and intracardiac thrombus
4. LGE for infarct scar and MVO

CMR Versus Other Imaging Modalities

CMR is the most versatile imaging modality for assessment of acute myocardial infarction. Its main drawback is that CMR scanners are usually remote from cardiology wards and unstable patients will not be suitable for CMR assessment. The role of echocardiography for bedside assessment of acute MI is therefore unchallenged by the emergence of CMR. However, stable patients with recent acute coronary syndromes can be safely scanned in a suitable CMR environment and important additional information can be obtained that is not available from other imaging modalities. Although no direct comparisons have been published in the context of acute infarction or other acute coronary syndromes, CMR is likely to be the most valuable second line test in their assessment, offering much more information than nuclear imaging studies.

Methods

Cine and LGE-CMR

The extent of myocardial infarction is a reliable predictor of clinical outcome and patients with large infarcts and poor contractile function are at substantially higher risk of malignant arrhythmia and heart failure than patients with limited infarction and preserved LV function. CMR is the most accurate test currently available for the measurement of LV function and infarct size, both in the acute, necrotic phase and in the late fibrotic stages of infarction. CMR has therefore become the imaging modality of choice in clinical trials assessing the effects of therapies in acute MI.

Oedema Imaging for Area at Risk Assessment

Prolonged ischaemia triggers an inflammatory response, which results in tissue oedema. Hence, oedema is one of the key features of viable myocardium at risk. T2- weighted CMR sequences are very sensitive to water-bound protons and, therefore, can delineate tissue oedema as regions of high signal intensity. T2-weighted CMR has been shown to successfully visualize infarct-related oedema (Fig. 29.6) and help differentiate acute from chronic infarction (Abdel-Aty et al. 2004). This CMR sequence can also help to diagnose acute myocardial ischaemia in the emergency setting (Cury et al. 2008). Acute inflammatory conditions such as acute myocarditis may also produce high signal intensity on T2-weighted imaging. However, the distribution of the oedema may not be consistent with a coronary artery territory as in the case of acute myocardial ischaemia.

Myocardial Salvage

The difference between the actual infarct size on LGE and area at risk, or potential infarct size, on T2-weighted CMR is a measure of myocardial salvage. This measure is important because it can be used to assess the effectiveness of strategies to optimize management of acute MI. Myocardial salvage can be measured by SPECT performed during coronary artery occlusion and after reperfusion. However, this is not a logistically practical option in clinical practice. CMR imaging performed several days after the index event provides similar estimates of salvage and may therefore become the method of choice for measurements of myocardial salvage, particularly in clinical trials.

Microvascular Obstruction

Microvascular obstruction (MVO) occurs early after acute myocardial infarction (AMI) and represents the angiographic appearance of "no-reflow". The presence of MVO predicts cardiovascular complications in the first two years after AMI and is associated with a significant reduction in event-free survival (Wu et al. 1998).

CMR can be used to detect MVO with early gadolinium enhancement (EGE). EGE uses the same sequence as LGE but images are acquired in the first 1–min after administration of the contrast agent. A fixed inversion time (TI) is usually set to ensure that the myocardium is bright. We recommend a TI of 400–500 ms. MVO appears as black areas within the infarct territory. MVO will be evident on LGE images as black areas within the bright white region of infarcted tissue.

MVO can also be detected on first-pass perfusion imaging. The volume of MVO measured by these three methods may differ because contrast agent diffusion into the MVO reduces its apparent extent over time following contrast injection. Theoretically, first-pass perfusion CMR should be the most accurate method to measure MVO, but this technique has been limited by lower spatial resolution than EGE and LGE as well as incomplete cardiac coverage. A recent study compared these three techniques and concluded that MVO detected by LGE is the best prognostic marker of LV remodelling and that the contrast to noise ratio between the infarct and MVO areas is highest with LGE imaging (Nijveldt et al. 2009).

Myocardial Haemorrhage

Myocardial haemorrhage is another feature of reperfusion injury. The extent of haemorrhage is strongly correlated to infarct size and the presence of haemorrhage is a marker of poor prognosis following acute MI. Haemorrhage can be assessed by T2-weighted and T2* imaging. The appearance of haemorrhage on MRI is dependent on the paramagnetic effects of haemoglobin degradation products. Initially, haemorrhage may consist of oxyhaemoglobin, which lacks paramagnetic effects. However, within the first few days after acute MI, oxyhaemoglobin denatures into deoxyhaemoglobin, which does exhibit paramagnetic properties and significantly reduces T2 relaxation time. Deoxyhaemoglobin is then converted to methaemoglobin, which is strongly paramagnetic. Haemorrhage can therefore be visualised on CMR as hypoenhanced regions surrounded by hyperintense signal intensity representing oedema, on T2-weighted imaging. Haemorrhage is most often seen in areas of MVO. Direct T2 quantification with T2 mapping may improve the ability of CMR to differentiate MVO with and without haemorrhage.

T2* decay is caused by a combination of spin-spin relaxation and magnetic field inhomogeneity. Iron deposits and blood products cause magnetic field inhomogeneities, therefore, T2* imaging has been used to detect myocardial iron deposition in the context of iron overload cardiomyopathies and more recently to detect haemorrhage in the setting of acute reperfused MI. The paramagnetic effects of haemoglobin byproducts are stronger on T2* than T2, and therefore, T2*-weighted imaging should exhibit higher sensitivity for the detection of haemorrhage.

Complications of Acute MI

Ventricular thrombus is a recognized complication of acute myocardial infarction. Thrombus tends to occur at the site of scarred myocardium as detected by LGE and often the myocardium in this area appears dyskinetic or aneurysmal on cine imaging. Thrombus is best visualized with EGE images. The blood pool will have high signal intensity due to the contrast agent but the thrombus will demonstrate low signal intensity and will appear as a dark mass in the bright ventricular cavity (Case 10). Perfusion imaging sequences can also be performed if there is any doubt about the ventricular mass. Thrombus will not take up contrast on perfusion imaging unlike a tumour, which will have a vascular supply. Post-infarction VSDs can be assessed by cine imaging (Case 11) which will demonstrate the anatomy of the defect as well as highlight signal loss in the right ventricle due to flow of blood through the VSD. The ventricular short axis cine stack can be used to measure the difference in stroke volumes between left and right ventricles. This information can then be used to assess the shunt ratio. Shunt ratio can also be calculated from the comparison of flow measurements of the pulmonary and systemic circulations.

Tips and Tricks

1. T2-weighted images must be acquired **before** the administration of any contrast agents.
2. Thrombus and MVO are best seen on early gadolinium enhanced images (within 2 minutes of contrast application) with a fixed TI of 400–500 ms.

The Role of CMR in ACS

1. Assess global and regional contractile function
2. Delineate area at risk and myocardial salvage
3. Provide risk stratification based on assessment of infarct size, LV function and presence of MVO and haemorrhage
4. Further assess complications of MI such as thrombus or VSD.

Case Examples

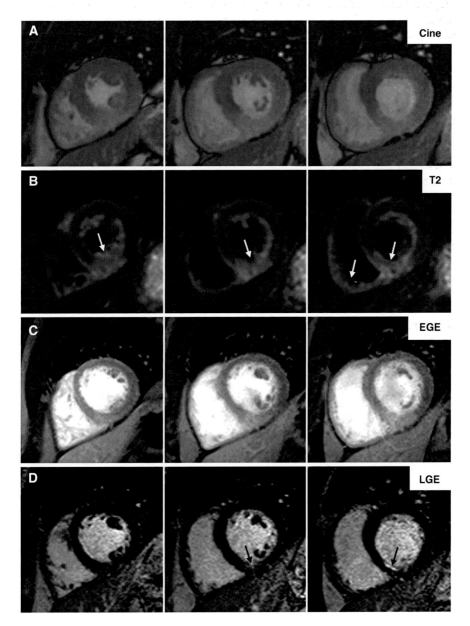

Case 7 39 year-old male presented with an acute inferior myocardial infarction and was successfully treated with primary PCI within two hours of symptom onset. Cine imaging demonstrated only mild hypokinesia in the inferior wall (*row A*). T2-weighted imaging highlighted myocardial oedema in the inferior walls of both left and right ventricles (*row B*, see *arrows*). Early gadolinium enhancement did not demonstrate any microvascular obstruction (*row C*). Late gadolinium enhancement showed only minimal scar in the inferior wall of the left ventricle (*row D*, see *arrows*)

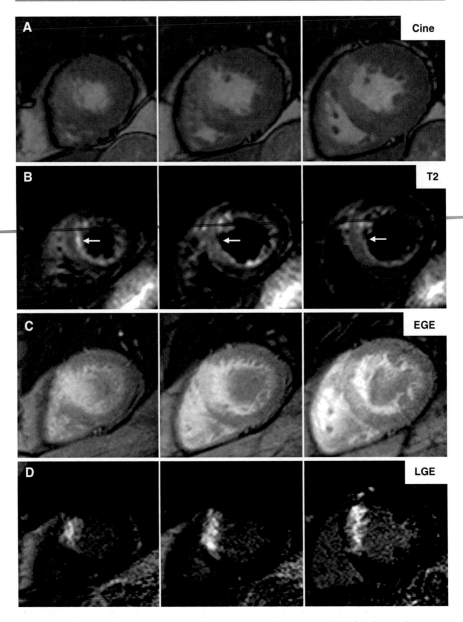

Case 8 A 59 year-old male presented with an acute anterior myocardial infarction and was successfully treated with primary PCI six hours after the onset of chest pain. Cine imaging demonstrated hypokinesia of the mid-interventricular septum (*row A*). T2-weighted imaging highlighted myocardial oedema in the mid-septum (*row B*, see *arrows*). Early gadolinium enhancement did not demonstrate any microvascular obstruction or intracardiac thrombus (*row C*). Late gadolinium enhancement revealed transmural myocardial infarction in the mid-septum (*row D*)

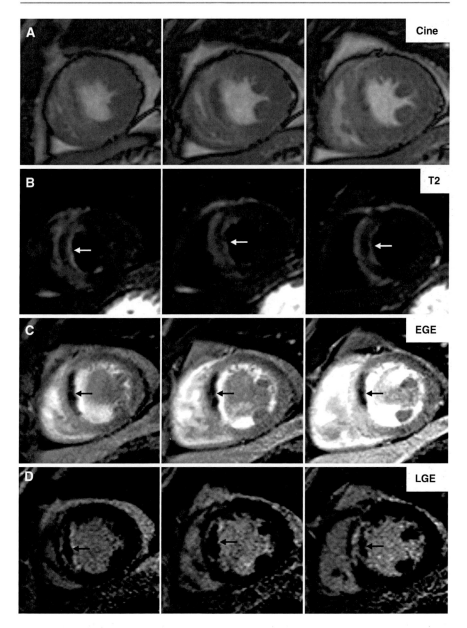

Case 9 A 36 year-old male presented with an acute anterior myocardial infarction and was successfully treated with primary PCI five hours after the onset of symptoms. Cine imaging demonstrated hypokinesia in the mid-interventricular septum (*row A*). T2-weighted imaging highlighted myocardial oedema in the mid-septum (*row B*, see arrows). Early gadolinium enhancement demonstrated significant microvascular obstruction (*row C*, see *arrows*). Late gadolinium enhancement confirmed the presence of microvascular obstruction within an area of infarcted myocardium (*row D*, see *arrows*)

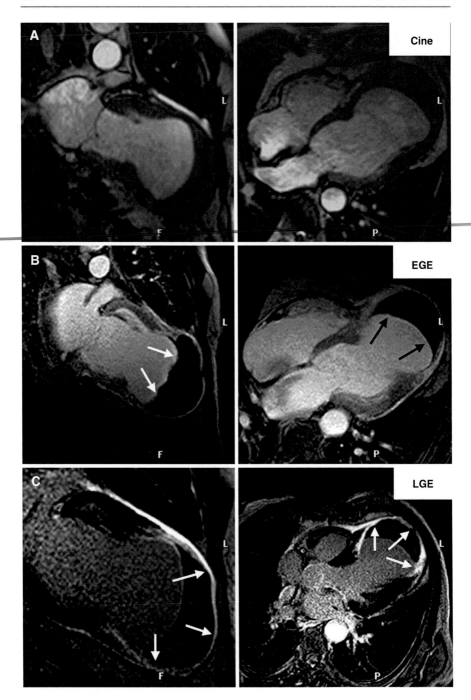

Case 10 A 60 year-old male presented with breathlessness after suffering an anterior myocardial infarction. Cine imaging demonstrated that the left ventricular apex was aneurysmal and akinetic (*row A*). Early gadolinium enhancement revealed a large mass of thrombus in the apex (*row B*, see *arrows*). Late gadolinium enhancement confirmed the presence of apical thrombus surrounded by transmural scar (*row C*, see *arrows*)

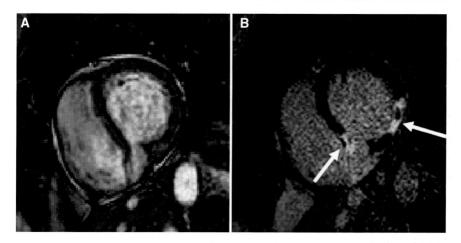

Case 11 A 78 years old lady presented several days after severe chest pain and ECGs suggested recent inferior MI. (**a**) SA cine imaging revealed a ventricular septal defect in the inferior septum. (**b**) LGE confirmed the VSD within the region of infarcted myocardium and associated MVO

Raised Cardiac Enzymes and Normal Coronary Arteries

With the development of increasingly sensitive markers of myocardial necrosis, larger numbers of patients are being labelled as having an acute coronary syndrome and undergo coronary angiography. In a proportion of this group, the coronary arteries are found to be normal, raising questions as to the cause of the biomarker rise. Potential explanations include:

- Myocardial infarction with subsequent recanalisation of the artery
- Myocarditis or other cardiomyopathy
- Non-cardiac causes

Given its ability to detect myocardial infarction and oedema, CMR represents an ideal method to investigate this patient group. Assomull et al. investigated the use of CMR in a group of 60 patients with raised troponin levels and normal coronary angiography. They were able to establish a diagnosis in 65 % of patients, the details of which are shown in Table 29.3 (Assomull et al. 2007).

Table 29.3 CMR findings in patients with raised cardiac enzymes and normal coronary angiogram (n = 60) (Assomul et al. 2007)

CMR findings	n (%)
Myocarditis	30 (50 %)
Acute	19 (31.7 %)
Chronic	11 (18.3 %)
Myocardial infarction	7 (11.6 %)
Takotsubo cardiomyopathy	1 (1.7 %)
Dilated cardiomyopathy	1 (1.7 %)
Normal CMR findings	21 (35 %)

These results make a strong case for the use of CMR in this clinical situation. It is particularly interesting to note the 11.6 % of patients that had evidence of myocardial infarction at CMR despite normal coronaries at angiography. By identifying this group with CMR, prognostically important secondary prevention therapy could be commenced with confidence.

Case Example

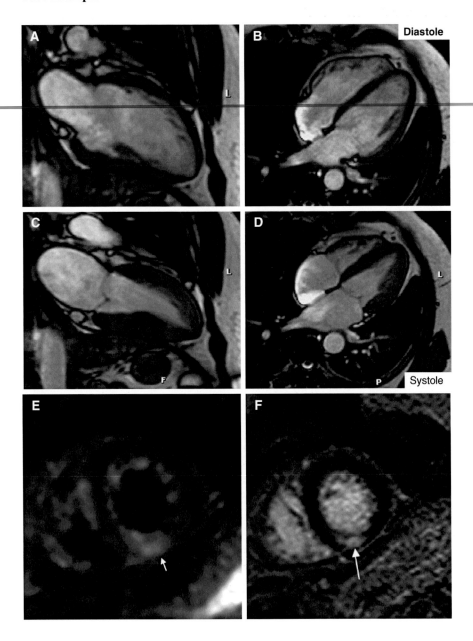

Potential Future Developments

The future of CMR imaging in IHD will be guided by software and hardware-led refinements of existing CMR techniques, and by the introduction of new methods that will provide a different perspective on the heart.

Hardware Development

The greatest potential for improvement exists in the hardware field, where the introduction of many-element cardiac receiver coils and 3 T scanners has allowed the use of significantly higher degrees of acceleration by parallel imaging, which in turn translates into improved image resolution, with consequent benefits for both CMR perfusion and coronary imaging.

The use of CMR to help guide coronary and non-coronary interventions has led to the emergence of combined MR and x-ray suites, so-called XMR interventional suites. These facilities are likely to become more popular as the role of CMR imaging expands.

Software Development

From a software perspective, advanced acceleration methods (eg. *k-t* BLAST and T-SENSE, Compressed sensing) are now allowing higher resolution perfusion images to be generated using existing hardware (Fig. 29.8). Most of these techniques are also applicable to the more advanced hardware outlined above.

New Methods

Non-invasive Arterial Wall Imaging

Intravascular ultrasound (IVUS) is now a widely used, but invasive, method of assessing the characteristics and extent of coronary artery atherosclerosis. There have been several promising reports using black blood MRI to assess vessel wall thickness. However, the spatial resolution of this technique is still significantly less than IVUS and the method is challenging to apply in many patients.

Case 12 46 year old female presenting with a Troponin-positive acute coronary syndrome. Coronary angiography revealed no detectable stenosis. LV cine imaging revealed good LV systolic function. T2-weighted imaging revealed transmural oedema of the inferior LV wall (*arrow*). Late gadolinium enhancement imaging revealed a small focal transmural inferior wall infarction. The patient was therefore informed that she had sustained a small myocardial infarction and started on secondary prevention therapy

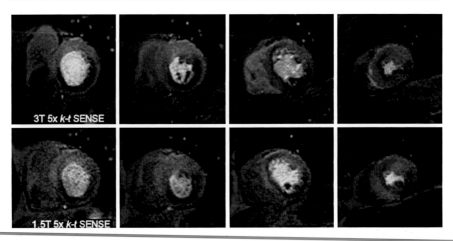

Fig. 29.8 CMR myocardial perfusion images of the same patient at 1.5 T and 3 T field strengths, using the advanced acceleration technique, *k-t* SENSE. Note the improved image quality at the higher field strength (From Plein et al. 2008))

Myocardial Perfusion Imaging Without Contrast?

There have been some initial investigations into MRI myocardial perfusion imaging using arterial spin labelling (ASL), where arterial water is used as a tracer and gadolinium-based contrast is not therefore required (Northrup et al. 2008). Although this technique may hold promise for the future, it is not yet a practical proposition for the clinical setting.

Targeted (Molecular) Contrast Agents

There is growing interest in the use of targeted contrast agents to help investigate specific disease processes. For example, fibrin-specific agents may be used to highlight ruptured coronary artery plaques, thereby aiding the non-invasive detection of acute coronary syndromes.

Key Points CMR in IHD

1. Adenosine myocardial perfusion and dobutamine stress wall motion imaging have similarly high accuracies for the detection of myocardial ischaemia.
2. The diagnostic accuracy and prognostic value of both techniques is at least comparable to other non-invasive modalities
3. Comprehensive CMR protocols provide greater information than any other single non-invasive imaging modality alone
4. Late gadolinium enhancement imaging by CMR is the reference standard for in-vivo detection of myocardial scar

5. The extent of myocardial scar on LGE imaging is a good predictor of functional recovery following revascularisation
6. T2-weighted imaging may differentiate acute from chronic myocardial injury
7. CMR may be used to detect many IHD-related complications and is an ideal modality for the investigation of patients with chest pain, raised myocardial enzymes and normal epicardial coronary arteries.

References

2014 ESC/EACTS Guidelines on myocardial revascularization: The Task Force on Myocardial Revascularization of the European Society of Cardiology (ESC) and the European Association for Cardio-Thoracic Surgery (EACTS) Developed with the special contribution of the European Association of Percutaneous Cardiovascular Interventions (EAPCI). Authors/Task Force members.

Abdel-Aty H, Zagrosek A, Schulz-Menger J, Taylor AJ, Messroghli D, Kumar A, et al. Delayed enhancement and T2-weighted cardiovascular magnetic resonance imaging differentiate acute from chronic myocardial infarction. Circulation. 2004;109(20):2411–6.

Assomull RG, Lyne JC, Keenan N, Gulati A, Bunce NH, Davies SW, et al. The role of cardiovascular magnetic resonance in patients presenting with chest pain, raised troponin, and unobstructed coronary arteries. Eur Heart J. 2007;28(10):1242–9.

Beek AM, Kuhl HP, Bondarenko O, Twisk JW, Hofman MB, van Dockum WG, et al. Delayed contrast-enhanced magnetic resonance imaging for the prediction of regional functional improvement after acute myocardial infarction. J Am Coll Cardiol. 2003;42(5):895–901.

Bhave NM, Freed BH, Yodwut C, Kolanczyk D, Dill K, Lang RM, et al. Considerations when measuring myocardial perfusion reserve by cardiovascular magnetic resonance using regadenoson. J Cardiovasc Magn Reson. 2012;14:89.

Cerqueira MD, Weissman NJ, Dilsizian V, Jacobs AK, Kaul S, Laskey WK, et al. Standardized myocardial segmentation and nomenclature for tomographic imaging of the heart: a statement for healthcare professionals from the Cardiac Imaging Committee of the Council on Clinical Cardiology of the American Heart Association. Circulation. 2002;105(4):539–42.

Cury RC, Shash K, Nagurney JT, Rosito G, Shapiro MD, Nomura CH, et al. Cardiac magnetic resonance with T2-weighted imaging improves detection of patients with acute coronary syndrome in the emergency department. Circulation. 2008;118(8):837–44.

Greenwood JP, Maredia N, Younger JF, Brown JM, Nixon J, Everett CC, et al. Cardiovascular magnetic resonance and single-photon emission computed tomography for diagnosis of coronary heart disease (CE-MARC): a prospective trial. Lancet. 2012;379(9814):453–60.

Heijenbrok-Kal MH, Fleischmann KE, Hunink MG. Stress echocardiography, stress single-photon-emission computed tomography and electron beam computed tomography for the assessment of coronary artery disease: a meta-analysis of diagnostic performance. Am Heart J. 2007;154(3):415–23.

Jaarsma C, Leiner T, Bekkers SC, Crijns HJ, Wildberger JE, Nagel E, et al. Diagnostic performance of noninvasive myocardial perfusion imaging using single-photon emission computed tomography, cardiac magnetic resonance, and positron emission tomography imaging for the detection of obstructive coronary artery disease: a meta-analysis. J Am Coll Cardiol. 2012;59(19):1719–28.

Jose TO-P, Jose R, Sheridan NM, Daniel CL, Charles D, Edwin W. Correspondence between the 17-segment model and coronary arterial anatomy using contrast-enhanced cardiac. Magn Reson Imaging. 2008;1(3):282–93.

Kim RJ, Wu E, Rafael A, Chen EL, Parker MA, Simonetti O, et al. The use of contrast-enhanced magnetic resonance imaging to identify reversible myocardial dysfunction. N Engl J Med. 2000;343(20):1445–53.

Kramer C, Barkhausen J, Flamm S, Kim R, Nagel E. Standardized cardiovascular magnetic resonance imaging (CMR) protocols, society for cardiovascular magnetic resonance: board of trustees task force on standardized protocols. J Cardiovasc Magn Reson. 2008;10(1):35.

Lipinski MJ, McVey CM, Berger JS, Kramer CM, Salerno M. Prognostic value of stress cardiac magnetic resonance imaging in patients with known or suspected coronary artery disease: a systematic review and meta-analysis. J Am Coll Cardiol. 2013;62(9):826–38.

Nagel E, Lehmkuhl HB, Bocksch W, Klein C, Vogel U, Frantz E, et al. Noninvasive diagnosis of ischemia-induced wall motion abnormalities with the use of high-dose dobutamine stress MRI: comparison with dobutamine stress echocardiography. Circulation. 1999;99(6):763–70.

Nandalur KR, Dwamena BA, Choudhri AF, Nandalur MR, Carlos RC. Diagnostic performance of stress cardiac magnetic resonance imaging in the detection of coronary artery disease: a meta-analysis. J Am Coll Cardiol. 2007;50(14):1343–53.

Nijveldt R, Hofman MB, Hirsch A, Beek AM, Umans VA, Algra PR, et al. Assessment of micro-vascular obstruction and prediction of short-term remodeling after acute myocardial infarction: cardiac MR imaging study. Radiology. 2009;250(2):363–70.

Northrup BE, McCommis KS, Zhang H, Ray S, Woodard PK, Gropler RJ, et al. Resting myocardial perfusion quantification with CMR arterial spin labeling at 1.5 T and 3.0 T. J Cardiovasc Magn Reson. 2008;10(1):53.

Plein S, Greenwood JP, Ridgway JP, Cranny G, Ball SG, Sivananthan MU. Assessment of non-ST-segment elevation acute coronary syndromes with cardiac magnetic resonance imaging. J Am Coll Cardiol. 2004;44(11):2173–81.

Plein S, Schwitter J, Suerder D, Greenwood JP, Boesiger P, Kozerke S. k-Space and time sensitivity encoding-accelerated myocardial perfusion MR imaging at 3.0 T: comparison with 1.5 T. Radiology. 2008;249(2):493–500.

Thomson LEJ, Fieno DS, Abidov A, Slomka PJ, Hachamovitch R, Saouaf R, et al. Added value of rest to stress study for recognition of artifacts in perfusion cardiovascular magnetic resonance. J Cardiovasc Magn Reson. 2007;9(5):733–40.

Wu KC, Zerhouni EA, Judd RM, Lugo-Olivieri CH, Barouch LA, Schulman SP, et al. Prognostic significance of microvascular obstruction by magnetic resonance imaging in patients with acute myocardial infarction. Circulation. 1998;97(8):765–72.

Windecker S, Kolh P, Alfonso F, Collet JP, Cremer J, Falk V, Filippatos G, Hamm C, Head SJ, Jüni P, Kappetein AP, Kastrati A, Knuuti J, Landmesser U, Laufer G, Neumann FJ, Richter DJ, Schauerte P, Sousa Uva M, Stefanini GG, Taggart DP, Torracca L, Valgimigli M, Wijns W, Witkowski A; Authors/Task Force members. Eur Heart J. 2014;35(37):2541–619.

Basic Adult Congenital Heart Disease (ACHD)

30

Andrew M. Crean and Bernhard A. Herzog

Abstract

There are an increasing number of patients with congenital heart disease surviving into adult life. Many of these patients have survived corrective procedures that have fixed but not cured their underlying condition. These patients are frequently at risk of complications and require lifelong surveillance. Others present for the first time in adult life with previously unknown conditions – often shunt lesions, which lead to insidious ventricular enlargement that may go unnoticed for years. All of these patients require anatomic and physiologic delineation of their lesions whether repaired or unrepaired. Cardiovascular MR (CMR) is the ideal tool for this with its unique ability to image clearly regardless of body size and to demonstrate not only ventricular size and function but also vascular flow/stenosis/regurgitation as well as provide information about tissue properties. Finally, the lack of ionizing radiation makes CMR a particularly appropriate tool for the surveillance of this often young and radiation-sensitive population.

Keywords

Cardiac MR (CMR) • ACHD • Cardiac situs • Coarctation • Bicuspid aortic valve • Tetralogy of Fallot • Transposition of the Great Arteries • Mustard • Senning • Arterial switch • Coronary anomalies • Partial anomalous venous return (PAPVR) • Sinus venosus defect • Structured reporting • Steady state free precession (SSFP) • Whole heart navigator • Magnetic resonance angiogram (MRA) • Phase contrast/velocity • QpQs

A.M. Crean, BSc, BM, MRCP, MSc, MPhil, FRCR (✉)
Department of Cardiology, University of Cincinnati Medical Center & Cincinnati Children's Hospital, 222 Piedmont Avenue #4300, Cincinnati, OH 45219, USA
e-mail: andrewcrean@gmail.com

B.A. Herzog, MD
Cardiac Imaging, University Hospital Zurich, Zurich, Switzerland
e-mail: andrewcrean@gmail.com

© Springer International Publishing 2015
S. Plein et al. (eds.), *Cardiovascular MR Manual*,
DOI 10.1007/978-3-319-20940-1_30

CMR in Adult Congenital Heart Disease
1. Is ideally suited to long-term follow up of anatomy and function in older children and adults
2. Represents the reference standard for measurement of LV and RV size and function
3. Is invaluable for examination of the systemic thoracic arteries, veins and surgical conduits which are not readily accessible to echo
4. Is the only technique sufficiently sensitive for detection of myocardial scar, particularly in the subpulmonic ventricle

CMR Protocol in ACHD

Core clinical components
1. LV and RV function (page 206–209)
2. MR angiography (page 214)
3. Phase velocity mapping (page 211) – selected vessels as indicated eg for Qp:Qs, differential pulmonary flow, or peak velocity measurements across stenoses

Optional clinical components
4. Late-gadolinium enhancement module (page 222) for ventricular scar or to rule out thrombus (in a Fontan circuit for example)
5. Coronary MR angiography module (page 228–233)
6. Stress perfusion imaging for coronary anomalies, reimplanted coronary arteries and Kawasaki disease
7. Thin slice cine imaging in non-standard planes to answer specific questions eg LVOT, RVOT obstruction?

Research components
8. T1 and T2 tissue mapping
9. Four dimensional flow imaging

Tips and Tricks
1. There is no substitute for planning in advance. Access to clinical notes or letters is **essential** if the correct study to answer the clinical question is to be performed.
2. All first time examinations should ideally be monitored by a CMR physician to allow for protocol modifications if unsuspected pathology is detected

3. An MRA is advised for a first-time examination since anatomy is often more complex than suspected (and follow with a venous phase acquisition to collect 'free' additional data at a cost of just one extra breath-hold)
4. Areas of dephasing on the cine images are important – these often indicate the presence of unsuspected shunts or areas of static or dynamic obstruction often requiring further focused imaging

Thinner slices resolve areas of confusion in many cases

Key Points CMR in ACHD
1. Congenital heart patients require lifelong surveillance for all but the most simple repaired lesions
2. CMR is the method of choice for assessment of complex anatomy, ventricular function, surgical / interventional planning and post-operative surveillance.
3. CMR for ACHD can not be entirely driven by protocol and in many cases requires protocol modification 'on the fly' for adequate assessment of pathology
4. Terminology is all-important in ACHD reporting – care is required in the naming of ventricles and AV valves especially where anatomy is complex or confusing.
5. An understanding of the types of anatomic and physiologic repairs (complete and palliative) performed in infancy is vital
6. The MR imager plays a key role in the ACHD team and should be available to present imaging data at regular multidisciplinary meetings to aid management planning
7. CMR is relatively insensitive for the presence of calcium – there are rare occasions where cardiac CT may be required to complement the CMR data acquired

Introduction

Over the last 15 years CMR has indisputably become the reference standard for the anatomical and functional assessment of the heart in adult congenital heart disease (ACHD). The number of children with congenital heart disease surviving to adulthood continues to increase, with many having had complex repairs in childhood. Indeed, there are now more adults alive with congenital heart disease than children and this number continues to grow. Many will develop problems relating to their underlying diagnosis and some will suffer late complications of remote surgery – patients with all but the simplest lesions are often 'fixed but not cured'. The role of the CMR physician is to provide: a complete description of the anatomical and physiological findings; an accurate assessment of ventricular size and function; an appraisal of the imaging appearances post-surgery; and – by integrating all of the above – to make a valuable contribution to the management of these complicated patients. What follows is a description of several of the commoner congenital lesions – such as might be encountered in non-specialist imaging practice – to illustrate general imaging principles. More complex anatomy, particularly single ventricle lesions are not covered here.

Sequential Segmental Analysis in ACHD

ACHD can be complicated, particularly when starting out. A sequential segmental approach to the anatomy is invaluable in helping the reporting clinician and the referring specialist understand what is going on. Cardiac situs, position, segments and connections should be clearly described at the start of the report. Further details are given in Figs. 30.1, 30.2, 30.3, and 30.4.

Coarctation of the Aorta

This is one of the commonest forms of congenital aortic anomaly and amongst the most straightforward to image by CMR. The majority of patients will have had surgical repair in childhood and are being followed routinely for evidence of recoarctation. A much smaller proportion will present in adult life, with a suspicion of coarctation from chest xray appearances (Fig. 30.5a) and/or clinical findings.

Key imaging features to assess are given in Table 30.1. Recognition of coarctation is generally not difficult. Either MRA or sagittal oblique cine imaging ('candy cane view' – see Chap. 23) may be used to assess the thoracic aorta. The former has the advantage that a 3D volume render may be performed and is particularly helpful in understanding and demonstrating the tortuosity of the coarct segment to physicians less-trained in mentally integrating multiple thin slice data sets (Fig. 30.5b). Cine imaging, however, has the advantage of revealing flow disturbance secondary to focal stenosis.

It may sometimes be surprisingly difficult to establish whether the visualized stenosis is of functional significance or represents a 'pseudocoarct'. The presence of large collaterals (Fig. 30.5b), a peak velocity on phase contrast imaging of >3 m/s (Fig. 30.2c), or elevated LV mass all point to the former. Some patients with coarctation also have hypoplasia of the aortic arch. This is worth comment – particularly if a stent dilatation of the aorta is planned – since relief of stenosis at the coarct site alone may not lead to significant reduction in LV pressure

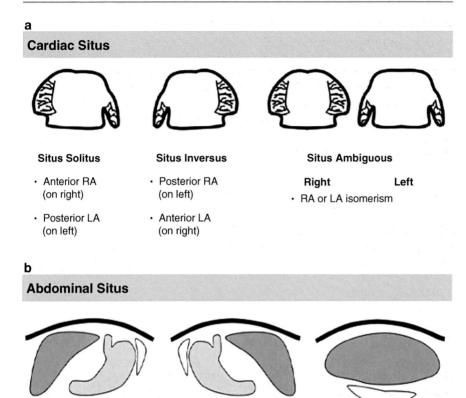

Fig. 30.1 Understanding cardiac & abdominal situs. (**a**) A schematic depiction of the atrial appendages is shown with a broad-based right atrial appendage and a narrow finger-like left atrial appendage.
Note that in right or left atrial isomerism there will be two right or two left atrial appendages respectively. (**b**) The liver, stomach and spleen are depicted according to situs. Note that in right isomerism
the spleen may be absent and that in left isomerism there may be multiple spleens present

overload or systemic blood pressure. Such cases are difficult to manage successfully and in extreme cases extra-anatomic bypass of the arch may be required
(Fig. 30.5d).

Common ancillary findings include bicuspid aortic valve and associated ascending aortopathy (see Chap. 23). In the context of a prior coarctation repair with either
a flap of the subclavian artery or a Dacron patch, it is important to exclude a focal
weakness in the material used which may give rise to focal aneurysmal dilatation
years after surgery. Both true and false aneurysms may develop – distinction is
rarely possible except at surgery.

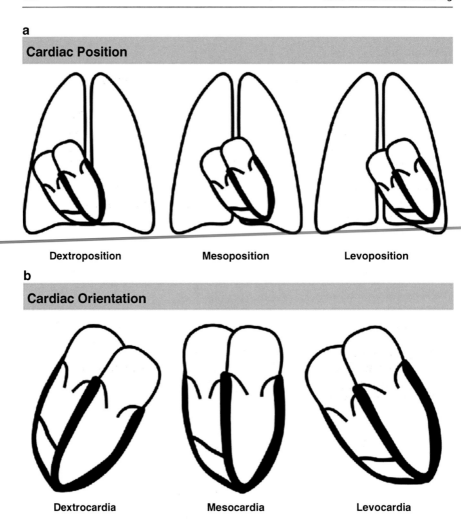

Fig. 30.2 Understanding cardiac position. (**a**) Position and orientation are often confused. "Position" refers to the physical location of the entire cardiac mass within the thorax. (**b**) "Orientation" or "-cardia" refers to the direction in which the dominant ventricle (usually the *left*) points. Therefore any combination of position and orientation may occur and both should be described independently

Tetralogy of Fallot

By congenital standards this is another common condition – and one in which CMR surveillance has a major role to play. The cardinal tetrad of infundibular RV stenosis, over-riding aorta, VSD and RV hypertrophy (Fig. 30.6) are rarely seen since most patients will have been repaired in childhood. The occasional

a

Atrial Segment

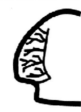 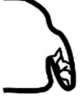

Right atrium

- Broad, based, triangular appendage
- Short and verticular bronchus arrangement

Left atrium

- Narrow, tubular appendage
- Long and horizontal bronchus arrangement

b

Ventricular Segment

Right ventricle

- Trabeculated
- TV associated, TV attachments to the septal moderator band
- Muscular infundibulum between inlet and outlet

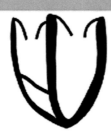

Left ventricle

- Smooth walled
- MV associated, MV attachments to papillary muscles

c

Arterial Segment

Pulmonary Trunk

- Bifurcation to RPA and LPA

Aorta

- Left- or right-sided
- Coronary arteries
- Regular branches

Fig. 30.3 Understanding atrial and ventricular segmentation. Atria and ventricles both have defining characteristics which should be used to identify them. Relying simply on anatomic position can be misleading in ACHD and it is safer to recognize these structures by their fundamental morphologic features as shown here. Bronchial anatomy is often challenging for novices but can usually be very readily determined from inspection of coronal magnetic resonance angiography images. (**a**) Features of morphological right and left atria. (**b**) Features of morphological right and left ventricles. (**c**) Arterial segmental anatomy – should be determined by direct inspection and not by virtue of their ventricular connections

a

Veno-Atrial Connection

- IVC and SVC connections
- Prescence of left SVC (90% left SVCs drain to RA via coronary sinus)
- Normal, partial or anomalous pulmonary venous drainage

b

Atrio-Ventricular Connection and Inlets

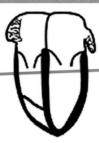
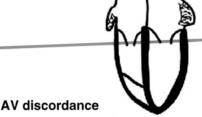

AV concordance

- RA is connected to RV, LA to LV

  The valves go with the ventricles

  Double inlet, mitral atresia, tricuspid atresia, AVSD

AV discordance

- RA is connected to LV, LA to RV

c

Ventricular-Arterial Connection

VA concordance

- LV is connected to Ao
- RV to MPA

Double outlet, single outlet

(e.g. pulmonary atresia or truncus arteriosus)

VA discordance

- LV is connected to MPA
- RV to Ao

Fig. 30.4 Understanding segmental connections. Description of segmental anatomy is vital so that both reporting and referring physicians understand the patient's underlying condition fully. (**a**) Veno-atrial connections. (**b**) Atrio-ventricular connections. (**c**) Ventriculo-arterial connections.

adult patient presents unrepaired and often cyanotic secondary to Eisenmenger complex. In most cases however the role of CMR is to demonstrate the almost invariable late consequences of surgery. In the past relief of infundibular obstruction was performed by resection and patch enlargement of the RVOT. In most cases a trans-annular style of repair meant that the pulmonary valve was either severely disrupted or completely excised. Unrecognised, in that era, were the late consequences of free pulmonary regurgitation, which in most patients leads to progressive RV dilatation, impairment of function and secondary effort intolerance, or even ventricular arrhythmia.

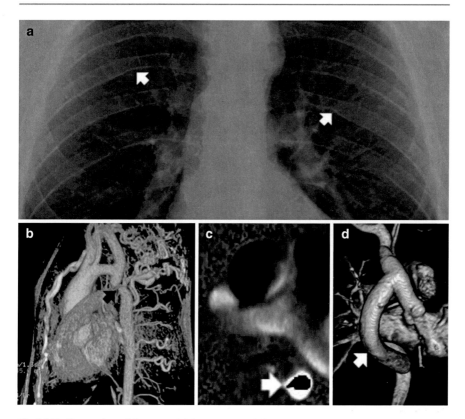

Fig. 30.5 Coarctation of the aorta. (**a**) Appearance of rib-notching (*arrows*) on frontal chest xray. (**b**) Volume rendered image of aorta MR angiogram shows coarct segment (*black arrow*) and multiple enlarged collaterals and a hypoplastic transverse arch. (**c**) Phase velocity image at the level of the coarctation; the encoding velocity has been set lower than the actual velocity and aliasing has occurred. The image should be re-acquired with a higher encoding velocity. (**d**) Volume rendered image of the aorta post surgery for relief of arch obstruction. An extra-anatomic bypass has been performed with creation of a surgical conduit (*arrow*) between the ascending and descending portions of the thoracic aorta – this is usually done for situations of extreme arch hypoplasia which can not be surgically reconstructed

The principal role of CMR is to monitor serial change in RV size and function. End diastolic volume should be indexed to body surface area for meaningful interpretation and a standardized method of contouring the endocardial surface on cine images is required to avoid spurious changes in volume from being reported. It matters less whether measurements are made from an axial or short axis oblique cine stack as long as a consistent approach is taken for subsequent examinations. The goal of monitoring is to alert the ACHD physician to any genuine deterioration in RV size or function so that the optimal timing of pulmonary valve replacement (PVR) can occur (Fig. 30.7a). Many centers will consider PVR at a threshold volume of between 150 and 170 ml/m^2 even

Table 30.1 CMR in ACHD

Potential findings in coarctation to include in CMR report
Repaired or unrepaired? (will probably not have had sternotomy – thoracotomy more usually which can be difficult to recognize)
Evidence of prior subclavian flap repair? (Absent left subclavian beyond origin from arch)
Evidence of restenosis
Evidence of hypoplastic arch?
Evidence of collateral flow (large internal mammary or intercostal arteries)
Peak velocity across narrowing
Bicuspid aortic valve? Stenotic?
Evidence of ascending aortopathy (associated with bicuspid valve)
Patch aneurysm? (if subclavian flap or Dacron patch repair)
Left ventricular hypertrophy if stenosis tight/longstanding (measure LV mass)
Multiple levels of left heart or aortic obstruction (Shone complex)?

Possible CMR findings in coarctation of the aorta

in minimally symptomatic patients, with the goal of preserving long term RV function.

Phase velocity mapping quantitates the pulmonary regurgitant fraction with precision (Fig. 30.7b) but in reality adds little to echocardiographic assessment of the valve. MR angiography has a place at the initial examination since a significant minority of these patients will have unsuspected proximal pulmonary arterial stenoses (Fig. 30.7c). Angiographic data facilitate interventional planning both at this site and also more proximally in the main pulmonary artery when stent-mounted percutaneous pulmonary valve replacement is being contemplated. Here, cardiac CT angiography may also be required for clear identification of the proximal coronary tree in relation to the site of proposed stent implantation.

Transposition of the Great Arteries

It is now rare to see **unrepaired** *d*-TGA in an adult CMR practice. Repaired patients fall into two quite different groups: those having had surgery more than 15–20 years ago are likely to have had an *atrial switch* procedure – often known eponymously as a Mustard or a Senning procedure. In this operation a physiologically-corrected circulation is restored by means of an inter-atrial baffle which directs blue blood to the lungs and pink blood to the body. Unfortunately the procedure leaves the patient with the pre-existing ventriculo-arterial discordance such that the RV remains in place as the systemic ventricle facing systemic arterial pressure. Although the initial RV response is to hypertrophy in response to increased afterload, eventual symptomatic decline of RV function is the norm. In the context of discordant connections it is prudent to use terminology carefully so that the referring clinician understand what is being described. Terms such as 'right' and 'left' ventricle should be replaced

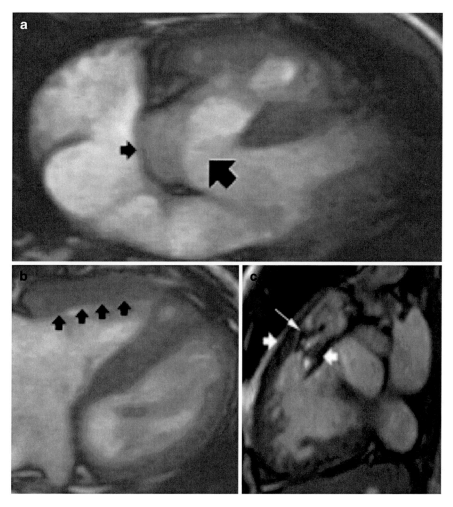

Fig. 30.6 The features of unrepaired tetralogy of Fallot. (**a**) Large non-restrictive VSD (*big arrow*), over-riding aorta (*small arrow*); (**b**) RV hypertrophy; (**c**) Infundibular obstruction due to muscle bundles (*thick arrows*) – evidence of flow disturbance is seen as a linear black jet of spin dephasing (*thin arrow*)

with the more precise 'subpulmonic (morphological left) ventricle' and 'subaortic (morphological right) ventricle'.

Mustard/Senning patients are monitored by CMR not only for RV dysfunction and dilatation but also for late surgical complications such as baffle stenosis or leak. The former is readily detected by either MRA or thin slice cine imaging (Fig. 30.8). The latter is more challenging and requires careful planning of phase velocity maps parallel to the superior and inferior systemic venous baffles – even in expert hands leaks may go unrecognized and this is one of the few areas where invasive catheter angiography retains a degree of superiority.

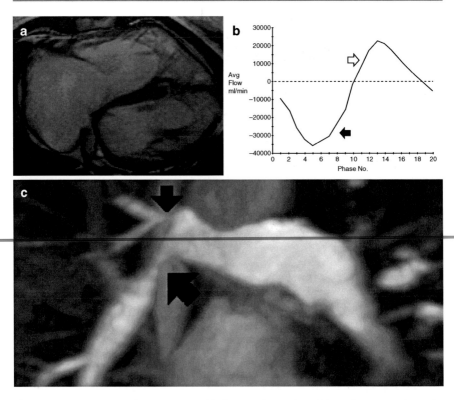

Fig. 30.7 Features of repaired tetralogy of Fallot. (**a**) Disruption of the pulmonary valve at the time of initial repair leads to free pulmonary incompetence which results in progressive RV dilatation (moderately enlarged in this example). (**b**) Phase velocity mapping at the level of the main pulmonary artery demonstrates normal forward flow in systole (*black arrow*) but with significant reverse flow (*grey arrow*) in diastole. (**c**) Maximum intensity projection image from a coronal MRA in a tetralogy patient. Several branch pulmonary artery stenoses are apparent (*arrows*). Central and proximal branch PA stenoses are not infrequent in tetralogy, may be amenable to stent therapy, and should be sought as the resultant pressure overload may worsen the degree of pulmonary regurgitation

Since the 1980s the technique of *arterial switch,* (Jatene operation), has been widely adopted. This involves restoration of ventriculo-arterial concordance so that the patient is corrected both physiologically and anatomically. Potential complications include narrowing of the RVOT/MPA as it straddles the anterior aspect of the aorta as well as myocardial ischaemia due to stenosis formation at the coronary reimplantation sites. The neo-aortic root (i.e., the unswitched pulmonary stump containing the pulmonary valve) is also at risk of progressive dilatation and regurgitation (Fig. 30.9).

Less common but not rare in any significant ACHD practice, is *l*-TGA or congenitally corrected transposition (Fig. 30.10). The term is in truth a misnomer: in this situation both the AV and VA connections are discordant and thus – like the atrial switch population – they are physiologically **but not anatomically** corrected.

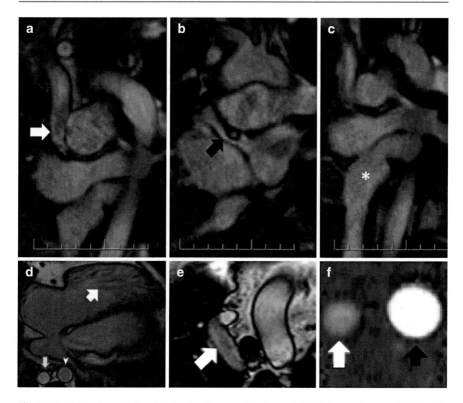

Fig. 30.8 Baffle stenosis in a Mustard patient. (**a, b**) Coronal SSFP frame showing SVC baffle (*white arrow*) which narrows as it enters the heart (*black arrow*). (**c**) Unobstructed IVC baffle (*asterisk*). (**d**) Axial SSFP image demonstrating dilatation and hypertrophy of the systemic RV (*large white arrow*). Note the size of the azygous vein (*small white arrow*) which is distended because of the distal baffle obstruction (azygous drains into SVC baffle) and is almost as large as the descending thoracic aorta (arrowhead). (**e**) extent of azygous engorgement is shown at level of azygous arch (*arrow*) close to its insertion into the SVC. Antegrade flow can not occur through the stenosed baffle. (**f**) phase velocity mapping of the azygous (*white arrow*) and descending aorta (*black arrow*) – normal cephalad azygous flow would be encoded black but here it is the same colour as the descending aorta indicating reverse flow

A proportion of these patients will have come to medical attention late in the absence of any other associated defect. Their main problem is progressive systemic RV decline, particularly when severe systemic AV valve regurgitation develops. Many ccTGA patients have an element of subpulmonic obstruction – if not too great this may actually be helpful, since the elevated subpulmonic ventricular pressure displaces the septum towards the systemic ventricle and may help to lessen the degree of systemic AV regurgitation. The same effect can be achieved by banding the main pulmonary artery, which is occasionally contemplated as destination therapy to slow systemic ventricular decline from volume loading.

PA banding is also occasionally performed to 'train' the subpulmonic LV prior to performing a double switch operation. The double switch procedure restores

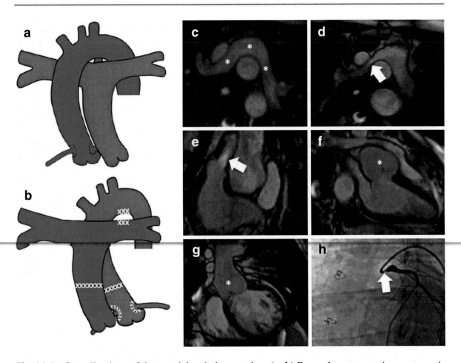

Fig. 30.9 Complications of the arterial switch operation. (**a**, **b**) Pre and post operative anatomy is demonstrated. Note that the arterial trunks are switched *above* the level of the valves so that the native pulmonary valve becomes the neo-aortic valve and vice versa. (**c**) Axial SSFP image showing the normal ventral appearance of unobstructed pulmonary arteries (*asterisks*), straddling the ascending aorta following the Le Compte manoeuvre. (**d**) Significant right pulmonary artery compression (*arrow*) as it passes between the SVC and ascending aorta. (**e**) sagittal SSFP image demonstrating systolic flow disturbance in the RVOT (*arrow*) – often seen to some degree due to the relatively small space between the sternum and the ascending aorta. (**f**, **g**) SSFP views of a dilated neo-aortic root (*asterisk*). (**h**) Angiographic shot of an ostial coronary stenosis (*arrow*) in a young adult arterial switch patient with exertional chest pain. Since coronary reimplantation is part of the original surgery, coronary distortion is a feared, but fortunately relatively rare, complication

anatomical continuity and although performed in children, is seldom performed in adults. In the few reported cases, the deconditioned subpulmonic (morphological left) ventricle is prepared to face systemic afterload during a period of progressively tighter pulmonary arterial banding. CMR may be used to estimate serial change in ventricular mass as a result of this 'training' and hence guide timing of the operation. This approach remains controversial.

Coronary Anomalies

There are many described anomalies of coronary artery origin, course or termination. Although CMR does not have the spatial resolution of conventional angiography, its 3D nature allows the course of the vessel to be more readily understood and image

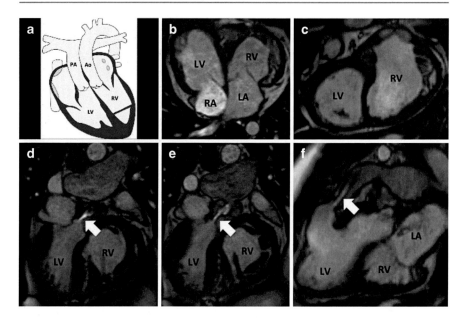

Fig. 30.10 Congenitally corrected transposition. (**a**) Schematic depiction of the segmental anatomy in ccTGA. Note the parallel arrangement of the great vessels. (**b**) Axial SSFP image demonstrating atrioventricular discordance. (**c**) Short axis SSFP image demonstrating ventricular relationships and the hypertrophy of the systemic RV. (**d**, **e**) Two contiguous SSFP slices to demonstrate narrowing and turbulent flow (*arrows*) in the region of the subpulmonic outflow tract (a common finding to some degree in ccTGA). (**f**) Oblique SSFP image to demonstrate a surgical conduit from LV to PA that was created in this case because of the obstruction to the native outflow tract shown in the two prior images. Unfortunately this surgical conduit has also developed proximal stenosis with associated flow turbulence (*arrow*)

quality is certainly sufficient for demonstration of coronary origin and proximal components. When a coronary arises from an aberrant location it frequently has a slit-like origin, which may predispose to ischaemia. Coronaries that pass between the aorta and RVOT are referred to as having a 'malignant' course – the implication being that they may suffer dynamic compression between the two outflow tracts, again resulting in myocardial ischaemia. Both mechanisms have been invoked to explain the increased risk of sudden death that such anomalies bestow. Rarer anomalies including coronaries with a connection to the pulmonary artery and post inflammatory coronary disease such as Kawasaki may also occasionally be encountered.

The two key attributes of an ideal coronary imaging sequence are isotropic voxel sizes and a short acquisition window (to prevent motion-related blurring). There are dedicated sequences that come close to achieving this in a breath hold (for a small targeted coronary volume) (Fig. 30.11a) or using a navigated free-breathing sequence over 10–15 min (Fig. 30.11b). Although these sequences may require considerable experience, in reality adequate assessment of coronary origin and initial course can be made by black blood or cine imaging as long as the matrix is optimized and the *z* axis resolution is increased by reducing slice thickness to 3–4 mm (Fig. 30.11c).

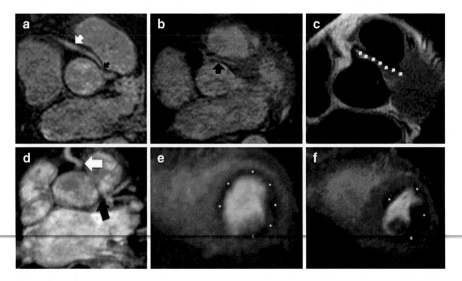

Fig. 30.11 Assessment of coronary anomalies. (**a**) Breath-held targeted coronary acquisition demonstrating an anomalous RCA (*white arrow*) arising from the left coronary sinus and taking a malignant course between the aortic root and RVOT. Note the narrow origin (*black arrow*), a finding suggestive of an intramural proximal segment. (**b**) Free breathing navigated whole heart acquisition of a patient with a malignant left main coronary artery (*arrow*). (**c**) Standard double inversion recovery black blood 3 mm thick slice clearly shows the malignant left main coronary artery (*arrows*). (**d**) Absence of the left main segment (*black arrow*) with retrograde flow via an enlarged right coronary artery (*white arrow*). This patient was born with the left main coronary artery arising from the pulmonary artery (ALCAPA) which was corrected by surgical reimplantation to the aorta in neonatal life. Unfortunately the reimplanted segment thrombosed shortly after surgery. (**e, f**) Stress perfusion images demonstrate a substantial subendocardial stripe of hypoperfusion (*asterisks*) in the left coronary territory (same patient as **d**)

Since surgical decision-making relates in part to the suspected physiological effects of the lesion, it may be worth performing stress imaging as part of the protocol (Fig. 30.11d–f). Some favour dobutamine for assessment of inter-arterial vessels, arguing that the mechanism of ischemia is due to compression of the vessel between aorta and MPA which should be exacerbated at the higher cardiac outputs produced by inotropic versus vasodilator stress. Practical experience at many centers, however, has suggested that vasodilator stress is reasonably robust despite the relatively minor changes in heart rate and contractility that occur.

Partial Anomalous Pulmonary Venous Return (PAPVR)

Unexplained right heart dilatation in a young or middle-aged individual should prompt a search for left-to-right shunting. One of the most frequently missed causes is PAPVR (Fig. 30.12). Even when the diagnosis is made, its frequent concomitant – sinus venosus defect – is not always appreciated. The most frequent type of PAPVR involves drainage of the right upper and middle lobes to the SVC. Second

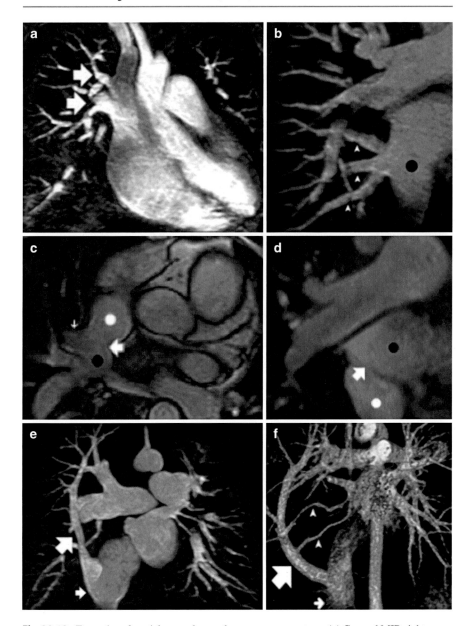

Fig. 30.12 Examples of partial anomalous pulmonary venous return. (**a**) Coronal MIP, right upper and middle lobe veins drain to SVC (*arrows*); (**b**) Coronal MIP (different patient), right lower lobe veins (*arrowheads*) drain to IVC (*black dot*); (**c**) Axial SSFP image, superior sinus venosus defect (*large arrow*) between lower SVC (*white dot*) and upper left atrium (*black dot*) with anomalous middle lobe vein (*small arrow*) draining at site of defect; (**d**) Coronal SSFP image, inferior sinus venosus defect (*arrow*) between left atrium (*black dot*) and IVC (*white dot*); (**e**) Coronal MIP demonstrating Scimitar vein (*large arrow*) draining to IVC (small arrow). (**f**) Coronal volume render of a different case of Scimitar syndrome. Note the presence of small bridging veins (*arrowheads*) between the scimitar vein (*large arrow*) and the left atrium

most common is drainage of part (or all) of the left lung to the left innominate vein. Sinus venosus defect is related to the former and may either occur superiorly (common) or inferiorly (rare). Diagnosis prior to the development of pulmonary arterial hypertension is essential if surgical intervention is to be successful.

The anomalous drainage is easily detectable with a coronal MRA. Less straight-forward is the superior sinus venosus defect, which is easy to miss unless specifically searched for. The author's practice is to use thin slice (5 mm) cine imaging in the axial plane through the region of the SVC/right upper pulmonary vein since this is where a superior defect is located. Measurement of Qp:Qs allows for non-invasive assessment of size of shunt. Indirect evidence of pulmonary hypertension should be sought (enlarged pulmonary arteries with tortuous segmental branches). RV volume and function should be formally quantitated.

Significant RV dilatation is only rarely caused by right isolated PAPVR and usually indicates the presence of a concomitant sinus venosus defect.

Reporting Guidelines

In general structured reports are to be favoured over paragraphs of text. With this method, complicated information may be conveyed swiftly and in logical anatomic order. An example of a structured report is given below. This is intended to be illustrative rather than definitive – individual adaptation will be required on a case-by-case basis:

STUDY INDICATION: Reason cardiac MR has been requested together with any relevant background information on underlying congenital diagnosis, prior surgical repairs and any interventional procedures
COMPARISON: Prior imaging (with dates) with which the current study is compared.
SCANNER: Manufacturer, field strength
PRE-MEDICATION: if any (type, dose)
TECHNIQUE: Sequences used eg black blood, cine steady state free precession, first pass perfusion, time-resolved or static angiography, first pass perfusion (stress/rest/both), T2 weighted imaging, late gadolinium enhancement

Cardiovascular

GENERAL: Situs, levo/dextrocardia, left/right aortic arch (cervical branching pattern)
PRIOR CONGENITAL REPAIR: e.g., Mustard procedure, arterial switch operation, Bentall procedure, coarctation repair (subclavian flap, interposition graft, end to end anastomosis)
SYSTEMIC VEINS: Connection and drainage of SVC, IVC, coronary sinus. Presence/absence sinus venosus defects. IVC interruption/azygous continuation. Location of candidate veins for CRT if appropriate.

RIGHT/SYSTEMIC VENOUS ATRIUM: Size, presence/absence of thrombus

RIGHT/SUBPULMONIC AV VALVE: Location (Ebstein), thickening, bridging leaflet anatomy, stenosis, prolapse regurgitation, masses

RIGHT/SUBPULMONIC VENTRICLE: Size, function, ventriculotomy site, trans-annular patch, regional dysfunction, outflow tract obstruction

PULMONARY ARTERIES: Size, connections (confluence, shunt connections), stenosis, dilatation, pulmonary valve stenosis/regurgitation, stent presence/ in-stent restenosis, conduit stenosis, conduit valve calcification, valve masses

PULMONARY VEINS: Size, drainage, flow volumes per vein, stenosis, presence of systemic-to-pulmonary venous collaterals

INTERATRIAL SEPTUM: Presence/absence, secundum defects, primum defects, AV canal defects, presence of patch/device, patch leak

PULMONARY VENOUS ATRIUM: Size, presence/absence of thrombus

LEFT/SYSTEMIC AV VALVE: Thickening, clefts/bridging leaflet anatomy, stenosis, prolapse, regurgitation, masses

INTERVENTRICULAR SEPTUM: Defects – membranous, subarterial, muscular, patch/device, patch leak

LEFT/SYSTEMIC VENTRICLE: Size, function, mass, regional wall motion abnormality, thinning, fatty metaplasia/calcification of scar, thrombus, LVOT size/narrowing/membrane

PERICARDIUM: Presence/absence, thickening, calcification, effusion, any associated features of constriction

AORTA & BRANCHES: Aortic valve morphology (tricuspid, bicuspid, unicuspid, dysplastic), masses, aortic stenosis/regurgitation, trans-sinus diameters, other diameters (sinotubular junction, ascending aorta, mid arch, descending aorta), arch hypoplasia, supravalvar aortic stenosis (site/severity), coarctation (site/ severity), aortic aneurysm, patch aneurysm, branch vessel origins and patency

CORONARY ARTERIES: Origin (normal, slit-like) and course (normal, inter arterial, intramural, transeptal, retro-aortic, pre-pulmonic), stenosis, occlusion

EDEMA IMAGING: Presence/absence, location, correlation with wall motion and late gadolinium enhancement)

PERFUSION IMAGING: Resting defects, stress-induced (adenosine/ dipyridamole/dobutamine dose schedule) defects, correlation with late gadolinium enhancement)

LATE GADOLINIUM IMAGING: Presence, location, transmurality, correlation with wall motion abnormality/wall thinning/perfusion defects

---

Pulmonary

AIRWAYS: Central airway anatomy (normal left-right anatomy, bilateral right lungs, bilateral left lungs), prior lobectomy/pneumonectomy. Bronchial compression (tetralogy with absent pulmonary valve). Plastic bronchitis (Fontan).

PLEURAL SPACES: Thickening, effusion, pleural enhancement, transpleural collaterals

PARENCHYMA: Parenchymal blush (MRA or perfusion) – uniform, lobar abnormality, segmental abnormality. Air trapping. Parenchymal abnormality – fibrosis, nodules, septal thickening (edema – heart failure, pulmonary venous obstruction)

Musculoskeletal

BONES: Deformity (scoliosis, kyphosis, pectus), fracture, destructive lesions
SOFT TISSUES: Masses, anasarca, abscess (endocarditis)

Other Findings

Eg arrhythmia such as 2:1 heart block occasionally seen on cine SSFP (two atrial appendage contractions to each ventricular contraction)
Eg features of heterotaxy in the abdomen

Opinion

1. Point form….
2. ……..is usually preferable ……..
3. ………………………..for clarity

Recommendations for Further Imaging

E.g. formal catheterization to assess systemic to pulmonary venous collaterals or look for small AVMs
E.g. stress perfusion CMR to assess the significance of congenital coronary anomalies

Summary

CMR is invaluable in the assessment of ACHD patients, unique in its large field of view and lack of ionizing radiation. With the three basic techniques of CMR – cine imaging, MRA and phase velocity mapping – 99 % of all the necessary information to enhance patient management can be acquired. Structured reporting enforces a logical approach to a large amount of data and is a clear and consistent method for presenting findings and interpretation back to the referring clinician.

CMR and Implantable Devices

31

Matthias Schmitt and Mark Ainslie

Abstract

Implantable cardiac device technology plays an ever increasing role in modern medicine and the probability of a cardiac device patient to benefit from MRI has been estimated to be 50–75 % over the lifetime of the device. Consequently the issue of MRI in patients with cardiac devices will be encountered with increasing frequency. However, in clinical practise scanning cardiac device patients is associated with logistic challenges and requires both an understanding of device indication and technology to facilitate safe scanning. This chapter will equip the interested reader with the required knowledge to set out in this interesting and expanding field.

Keywords

IPG • Pacemaker • MR-conditional • MR-unsafe • Cardiac devices • Image quality

Introduction

Implantable cardiac device-technology plays an ever-increasing role in modern medicine. The vast majority of patients benefitting from such devices however have co-morbidity profiles, including neurological, oncological and musculoskeletal disorders, which warrant magnetic resonance imaging (MRI) as a diagnostic tool.

M. Schmitt, MD, PhD (✉)
Cross-Sectional Cardiac Imaging Unit, Cardiovascular Division,
University Hospital of South Manchester, Office 4, North West Heart Centre,
UHSM, Southmoor Road, Wythenshawe, Manchester M23 9LT, UK
e-mail: Matthias.Schmitt@uhsm.nhs.uk

M. Ainslie, MBChB (Hons), BSc (Hons), MRCP
Department of Cardiology, University Hospital of South Manchester, Manchester, UK

© Springer International Publishing 2015
S. Plein et al. (eds.), *Cardiovascular MR Manual*,
DOI 10.1007/978-3-319-20940-1_31

Indeed it has been estimated that the probability of a *Device patient* to benefit from MRI over the lifetime of their device is ~ 50–75 % (Kalin and Stanton 2005). Worldwide >5 million patients are implanted with cardiac devices (CD) and currently there are over 250,000 patients with implantable pulse generators (IPGs) and implantable cardiac defibrillators (ICDs) in the UK alone, with 50,000 patients undergoing implantation in 2011 (Cunningham and Whittaker 2011). Consequently the issue of MRI in patients with CD will be encountered with increasing frequency. In total it has been estimated that ~200,000 patients with CD had an indication for an MRI scan in 2004 (Jung et al. 2012).

However, serious adverse events during MRI of patients with CD, including asystole and ventricular fibrillation, albeit rarely, have been reported (Gimbel et al. 2005; Gimbel 2009; Kalin and Stanton 2005), and therefore awareness of the safety issues is paramount in order to facilitate safe scanning in this patient group. This in turn requires an additional basic understanding of modern device technology, not least knowledge of the differences between so called MR conditional and non-MR conditional (i.e., MR unsafe) devices.

MRI Safety Terminology

This has been described in Chap. 2 (page 13). In this chapter the terms *non-MR conditional* and MR unsafe (ASTM terminology) are used interchangeably.

While MRI is an inherently safe imaging modality, the MRI environment harbours the potential for even fatal accidents, particularly in patients with CD. The theoretical effects of the three principal magnetic fields on device function are summarised in Table 31.1.

The practise of scanning MRI patients with MR unsafe devices operates outside of the Pacemaker license and is not endorsed by either professional bodies or manufacturers. The greatest risk exists in so called legacy devices, CD manufactured before the year 2000. Yet it is increasingly recognised that MRI and even CMR scanning of newer generation devices, i.e., manufactured post 2000, including MR unsafe IPGs and ICDs can, under certain circumstances be in the best interest of

Table 31.1 Potential harmful effects of static magnetic field, gradient magnetic fields and radio-frequency energy on CD

	Static	Gradient	Radiofrequency
Case heating		✓	✓
Force and torque	✓		
Vibration	✓	✓	
Device interactions including component damage and altered pacing function	✓	✓	✓
Lead Heating			✓
Myocardial stimulation		✓	✓

the patient, be performed with an acceptably low risk, and can indeed compare favourably to the risk of lead extraction and temporary device removal in non PPM dependent patient with a strong need for MRI investigation. While the majority of older studies assessing non-thoracic MRI in patients with MR unsafe IPGs have reported no adverse events, isolated incidents of asystole, ventricular fibrillation, and death have been described independently in several patients (Roguin et al. 2008). Moreover it can reasonably be assumed that case fatalities of CD patients during MRI scanning is significantly underreported. In a more contemporary review of the literature including 15 studies and ~1400 PPM recipients, no fatalities were reported in association with MRI examinations (Zikria et al. 2011). It should be noted that the vast majority of these studies were extra-thoracic and few patients were pacing dependent. In one of the largest prospective studies Nazarian et al. (2011) performed 555 MRI scans (40 % brain, 22 % spine, 16 % heart, 13 % abdominal, 9 % extremities) on 438 patients with either IPG (54 %) or ICD (46 %) from various manufacturers. Three patients experienced electrical reset during scanning but there was no device dysfunction on long-term (up to 5 years) follow up. Minor changes in atrial and ventricular lead impedance were seen, but no significant changes in pacing capture thresholds were noted. However, thoracic imaging was noted to be associated with decreased acute and chronic (3 months) R wave amplitudes and battery voltage compared to non-thoracic scans, supporting the intuitive notion that thoracic scans carry a higher risk. Similar findings with respect to small changes in lead impedance and small but significant device parameter changes were found in a study by Cohen et al. in 109 PPM and ICD patients (Cohen et al. 2012). Furthermore, a study by Junttila et al. in ten patients with a variety of MR unsafe ICDs undergoing three MRI scans each over a 12 months period found no significant changes in device parameters, pacing capture thresholds or battery voltage implying that serial investigations, as for example required for treatment monitoring in a patient with demyelinating disease, may not necessarily pose a greater risk than a single scan (Junttila et al. 2011). The MagnaSafe registry, a multi-centre prospective study, has been designed to assess the safety of non-thoracic MRI scanning in patients implanted with MR unsafe IPGs and ICDs undergoing clinically indicated scans at 1.5 T (Russo et al. 2012; Russo 2013). So far in excess of 600 scans across 12 sites have been performed without any occurrence, of loss of pacing capture, device failure or death. Despite these encouraging findings, it should be noted that decreases in battery voltage, R and P wave amplitudes did occur and the frequency of clinically relevant device changes occurred in 13 % of IPGs and 31 % of ICDs. Therefore MRI scanning in patients with MR unsafe devices should a priori not be considered as safe and pre-and post-scan device checks should be considered as mandatory.

From a pragmatic point of view the interaction between the magnetic fields operational during an MRI study and cardiac devices can be sub-grouped into three categories whereby it should be acknowledged that it is at times the unpredictable co-occurrence of multiple device-magnetic field interaction that may lead to biological and ultimately patient harm.

Pacemaker and or Lead Displacement/Force and Torque

CD contain variable degrees of ferromagnetic material which are subject to force and torque induced by the static and gradient magnetic fields this can lead to movement and vibration of the device and leads. These forces are directly related to mass of ferromagnetic material, the strength of the magnetic field and the positioning within the static magnetic field (Shellock et al. 2003). Whilst Phantom studies have demonstrated the potential for IPGs to move when placed within the static magnetic field of an MRI unit (Pavlicek et al. 1983), and while there are anecdotal reports of pull and drag in legacy devices, modern (i.e., manufactured after 2000) IPGs with their reduced ferromagnetic content appear safe with regards to force and torque in the 1.5 T environment beyond the first 6 weeks following implantation, after which time healing around the IPG and the lead tip is thought to provide sufficient anchorage (Ainslie et al. 2013). Studies conducted at 1.5 T found that the force in IPGs and ICDs at this field strength ranges from 0.05 to 3.6 N and 1.0–5.9 N (Luechinger et al. 2001).

Modern pacing leads are constructed from materials that are less magnetically susceptible (MP35N or drawn brazen strand) and as such pose little risk of movement or dislodgement (Ahmed et al. 2013). Indeed, in our experience leads such as the Medtronic CapSureFix MRI 5086, CapSureFix Novus 5076 or the St Jude Tendril MRI display no visible deflection of their gravitational behaviour when brought into the bore of a 1.5 T scanner.

Tissue Heating

Pacing leads can act as antennae, concentrating electromagnetic energy at the un-insulated points of the lead cathode, anode or active fixation helix, which can lead to heating of the surrounding tissue where the energy is dissipated and potentially cause localised oedema and/or fibrosis. Theoretically this could result in an increase in pacing thresholds, loss of pacing capture and cardiac perforation (Achenbach et al. 1997; Fetter et al. 1984; Nazarian and Halperin 2009; Roguin et al. 2004; Tandri et al. 2008). The potential for heating depends on the resonant frequency of the lead (dependent on lead length and diameter), the trajectory of the pacing leads, presence of lead loops, lead or insulation fractures, patient size and position within the scanner (Bottomley et al. 1985; Bottomley and Edelstein 1981; Chou et al. 1996; Cline et al. 2004; Wilkoff et al. 2011).

In-vitro studies without lead tip irrigation, have demonstrated lead temperature increases in excess of 60 °C during MRI scanning although such extreme temperature variations have not been observed in more sophisticated models with lead tip irrigation. One in-vivo study in pigs found an increase of 20.4 °C at the electrode tip in the setting of a SAR approaching 3.8 W/kg, considerably higher than that in routine clinical scanning (Roger Luechinger et al. 2005). In another study, a small rise in serum troponin was seen following 4 out of 114 scans performed at 1.5 T in patients implanted with a variety of conventional (i.e., MR-unsafe) IPGs, which the authors hypothesised likely reflected tissue necrosis secondary to lead tip heating (Sommer et al. 2006). To minimise the above effects, specifically designed MR conditional pacing leads have altered Lead diameter and pitch of the coils to remain inert to the resonant frequency and also contain 64 MHz Bandstop filters.

Device Malfunction

Reed Switches

Magnetic-operated reed switches were originally incorporated into IPGs to allow device interrogation. Magnet application activates the reed switch which inhibits demand functions and most commonly, but not consistently, sets an IPG to an asynchronous mode (Gimbel et al. 2005; Sommer et al. 2006). The position of the reed switch has been shown to be inconsistent within the MRI environment leading to potential malfunction (Luechinger et al. 2002). Variable reed switch responses to MRI have been demonstrated across different IPG models including asynchronous pacing, transient loss of pacing or continuous loss of pacing (Irnich et al. 2005; Luechinger et al. 2002; Sommer et al. 2006). Loss of pacing in a pacing-dependent patient could have significant consequences, whilst asynchronous pacing in individuals with an underlying rhythm could heighten the theoretical risk of R on T phenomenon and induce ventricular arrhythmias. In ICDs, activation of the reed switch commonly leads to deactivation of therapies whilst not affecting backup pacing Bovenschulte et al. 2012). In MR conditional devices the Reed switch has been replaced with a solid state or hall sensor, which does not contain moving ferromagnetic parts.

Electrical Reset

'Electrical reset', 'power on reset' and 'factory reset' are interchangeable terms for the emergency/backup mode that a device reverts to when its battery nears depletion. It is conventionally a VVI pacing mode at the lower rate limit with all advanced functions turned off (Roguin et al. 2004). For ICDs, power on reset is a safety mechanism, which prevents inappropriate shocks from a damaged device. It is a VVI back up mode with no therapies. It cannot be reprogrammed and the device has to be changed. It should not be confused with the normal magnet response of ICDs. This is fixed rate pacing with therapies disabled, but functions return on removal of the magnet. Publications have quoted an MRI-related incidence of electrical reset as high as 6.1 % in conventional (i.e., MR unsafe) IPGs (Shellock et al. 2003). The conversion of asynchronous or fixed-rate pacing to VVI mode in an IPG-dependent patient without an underlying ventricular rhythm, in combination with radiofrequency energy pulses being wrongly interpreted as intrinsic electric activity is potentially life-threatening and several MRI-related deaths in IPG patients have been attributed to this mechanism.

Inappropriate Pacing and Inhibition of Therapies

Radiofrequency energy pulses can lead to asynchronous pacing, programming changes or battery depletion or be wrongly interpreted as underlying electrical activity or arrhythmias and thus lead to inhibition of demand pacing or at least theoretically to delivery of ICD therapy respectively (Lauck et al. 1995; Luechinger et al. 2002; Martin et al. 2004; Mollerus et al. 2009; Sommer et al. 2006). In an Ex-vivo study by Erlebacher on three IPGs no longer in use, radiofrequency interference caused total inhibition of atrial and ventricular output or resulted in atrial pacing at a high rate (Erlebacher et al. 1986). No ICD induced defibrillation therapies in the MR environment have so far been reported. This likely relates to the inability of the capacitor to sufficiently charge in the static magnetic field (see below). Nevertheless, repeated attempts by a defibrillator to charge itself could lead to battery depletion (Roguin et al. 2008).

Capacitor and Transformer

ICDs cannot charge the capacitor in the MRI environment because the electrical characteristics of the circuit are significantly altered by the strong MRI magnetic field. If the device attempts to charge the capacitor in the MRI it could lead to serious device damage, requiring explant (the Medtronic Evera ICD system, the only MR conditional ICD without chest exclusion, disables charging in Surescan mode). The circuits used to charge the capacitors commonly contain a transformer. A transformer uses magnetic fields to change voltage levels. The strong magnetic field of the MRI negatively impacts the magnetic field of the transformer to the point that device damage is likely to occur if the transformer is used in the MRI environment.

Image Quality

Whilst the clinical utility and safety of performing cardiac and non-cardiac MRI in patients with MR conditional and to a lesser extent MR unsafe IPGs has been investigated extensively, much less data is available on the impact of these devices on image quality. Yet estimating the likelihood of achieving diagnostic image quality is a fundamental part of assessing the risk benefit ratio especially in the setting of an MR unsafe device. A basic working knowledge of anticipated device induced field distortion is therefore important.

CD have magnetic susceptibilities different from human tissues and such disparities in magnetic susceptibility lead to significant distortion of the magnetic field homogeneity resulting in imaging artefacts. In general the presence of ferromagnetic materials within the Device creates a magnetic field inhomogeneity that alters the precessional frequency of the protons within the surrounding tissue leading to varying degrees of artefact, whereby the latter is related to both the type and size

Fig. 31.1 IPG related susceptibility artefacts

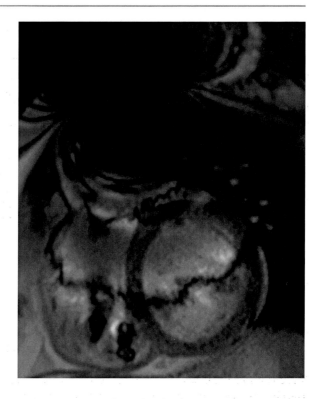

(volume) of the ferromagnetic object causing it. These metal susceptibility artefacts may appear as bright or dark bands due to either mis-registration or signal loss (Fig. 31.1).

In principal each metal has a different magnetic susceptibility, for example stainless steal has a much higher relative magnetic susceptibility than titanium hence producing more artefact (Suh et al. 1998). In addition to the volume and the relative magnetic susceptibility of the device material, the size and orientation of the artefact are also associated with the direction and strength of the magnetic gradient and field respectively, as well as the type of pulse sequence used. Sequences with the greatest sensitivity to magnetic field in-homogeneities are the balanced steady state free precession sequences (bSSFP), inversion recovery sequences with long echo times and those that use rapid K-space acquisition techniques such as EPI and spiral mode (Ferreira et al. 2013; Sasaki et al. 2011). On the other hand Spin echo sequences are less prone to metal susceptibility artefacts. Conventional gradient-echo sequence susceptibility is largely dependent on the TE setting. A shorter TE allows less time for dephasing to occur thereby limiting signal loss.

In practise cine image quality can be improved by either changing the centre frequency, which shifts the location rather than eliminating the artefact (Fig. 31.2a, b), or indeed changing to old fashioned gradient echo imaging which reduces artefact intensity but also image contrast (Fig. 31.3). Alternatively artefacts can also be

Fig. 31.2 (a) Still frame of SSFP cine at 0 Center frequency. Note the diffuse signal loss within the LV cavity. (b) Still frame of same SSFP cine with center frequency shift +75

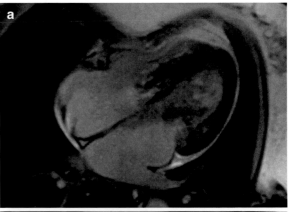

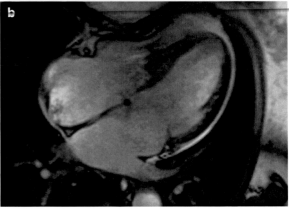

Fig. 31.3 Still frame of Spoiled gradient Echo cine image. Note less diffuse signal lose in LV cavity but also substantially lower signal contrast between blood and myocardium

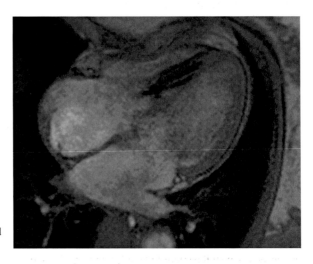

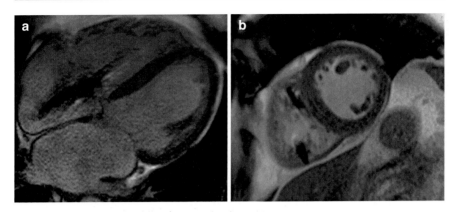

Fig. 31.4 (**a**) SSFP cine still frame of right sided IPG implant demonstrating no IPG related artefacts within LV cavity. (**b**) SSFP cine still frame of right sided IPG. Note generator artefact displays minimal projection into the FOV and causes no susceptibility artefact within LV/RV cavity and does not affect cardiac wall motion assessment

reduced theoretically by use of lower field strength and/or shorter Echo times, whereby both may have detrimental effects on overall image quality and contrast respectively.

Pragmatically, all of the following are associated with greater susceptibility artefacts; Larger generator size, lower BMI and smaller LVEDD, shorter distance between device and ROI (e.g., cardiac silhouette) on plain radiograph.

Concerning CMR, conventional left sided implants cause more relevant artefacts then right-sided implants, specifically affecting the anterior wall and apex (Figs. 31.1 and 31.4a, b = SAX and 4 chamber left and right implant).

Artefact size is substantially greater with Bivent/ICDs than with simple PPMs and differs in proportion to size difference (Fig. 31.5 a–c in ICD patient – with comparative pre- and post implant images in a patient with ALVC).

Assessment of cardiac function, both on global and regional level, of right sided PPM and ICDs is uncomplicated as the artefacts conventionally don't impede on the cardiac borders with optimised FOV settings. The same is largely true for left sided PPM implants, whereby applying above mentioned strategies, one is able to either shift the site of artefact projection temporarily away from a location (usually anterior wall) or alternatively render it less prominent by means of deploying an alternative sequence. In our limited experience left sided Bivent/ICDs can be rather challenging with respect to their artefact projection. However Sasaki et al. reported diagnostic cine imaging in >85 % of their cases.

The same investigators found that, as already stated above, in general the strongest predictors for diagnostic cine imaging again were BMI + LVEDD whereby both associations are likely mediated via the distance of generator and the heart which as stated can be estimated from an PA film projection.

For a detailed and quantified assessment of imaging artefacts on sequences relevant for cardiac assessment the interested reader is referred to the paper by Sasaki et al. (2011a).

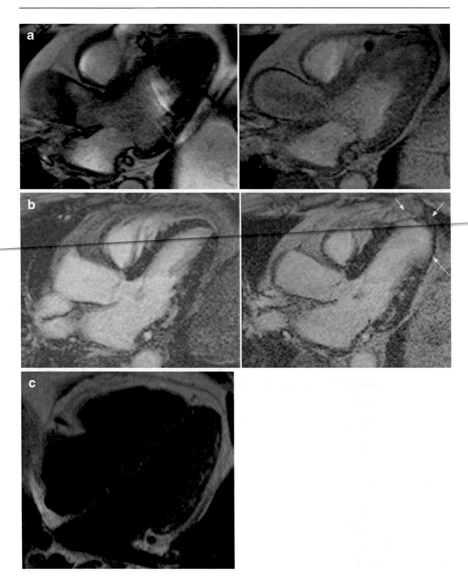

Fig. 31.5 (**a**) Patient with ALVC implanted with MR conditional EVERA ICD. The SSFP sequence shows significant apical artifact which is not present on SpGR sequence. (**b**) LGE images in same patient pre and post ICD. Apical "LGE" (*yellow arrows*) artifactual. Basal and mid infero-lateral LGE (*red arrows*) is true LGE and unaffected by presence of ICD. (**c**) T1 Weighted 4ch view with ICD showing fatty infiltration in lateral wall

In the ADVISA image quality sub-study, the only multi-centre study of an MR conditional pacemaker assessing cardiac image quality using a pre-specified image quality protocol, 95 % of the LV and 98 % of the RV cine long axis SSFP acquisitions were of diagnostic quality, with 84 and 93 % being of excellent or good quality. Overall, only 5 % of the LV and 2 % of the RV images were of non-diagnostic quality (Schwitter et al. 2013). The ADVISA imaging sub-study also specifically investigated the performance of CSPAMM tagging and HARP based post-processing in the presence of the Medtronic ADVISA MRI™ Pacing System to assess the performance of these technologies; Tagging points could be tracked into early diastole in all segments of a mid-ventricular short axis slice. In particular, systolic and early diastolic tracking was possible in the inter-ventricular septum, where the pacing electrode might be expected to interfere most with tagging data quality (Schwitter et al. 2013). Therefore, a CSPAMM/HARP based approach to the assessment of changes in myocardial deformation appears feasible even in the presence of an IPG.

With respect to Leads and lead tip related artefact these are usually minimal and don't affect clinical image interpretation. Whilst the leads are weakly ferromagnetic most spring coils and lead tips are made out of non-ferromagnetic alloys such as platinum that cause minimal artefacts. Indeed CMR related lead and especially lead tip artefacts are much less pronounced that those seen on CT which may be of clinical relevance when attempting to investigate the tip surrounding myocardium for perforation. In our own experience T1 values "normalise" in a distance of ~1 cm from the lead tip and body.

MR Conditional Devices

In recent years the device industry has invested significant effort into developing MR-conditional systems to address the discussed safety issues. Many new design features of both hardware and software have been incorporated into these devices to allow them to perform more reliably in a specified MRI environment (i.e., 1.5 T field strength). Hardware modifications have been made to both the generator and leads whereby some of these changes are manufacturer-specific (see Tables 31.2 and 31.3). Software changes include the incorporation of a dedicated MRI pacing mode that can be activated for the duration of the scan. In most instances this requires a trained individual, commonly a pacing technician, Cardiologist or Electrophysiologist, to activate and deactivate this mode. There are novel alternatives, with St Jude providing a hand held activator to perform this task before and after the scan, and Boston Scientific's Ingenio and Advantio devices having an MRI time-out mode negating the need to deactivate the safe mode manually post-scanning. Nevertheless current recommendations are that a full IPG interrogation is

Table 31.2 Common design features of MR conditional devices

Generator design
Ferromagnetic content reduced
Replacement of reed switch with solid state technology e.g., Hall sensor
Bandstop filter (64 Mhz) in casing to shield circuitry
Lead design
Lead pitch of the inner coil redesigned to alter resonant frequency of the lead
Lead diameter altered
Bandstop filter (64 Mhz) at lead tip (e.g., St Jude Tendril lead)

Table 31.3 Current MR-conditional pacemakers on market

	St Jude	Medtronic	Boston Scientific	Biotronik	Sorin
Device	Accent MRI	Advisa MRI Enrhythm MRI Ensura MRI	Ingenio MRI Advantio MRI	Evia MRI Estella MRI	Reply MRI KORA MRI
Leads	Tendril MRI	CapsureFix MRI Capsure sense	Fineline II	Safio/Solia	Filtrea
Lead fixation	Active	Active and passive	Active and passive	Active and passive	Active
Lead diameter	6.6 F	5.4 F	5.1 F	5.6 F	6.5 F
Thorax exclusion	No	No	No	Yes	No
Scan time limit	No	No	No	Yes	No
Static field strength limit	1.5 T	1.5 T	1.5 T	1.5 T	1.5 T
Max permitted scan time	None	None	None	30 min	None
SAR limit (w/kg)	4	2	2	2	4
Slew rate (T/m/s)	≤200	≤200	≤200	≤200	≤200
Manual programming required post MRI	(Activator operated)	Yes	No (automatic timer)	Yes	No
Device identifiers	Three radiopaque rings on the proximal portion of the lead identify it to be a Tendril MRI product. The radiopaque letters MRI are on the device.	Radiopaque wavy lines are present on the proximal portion of the capsurefix lead and ~symbol is present on MR conditional device.	A solid triangle followed by the letters BSC on MR conditional device.	Biontronik symbol followed by letters SF found on MR conditional device.	

carried out pre- and post-MRI (Ainslie et al. 2013; Saman Nazarian et al. 2011). Activation of the "MR Safe" mode switches off advanced functions and the IPG paces in an asynchronous fashion (i.e., no sensing) to reduce the risk of electromagnetic interference being misinterpreted as an intrinsic rhythm with the potential of suppressed pacing. In some models the pulse amplitude and pulse duration are also both increased (e.g., 5 V and 1 mS in the St Jude Accent), which increases the pacing stimulus and minimises the risk of loss of capture. Tables 31.3 and 31.4 outlined some of the features and restrictions of currently approved MR conditional IPGs and ICDs respectively.

Table 31.4 Current MR conditional ICDs

	Medtronic	Biotronik
Device	Evera MRI	Lumax 640 and 740 Iforia 5 & 7 Ilesto 5 & 7
Leads	6947 M/6935 M	Linox ProMRI
Lead fixation	Active	Active
Thorax exclusion	No	Yes
Scan time limit	No	Yes
Static field strength limit		1.5 T
Max permitted scan time	NA	30 min
SAR limit (w/kg)	2	2
Manual programming required post MRI	Yes	Yes

Scanning of IPG Patients

Current US guidelines for safe MRI scanning *strongly discourage* MRI of Pacemaker dependent patients ("very high risk" classification) and ICD patients and *discourage* MRI of non-dependent ("low risk") MRI unsafe devices except in case of urgent need (Levine et al. 2007). Similarly, current European Guidelines for safe MRI indicate that patients should have life threatening or *severely quality-of-life* limiting conditions (Roguin et al. 2008). Both guidelines however do not impose absolute contraindications and acknowledge that in certain clinical scenarios and under stringent conditions the risk-benefit ratio can be in favour of MRI.

In practise the conditions imposed by those guidelines / position papers are burdensome and costly with the net effect of severely restricting access to a potentially beneficial diagnostic modality in clinical important populations (Jung et al. 2011), see Table 31.5. However, from a safety point of view such recommendations are sensible and justified. Whilst it has been demonstrated that MRI of non-MR conditional IPGs can be performed safely when certain logistic, safety and monitoring requirements are adhered to, concerns remain not only about the unpredictable nature of malfunctioning of such devices in the MR environment, especially in pacing dependent patients, but possibly more so about what potential effects the lowering of the acceptance threshold for scanning IPGs would have in real world clinical practice in the long term. The greatest concern would possibly be that the minimum required standards for proceeding "safely" with such exceptional scans could subsequently become eroded, exposing patients to avoidable risk. The second less apparent, but in the long term equally important aspect is that such a lowering in threshold would remove the incentive for industry to bring their entire product range to MRI compatible standards. With respect to the latter the core question remains how safe is safe? In the meantime clinicians and implanters have to address the question which patients are most likely to benefit from such devices, which basically equates into estimating the lifetime likelihood of requiring an MRI scan.

Table 31.5 American College of Radiology Appropriateness Criteria of common comorbidities indicating that MRI is standard of care of many comorbidities

Condition	MRI Rating	CT Rating	CT radiation level
Chronic Neck Pain (Radiographs normal, Neurologic sings or symptoms present)[a]	9	5 CT/Myelogram	☢☢ ☢☢ ☢☢ ☢☢
Low Back pain (> 70 yrs old)[b]	8	6 Only if MRI contraindicated	☢☢ ☢☢ ☢☢
Soft Tissue Masses (Clinically suspected soft tissue mass: general)[c]	9	5	Varies
Stroke symptoms (New focal neurologic defect, fixed or worsening 3 to 24 hours)[d]	8	8-MRI preferred if not unreasonably delayed	☢☢ ☢☢ ☢☢
Possible or probable Alzheimer's disease[e]	8	6	☢☢ ☢☢ ☢☢

Relative Radiation Level Designations

Relative Radiation Level	Adult Effective Dose Estimate Range
○	0 mSV
☢	<0.1 mSV
☢☢	<0.1-1 mSV
☢☢☢	1-10 mSV
☢☢☢☢	10-30 mSV
☢☢☢☢☢	30-100 mSV

[a]*ACR Appropriateness Criteria® – Chronic Neck Pain – 2010*
[b]*ACR Appropriateness Criteria – Low Back Pain – 2011*
[c]*ACR Appropriateness Criteria – Soft Tissue Masses– 2009*
[d]De La Paz RL, et al. Expert Panel on Neurologic Imaging. *ACR Appropriateness Criteria cerebrovascular disease*. [online publication]. Reston (VA): American College of Radiology (ACR); 2010. 23 p. [129 references]
[e]*ACR Appropriateness Criteria – Dementia and Movement Disorders – 2010*

Who Should Receive an MR-Conditional Device?

Publications have started to address this issue (Jones and Rajappan 2011), but consensus and/or societal guidance is still lacking. Obvious candidates appear those with congenital heart disease, underlying heart muscle disorders, conduction disease at young age or occurring as part of a systemic illness, Neurological disorders and specifically demyelinating conditions, prior or current malignancy and or cardiotoxic chemotherapy, back pain, arthritis and musculoskeletal disorders and potentially the "pending epidemic" of Alzheimer patients. Whilst one may argue that all IPG implants should be MR-conditional because of the relative high lifetime likelihood of benefiting from MRI this line of argument ignores the fact that clinical scenarios in which only MRI will provide an adequate (as opposed to the best) answer are actually rare. Such scenarios, encountered by the authors, include IPG patients with query of thoracic spinal cord compression, patients with multiple sclerosis and rapidly demyelinating disease or surgical planning in a case of an osteosarcoma. According to our own analysis performed based on 2006–2007 data from the English Hospital Episode Statistics (HES) database and the Hospital Activity Statistics (HAS) the 1 year and lifetime risk for a 75–79 year old to require an outpatient MRI was 7.9 and 46 % respectively (Schmitt et al. 2009). Whilst there are patient groups that very apparently self-select for implantation of MR conditional devices, including those mentioned above, it may indeed be more appropriate to approach the subject of selection considering those patients who would not benefit from MR-conditional devices first. This logically would include those that have a definite contraindication to MRI, including claustrophobia, or are unlikely to require an MR due to extreme age or terminal disease. Table 31.5 outlines a head to head comparison between MRI and CT with respect to common comorbidities encountered in CD patients.

Decision Making/Flow Charts/Check Lists

When presented with an appropriate request to image a patient with an IPG in situ it is helpful to follow published flow charts. For an example see Fig. 31.6. The first fundamental question now is if the device is MR-conditional or not. In the former scenario the 2nd fundamental question is if the patient has a stabile underlying rhythm or is pacing dependent. If the former is the case scanning can be considered low risk but care must be taken that all other safety steps where checked and that the relevant Cardiologist and/or Radiologist is aware of the device specific scanning restrictions that are easiest obtained from the device manufacturer and that the device, including leads, have been identified as MR conditional. Sources of identification include the implant record, programmer interrogation as well as device specific radio-opaque markers detectable on plain chest radiograph (see Fig. 31.7). Most device manufacturers are now able to provide specific checklists that facilitate adherence to licensed procedures and patient safety. An example of such checklists is provided in Fig. 31.8. When first embarking scanning patients with MR conditional devices it is generally advisable to request presence of an expert technologist from the relevant device company.

In the scenario of a scanning request for a patient with a MR unsafe device and/ or no underlying rhythm the first question should be if there is alternative diagnostic pathway that could deliver the required information with a more favourable risk benefit ratio. If the answer to this question is No a series of further questions require careful consideration. The most pertinent are summarised in the below Safety checklist (Fig. 31.8).

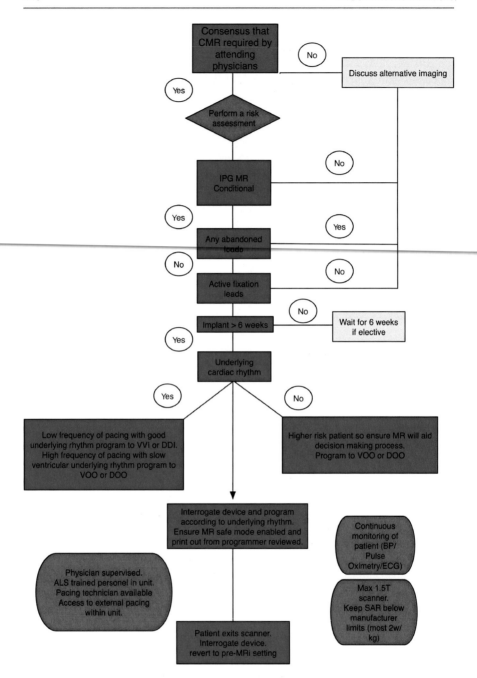

Fig. 31.6 Suggested MR scan pathway

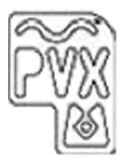

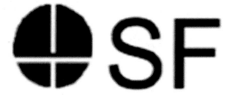

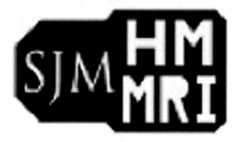

BSC011

Fig. 31.7 Radiographic markers located on header of pacemaker.

a Cardiologist Checklist:

> **Full Medtronic MRI SureScan**
> **Pacing or Defibrillation System implanted** ☐

SureScan Pacing and Defibrillation Systems Verification

Consult patient records to verify only Medtronic MR-Conditional Pacing and Defibrillation Systems constructed from the following components are implanted:

Medtronic SureScan leads

Medtronic Sprint Quattro Secure MRI™ leads (models: 6947M-55, 6947M-62, 6935M-55, 6935M-62)

Medtronic CapSure Sense MRI® leads (models: 4574-45, 4574-53, 4074-52, 4074-58)

Medtronic CapSureFix® 5086MRI leads (models: 5086-45, 5086-52, 5086-58)

Medtronic CapSureFix Novus MRI® leads (models: 5076-35, 5076-45, 5076-52, 5076-58, 5076-65, 5076-85)

Medtronic SureScan MRI pacemakers	Medtronic SureScan MRI defibrillators (ICDs)
Models: Advisa MRI® A3DR01 and A3SR01, Ensura MRI® EN1DR 01 and EN1SR01, EnRhythm MRI® EMDR01	Models: Evera MRI® DDMB2D4, DDMC3D4, DVMB2D4, DVMC3D4

Medtronic SureScan MRI pacemakers		Medtronic SureScan MRI defibrillators (ICDs)	
Implant > six weeks	☐	Post-lead maturation period	☐
Pectoral implant	☐	Pectoral implant	☐
Pacing Thresholds ≤ 2.0 V @ 0.4 ms	☐	Pacing Thresholds ≤ 2.0 V @ 0.4 ms	☐
Leads must be electrically intact (Pacing lead impedance 200-1,500 ohms)	☐	Leads must be electrically intact (Pacing lead impedance 200-3,000 ohms, Defibrillation lead impedance 20-200 ohms)	☐
No other devices, leads (including abandoned), adaptors, or extenders	☐	No other leads (including abandoned), lead extenders, or adaptors. Scanning patients who have multiple MR-Conditional devices present is acceptable when the MR labeling conditions for all implants are satisfied.	☐

> **Program MRI SureScan Mode ON before the scan**
> **(OFF after the scan)**

Pacemaker Patient Monitoring	Defibrillator Patient Monitoring
During the MRI scan, the patient's hemodynamic function must be monitored using at least 1 of the following systems: • pulse oximetry • electrocardiography • noninvasive blood pressure measurement	Patients must be monitored the entire time SureScan is programed ON. This includes visual and verbal monitoring as well as one of the following systems: • pulse oximetry • electrocardiography • noninvasive blood pressure measurements

For Defibrillator patients: In preparation for patient rescue, an external defibrillator must be immediately available while MRI SureScan is programmed to On.

> **Patient ready to get an MRI Scan**

Fig. 31.8 (**a, b**) Example of cardiology/radiology checklists for safe scanning of Medtronic MR conditional devices (Images courtesy of Medtronic)

ᵇ Radiologist Checklist:

A Full Medtronic MR-Conditional Pacing or Defibrillation System Confirmed by Cardiologist or Patient Records.

1.5 T closed bore MRI	☐
Maximum spatial gradient of ≤ 20 T/m (2,000 gauss/cm)	☐
Maximum gradient slew rate per axis ≤ 200 T/m/s	☐
Whole body SAR ≤ 2 W/kg	☐
Head SAR ≤ 3,2 W/kg	☐
Ensure with cardiology department that SureScan mode is programmed ON	☐
Pacemaker Patient Monitoring Patients must be monitored during the MRI scan **Defibrillator Patient Monitoring** Patients must be monitored the entire time SureScan is programed ON.	☐
Monitoring includes visual and verbal monitoring as well as one of the following systems: • pulse oximetry • electrocardiography • noninvasive blood pressure measurements	

For Pacemaker Patients: Keep an external defibrillator available during the MRI scan. The use of local transmit-only coils or local transmit-receive coils placed directly over the pacing system is contraindicated.

For Defibrillator patients: In preparation for patient rescue, an external defibrillator must be immediately available while MRI SureScan is programmed to On.

Perform the indicated scan

Cardiology to program the MRI SureScan Mode OFF

Fig. 31.8 (continued)

With respect to the actual procedure a number of established clinical protocols and algorithms have been proposed with physician led scans and pacing support readily available (Ainslie et al. 2013; Nazarian and Halperin 2009). It is good clinical practice to perform device interrogation before and after scanning to assess for battery depletion, programming changes or electrical reset. Patient monitoring throughout the scan period should include monitoring of pulse oximetry, ECG, blood pressure and verbal responsiveness. A suggested algorithm is given in Fig. 31.7. Indeed it should be emphasised that above mentioned European and American guidelines impose stringent monitoring requirements. In the European guidelines an advanced cardiac life support-certified health-care provider must be present during the entire exam to monitor the patient and perform cardiac life support if needed. A Cardiologist and a pacemaker/ICD programmer should be present during the scan. Monitoring requirements include ECG, pulse oximetry, and in some circumstances non-invasive BP and breathing sensors. Resuscitation equipment including a defibrillator must be present during the scan. Figure 31.9 outlines an example of a safety checklist that facilitates a safer environment in which to perform MRI of CD patients, especially those with no sufficient underlying rhythm and/or MR unsafe devices.

In general, 6 weeks is the recommended interval between implant and MR scan from published studies and this is also a mandatory stipulation for safe scanning of most of the MR-conditional devices. Lead dislodgment is more frequent in the first 6 weeks following an implant, and thus studies did not want to subject patients to MR scans and the theoretical risk of force and torque on the leads, whilst tissue encapsulation is not fully established. No studies exist that we are aware of that address scanning at shorter time intervals. In emergencies, particular spinal cord lesions, the benefit of an MR scan even within a week of implant may outweigh potential risks. A team discussion is essential, as is full patient consent and strict cardiac monitoring.

Summary

Worldwide over five Million patients (UK >250,000) are implanted with Cardiac devices.

It is estimated that the probability of a Device patient to benefit from MRI over the lifetime of their device is as high as 50–75 %.

Scanning MR-conditional IPGs in patients with stable underlying rhythm is now relatively straightforward and can be performed safely as long as device restrictions are adhered to and safety precautions are taken.

Scanning of MR unsafe IPGs and ICDs, especially legacy devices is considered high risk and discouraged by both European and American guidelines and consensus papers. However, it is acknowledged that it is not a contraindication and there are a number of clinical scenarios in which the risk benefit ratio can justify MRI. Indeed when published safety strategies are adhered to the risk benefit ratio is frequently favourable when compared to the accepted strategy of device extraction for the sole purpose of facilitating MRI.

MRI of pacemaker dependent patients, especially those with legacy devices is not infrequently ill conceived and is considered very high risk, particularly when the FOV includes the thorax. Scanning should only be considered under highly compelling circumstances and where an exit strategy in the event of device failure is firmly in place.

Left and right-sided IPGs and right sided ICDs frequently allow diagnostic studies including CMR imaging. Left sided ICDs can render certain thoracic studies including CMR investigations non-diagnostic.

Have all alternative imaging modalities been considered ? Specifically document why neither CT nor Nuclear imaging (where applicable) is likely to provide required information.	Date.................Physican(s) involved in decision making process;.. Explanation:.. ....
Is a diagnostic study likely to provide information that impacts significantly on the patients care, QoL and/or prognosis ?	....
Is study likely to be non-diagnostic? I.e. consider anatomic relationship of Bionic device and its likely field disturbance artifacts on ROI	....
Has a discussion with the referrer taken place specifically addressing risk benefit of MRI	Date.. ....
Has a discussion with patient taken place addressing risk benefit of MRI ?	Date.. ....
Has written patient consent been obtained ?	Date..
Are there any retained leads / wires / metal ?	....
Are there any other conventional contraindications ? Complete standard checklist.	....
Has the scan been protocolled by the relevant imaging specialist?	....
Monitoring logistics Has the device and leads been identified and is the appropriate equipment and trained technologist available for scanning period as well as pre- and post- scan checks?	Device;.. Implant date:.. Lead(s):.. Active / passive fixation:..
Have the device parameters been checked and documented? Battery near EOL ? Safety margin for Pacing capture thresholds ?	Document Battery status and Lead thresholds and impedance:.. ....
Has peri-scan Rhythm management been discussed with EP specialist / pacing doctor: General proposal: VOO/DOO (asynchronous pacing mode) in patients with slow rhythm and high frequency of pacing. VVI / DDI (inhibited pacing mode) in patients with good underlying rhythm and rare frequency of pacing.	Document underlying rate and rhythm, rational of chosen pacing mode, and switch off of advanced pacing features.. ....
Is CMR Cardiologist / Radiologist available to supervise scanning ?	....
Is sufficient ALS/ILS trained personnel available? Resus trolley checked;	....
Is external pacing equipment on site ?	....
All potentially required drugs available: A) Atropine [ ] B) Isoprenalline [ ] C) Midazolam [ ] D) Anexate [ ]	....
Additional requirement for **pacing dependent patients:** Is EP/pacing Cardiologist available / in building to provide exit strategy on the day in case of unexpected device failure? Is a lead compatible IPG on shelf? Has potential scenario been communicated to cath-lab manager.	....

Fig. 31.9 Checklist for MRI in patients with no underlying rhythm and/or MR unsafe IPGs/ICDs

Tips and Tricks
1. Purposeful centre frequency shifting; changes in imaging planes and frequency encoding can often shift the position of a susceptibility artefact away from a ROI.
2. Spoiled gradient echo cine imaging is less sensitive to the occurrence of susceptibility artefacts then b-SSFP cine imaging.
3. Patient selection for MR conditional devices is an unregulated area. Given the high probability of a device patient benefitting from MRI over the lifetime of their device it appears intuitive to ask which patient should not receive a MR conditional device (i.e., those with pre-existing contra-indications for MRI).

Future Perspective

If the progress in this field continues on its current trajectory and MR conditional devices become industry standard large patient groups currently denied the benefit of MRI will have access to the best as opposed to any diagnostic imaging modality for their specific condition.

With respect to cardiac MRI, CMR already plays a significant role in patient selection for device therapy. It is conceivable that CMR imaging might one day overcome the shortcomings of Echocardiography and help further refine device selection and optimisation with the ultimate goal of reducing the number of non-responders.

References

Achenbach S, Moshage W, Diem B, Bieberle T, Schibgilla V, Bachmann K. Effects of magnetic resonance imaging on cardiac pacemakers and electrodes. Am Heart J. 1997;134(3):467–73. Retrieved from http://www.ncbi.nlm.nih.gov/pubmed/9327704.

Ahmed FZ, Morris GM, Allen S, Khattar R, Mamas M, Zaidi A. Not all pacemakers are created equal: MRI conditional pacemaker and lead technology. J Cardiovasc Electrophysiol. 2013;24(9):1059–65. doi:10.1111/jce.12238.

Ainslie M, Miller C, Brown B, Schmitt M. Cardiac MRI of patients with implanted electrical cardiac devices. Heart (Br Cardiac Soc). 2013;1–7. doi:10.1136/heartjnl-2013-304324.

Bottomley PA, Edelstein WA. Power deposition in whole body NMR imaging. Med Phys. 1981.

Bottomley PA, Redington RW, Edelstein WA, Schenck JF. Estimating radiofrequency power deposition in body NMR imaging. Magn Reson Med: Off J Soc Magn Reson Med Soc Magn Reson Med, 1985;2(4): 336–49. Retrieved from http://www.ncbi.nlm.nih.gov/pubmed/4094551.

Bovenschulte H, Schlüter-Brust K, Liebig T, Erdmann E, Eysel P, Zobel C. MRI in patients with pacemakers: overview and procedural management. Dtsch Arztebl Int. 2012;109(15):270–5. doi:10.3238/arztebl.2012.0270.

Chou CK, Bassen H, Osepchuk J, Balzano Q, Petersen R, Meltz M, Cleveland R, Lin JC, Heynick L. Radio frequency electromagnetic exposure: tutorial review on experimental dosimetry. Bioelectromagnetics. 1996;17:195–208.

Cline H, Mallozzi R, Li Z, McKinnon G, Barber W. Radiofrequency power deposition utilizing thermal imaging. Magn Reson Med Off J Soc Magn Reson Med Soc Magn Reson Med. 2004;51(6):1129–37. doi:10.1002/mrm.20064.

Cohen JD, Costa HS, Russo RJ. Determining the risks of magnetic resonance imaging at 1.5 tesla for patients with pacemakers and implantable cardioverter defibrillators. Am J Cardiol. 2012;110(11):1631–6. doi:10.1016/j.amjcard.2012.07.030.

Cunningham D, Whittaker T. Cardiac Rhythm Management UK National Clinical Audit Report. 2011. http://www.hqip.org.uk/assets/NCAPOP-Library/CRM-2011-National-Clinical-Audit-Report-2010.pdf

Erlebacher JA, Cahill PT, Pannizzo F, Knowles RJ. Effect of magnetic resonance imaging on DDD pacemakers. Am J Cardiol. 1986;57(6):437–40.

Ferreira PF, Gatehouse PD, Mohiaddin RH, Firmin DN. Cardiovascular magnetic resonance artefacts. J Cardiovasc Magn Reson. 2013;15(1):41. doi:10.1186/1532-429X-15-41.

Fetter J, Aram G, Holmes Jr DR, Gray JE, Hayes DL. The effects of nuclear magnetic resonance imagers on external and implantable pulse generators. Pacing Clin Electrophysiol. 1984;7(4):720–7.

Gimbel JR. Unexpected asystole during 3 T magnetic resonance imaging of a pacemaker-dependent patient with a "modern" pacemaker. Europace. 2009;11(9):1241–2. doi:10.1093/europace/eup162.

Gimbel JR, Bailey SM, Tchou PJ, Ruggieri PM, Wilkoff BL. Strategies for the safe magnetic resonance imaging of pacemaker-dependent patients. Pacing Clin Electrophysiol. 2005;28(10):1041–6. PACE230 [pii] 10.1111/j.1540-8159.2005.00230.x.

Irnich W, Irnich B, Bartsch C, Stertmann WA, Gufler H, Weiler G. Do we need pacemakers resistant to magnetic resonance imaging? Europace. 2005;7(4):353–65. doi:10.1016/j.eupc.2005.02.120.

Jones M, Rajappan K. Implantable devices and cardiac MRI scans-no longer an absolute contraindication. Cardiol News. 2011;14(2):14–7.

Jung W, Zvereva V, Hajredini B, Jäckle S. Initial experience with magnetic resonance imaging-safe pacemakers: a review. J Interv Card Electrophysiol. 2011;32(3):213–9. doi:10.1007/s10840-011-9610-0.

Jung W, Zvereva V, Hajredini B, Jäckle S. Safe magnetic resonance image scanning of the pacemaker patient: current technologies and future directions. Europace. 2012;14(5):631–7. doi:10.1093/europace/eur391.

Junttila MJ, Fishman JE, Lopera G, Pattany PM, Velazquez DL, Williams AR, Trachtenberg BH, Sanina C, Mather J, Hare JM. Safety of serial MRI in patients with implantable cardioverter defibrillators. Heart (Br Cardiac Soc). 2011;97(22):1852–6. doi:10.1136/heartjnl-2011-300153.

Kalin R, Stanton MS. Current Clinical issues for MRI scanning of pacemaker and defibrillator patients. PACE. 2005;28:2878–91.

Lauck G, von Smekal A, Wolke S, Seelos KC, Jung W, Manz M, Luderitz B. Effects of nuclear magnetic resonance imaging on cardiac pacemakers. Pacing Clin Electrophysiol. 1995;18(8):1549–55.

Levine GN, Gomes AS, Arai AE, Bluemke DA, Flamm SD, Kanal E, Manning WJ, Martin ET, Smith JM, Wilke N, Shellock FS; American Heart Association Committee on Diagnostic and Interventional Cardiac Catheterization; American Heart Association Council on Clinical Cardiology; American Heart Association Council on Cardiovascular Radiology and Intervention. Safety of magnetic resonance imaging in patients with cardiovascular devices: an American Heart Association scientific statement from the Committee on Diagnostic and Interventional Cardiac Catheterization, Council on Clinical Cardiology, and the Council o. Circulation. 2007;116(24):2878–91. doi:10.1161/CIRCULATIONAHA.107.187256.

Luechinger R, Duru F, Scheidegger MB, Boesiger P, Candinas R. Force and torque effects of a 1.5-Tesla MRI scanner on cardiac pacemakers and ICDs. Pacing Clin Electrophysiol PACE. 2001;24(2):199–205. Retrieved from http://www.ncbi.nlm.nih.gov/pubmed/11270700.

Luechinger R, Duru F, Zeijlemaker VA, Scheidegger MB, Boesiger P, Candinas R. Pacemaker reed switch behavior in 0.5, 1.5, and 3.0. Tesla magnetic resonance imaging units: are reed switches always closed in strong magnetic fields? Pacing Clin Electrophysiol. 2002;25(10):1419–23.

Luechinger R, Zeijlemaker VA, Pedersen EM, Mortensen P, Falk E, Duru F, Candinas R, Boesiger P. In vivo heating of pacemaker leads during magnetic resonance imaging. Eur Heart J. 2005;26(4):376–83. doi:10.1093/eurheartj/ehi009; discussion 325–7.

Martin ET, Coman JA, Shellock FG, Pulling CC, Fair R, Jenkins K. Magnetic resonance imaging and cardiac pacemaker safety at 1.5-Tesla. J Am Coll Cardiol. 2004;43(7):1315–24.

Mollerus M, Albin G, Lipinski M, Lucca J. Ectopy in patients with permanent pacemakers and implantable cardioverter-defibrillators undergoing an MRI scan. Pacing Clin Electrophysiol. 2009;32(6):772–8. doi:10.1111/j.1540-8159.2009.02364.x.

Nazarian S, Halperin HR. How to perform magnetic resonance imaging on patients with implantable cardiac arrhythmia devices. Heart Rhythm. 2009;6(1):138–43. doi:10.1016/j.hrthm.2008.10.021.

Nazarian S, Hansford R, Roguin A, Goldsher D, Zviman MM. A prospective evaluation of a protocol for magnetic resonance. Ann Intern Med. 2011;155:415–24.

Pavlicek W, Geisinger M, Castle L, Borkowski GP, Meaney TF, Bream BL, Gallagher JH. The effects of nuclear magnetic resonance on patients with cardiac pacemakers. Radiology. 1983;147(1):149–53. Retrieved from http://radiology.rsna.org/content/147/1/149.abstract.

Roguin A, Zviman MM, Meininger GR, Rodrigues ER, Dickfeld TM, Bluemke DA, Lardo A, Berger RD, Calkins H, Halperin HR. Modern pacemaker and implantable cardioverter/defibrillator systems can be magnetic resonance imaging safe: in vitro and in vivo assessment of safety and function at 1.5 T. Circulation. 2004;110(5):475–82. doi:10.1161/01.CIR.0000137121.28722.33.

Roguin A, Schwitter J, Vahlhaus C, Lombardi M, Brugada J, Vardas P, Auricchio A, Priori S, Sommer T. Magnetic resonance imaging in individuals with cardiovascular implantable electronic devices. Europace. 2008;10(3):336–46. doi:10.1093/europace/eun021.

Russo RJ. Determining the risks of clinically indicated nonthoracic magnetic resonance imaging at 1.5 T for patients with pacemakers and implantable cardioverter-defibrillators: rationale and design of the MagnaSafe Registry. Am Heart J. 2013;165(3):266–72. doi:10.1016/j.ahj.2012.12.004.

Russo RJ, et al. Determining the risks of magnetic resonance imaging at 1.5 Tesla for patients with pacamakers and implantable cardioverter defibrillators (The Magnasafe Registry). Am Heart Assoc Sci Sess, 2012;126:A11726.

Sasaki T, Hansford R, Zviman MM, Kolandaivelu A, Bluemke DA, Berger RD, Calkins H, Halperin HR, Nazarian S. Quantitative assessment of artifacts on cardiac magnetic resonance imaging of patients with pacemakers and implantable cardioverter-defibrillators. Circ Cardiovasc Imaging. 2011a;4(6):662–70. doi:10.1161/CIRCIMAGING.111.965764.

Schmitt M, Busca R, Davidson NC. Risk of needing an MRI in pacemaker patients based on analysis of English Hospital statistics. ESMRMB Congress. Belek/Antalya; Turkey. 2009;491–2.

Schwitter J, Kanal E, Schmitt M, Anselme F, Albert T, Hayes DL, Bello D, Tóth A, Chang Y, van Osch D, Sommer T. Impact of the Advisa MRI™ Pacing System on the diagnostic quality of cardiac MR images and contraction patterns of cardiac muscle during scans: Advisa MRI randomized clinical multicenter study results. Heart Rhythm Off J Heart Rhythm Soc. 2013. doi:10.1016/j.hrthm.2013.02.019.

Shellock FG, Tkach JA, Ruggieri PM, Masaryk TJ. Cardiac pacemakers, Icds, and loop recorder: evaluation of translational attraction using conventional ("long-bore") and "short-bore" 1.5- and 3.0-Tesla Mr systems. J Cardiovasc Magn Reson. 2003;5(2):387–97. doi:10.1081/JCMR-120019424.

Sommer T, Naehle CP, Yang A, Zeijlemaker V, Hackenbroch M, Schmiedel A, Meyer C, Strach K, Skowasch D, Vahlhaus C, Litt H, Schild H. Strategy for safe performance of extrathoracic magnetic resonance imaging at 1.5 Tesla in the presence of cardiac pacemakers in non-pacemaker-dependent patients: a prospective study with 115 examinations. Circulation. 2006;114(12):1285–92. doi:10.1161/CIRCULATIONAHA.105.597013.

Suh J, Jeong E, Shin K, Cho J, Na J, Kim D, Han C. Minimizing artifacts caused by metallic implants at MR imaging: experimental and clinical studies. Am J Roentgenol. 1998;171: 1207–13.

Tandri H, Zviman MM, Wedan SR, Lloyd T, Berger RD, Halperin H. Determinants of gradient field-induced current in a pacemaker lead system in a magnetic resonance imaging environment. Heart Rhythm. 2008;5(3):462–8. doi:10.1016/j.hrthm.2007.12.022.

Wilkoff BL, Bello D, Taborsky M, Vymazal J, Kanal E, Heuer H, Hecking K, Johnson WB, Young W, Ramza B, Akhtar N, Kuepper B, Hunold P, Luechinger R, Puererfellner H, Duru F, Gotte MJ, Sutton R, Sommer T, EnRhythm MRI SureScan Pacing System Study Investigators. Magnetic resonance imaging in patients with a pacemaker system designed for the magnetic resonance environment. Heart Rhythm Off J Heart Rhythm Soc. 2011;8(1):65–73. doi:10.1016/j. hrthm.2010.10.002.

Zikria JF, Machnicki S, Rhim E, Bhatti T, Graham RE. MRI of patients with cardiac pacemakers: a review of the medical literature. AJR Am J Roentgenol. 2011;196(2):390–401. doi:10.2214/ AJR.10.4239.

Pulmonary Vein Assessment

32

Sven Plein and John P. Greenwood

Abstract

CMR of the pulmonary veins is useful for planning ablation procedures, during procedure and for assessment of complications with comparable measurements to CT. The pulmonary arteries are best identified from contrast-enhanced Magnetic Resonance Angiography complemented by phase contrast imaging through each pulmonary vein and SSFP cines in the axial and SAX orientation. LGE imaging can be used to identify ablation scars to comment on procedural success. 3D volume rendered images can be created to show the detailed anatomical arrangement of the left atrium and the pulmonary venous connections

Keywords

Cardiovascular • Magnetic resonance imaging • Pulmonary vein • Electrophysiology • Catheter ablation

---

CMR Protocol for Pulmonary Vein Assessment
1. LV structure and function module
2. Breath-hold non-gated contrast-enhanced MRA performed in the coronal projection encompassing the pulmonary veins and left atrium

---

S. Plein, MD, PhD (✉) • J.P. Greenwood, MBChB, PhD, FRCP
Division of Biomedical Imaging, Leeds Institute of Cardiovascular and Metabolic Medicine,
University of Leeds & Leeds Teaching Hospitals, Clarendon Way, Leeds LS1 9JT, UK
e-mail: s.plein@leeds.ac.uk, j.greenwood@leeds.ac.uk

© Springer International Publishing 2015
S. Plein et al. (eds.), *Cardiovascular MR Manual*,
DOI 10.1007/978-3-319-20940-1_32

3. Optional
   (a) in-plane cine imaging of each individual pulmonary vein
   (b) through-plane phase contrast flow analysis planned separately through
       each pulmonary vein
   Optional: LGE module (after ablation)

Introduction

There are two common clinical scenarios that generate a CMR referral specifically
for assessment of the pulmonary venous anatomy. These are: (1) suspicion of anomalous pulmonary venous drainage, usually in the setting of a dilated right heart. (2)
Assessment of the left atrial and pulmonary venous anatomy prior to an electrophysiological procedure. The former of these is fully covered in Chap. 30 p 424,
congenital heart disease, so this chapter will just focus on pre- and post-assessment
for radiofrequency ablation procedures.

Radiofrequency ablation (RFA) of the pulmonary veins (PVs) and the left
atrium has become a widely used procedure for the treatment of many forms of
cardiac arrhythmia, in particular atrial fibrillation (AF). The morphology of the
left atrium and the pulmonary veins is highly variable, and in around 1/3 of cases
an anomaly of the PV can be found, such as a common left or inferior truncus or
an additional right middle cardiac vein. Pre-procedural imaging by Computed
Tomography, Echocardiography and CMR is therefore today performed as a mat-
ter of routine to plan the interventional procedure, shorten its duration and minimize complications. The 3D imaging data generated by CMR or CT can be
integrated in clinical electrophysiological mapping systems to provide cardiac
electrical-anatomical maps during the ablation procedure. Increasingly, CMR is
used to delineate ablation lesions to measure procedural success and to assess
possible procedural complications such as pulmonary vein stenosis. PV stenosis
occurs in 1 or 2 % of cases and can be easily detected by CMR. The rare, but
severe complication of atrioesophageal fistula can also be delineated by CMR,
although CT is often preferred.

CMR Versus Other Imaging Modalities

In many institutions, cardiac CT is the commonest method for pre-procedural
assessment of the pulmonary veins because of ease of availability, fast data acquisition and high spatial resolution. However, the commercially available electrophysiological mapping software systems only produces low resolution 3D
eletcro-anatomimcal maps and so CMR imaging is perfectly adequate, if available.
Also, cardiac CT is associated with substantial radiation and iodinated contrast

exposure. As the main function of the 3D electro-anatomical mapping systems is to reduce procedural time and hence radiation exposure, CMR is likely to become an increasingly attractive alternative to acquire the 3D atrial maps.

CMR Protocol and Findings

The mainstay of CMR pulmonary vein assessment is contrast-enhanced Magnetic Resonance Angiography of the pulmonary veins. This is usually performed as a breath-hold, non-gated or ECG-gated acquisition in the coronal projection. Careful planning is essential to ensure that all of the pulmonary veins and left atrium are fully included in the field of view.

The following pulse sequence parameters are recommended for PV MRA:

(a) Gadolinium (0.1–0.2 mmol/kg) injected at 2–3 ml/s
(b) Slice thickness 1–2 mm; acquired spatial resolution in-plane 1–1.5 mm. If possible aim for isotropic voxels.
(c) 60–80 slices.
(d) Parallel acquisition used as available
(e) Single phase acquisition – breath-hold (typically 15–18 s), start the acquisition just after contrast leaves the RV as it is the pulmonary veins and LA that need optimal opacification.

Many CMR centres also perform through plane phase contrast imaging through each pulmonary vein. SSFP cines in the axial and SAX orientation can complement the imaging protocol. Following RF ablation, LGE imaging can be used to identify ablation scars to comment on procedural success.

CMR Analysis

Using advanced post-processing software, 3D volume rendered images can be created to show the detailed anatomical arrangement of the left atrium and the pulmonary venous connections (Fig. 32.1). In the CMR report it recommended to comment on the following:

1. Number of pulmonary veins (accounting for common trunks and accessory veins)
2. Exact anatomical arrangement in relation to the atria and/or systemic venous drainage (i.e., recognition of accessory or anomalous pulmonary veins). See Fig. 32.2.
3. Maximum and minimal ostial diameter of each pulmonary vein (dependant on cardiac and respiratory phase)
4. Presence or absence of stenosis in each PV, especially in reporting post-ablation CMR exams (Fig. 32.3). Pre- and post-ablation images should be compared side by side.

Fig. 32.1 3D volume
rendered image showing the
posterior aspect of the left
atrium and the pulmonary
venous connections

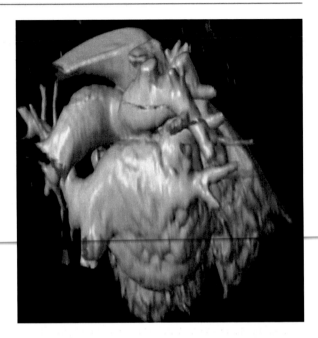

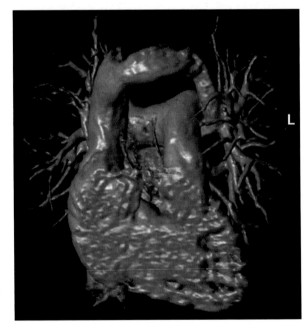

Fig. 32.2 3D reconstruction
showing partial anomalous
PV drainage (left upper
pulmonary vein connected to
the dilated innominate vein;
SVC is also clearly dilated)

Fig. 32.3 Post ablation MRA showing tight stenosis of the left lower pulmonary vein (see *arrow*)

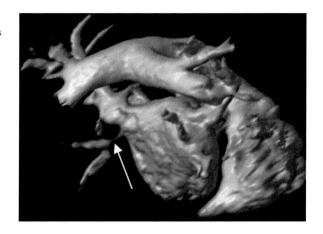

CMR Report for Pulmonary Vein Assessment

Morphology:

1. Number of pulmonary veins;
2. Exact anatomical arrangement of pulmonary vein return including recognition of accessory or anomalous pulmonary veins
3. Presence or absence of stenosis in each PV, especially in reporting post-ablation CMR exams.

Quantitative elements:

1. Maximum ostial diameter of each pulmonary vein;
2. Note the cardiac and respiratory phase during acquisition of images used for ostial measurements;
3. Minimum ostial diameter of each stenotic pulmonary vein
4. Imaging technique used for measurements

Key Points CMR in Pulmonary Vein Assessment

1. Useful for planning ablation, during procedure and for assessment of complications
2. Comparable measurements to CT

Interventional Cardiovascular Magnetic Resonance Imaging

33

Tarique M. Hussain, Kawal Rhode, and Gerald F. Greil

Abstract

Interventional CMR can be used to reduce the radiation burden during catheterization procedures or to improve image guidance for example in electrophysiology procedures. Interventional CMR is typically performed in hybrid CMR and x-ray suites. At present, the lack of devices that can be used in the CMR environment has limited the use of interventional CMR, but ongoing research including new guidance systems, real time imaging and faster post-processing promise a potential future clinical role for this method.

Keywords

Magnetic resonance imaging • Intervention • Interventional MRI • Catheter laboratory • X-ray angiography • Aorta • Fusion imaging

T.M. Hussain, MBBCHir, PhD
Research Fellow, Division of Imaging Sciences & Biomedical Engineering,
The Rayne Institute, King's College London, St Thomas' Hospital, London, UK

K. Rhode, PhD (✉)
Lecturer, Division of Imaging Sciences & Biomedical Engineering,
The Rayne Institute, King's College London, St. Thomas' Hospital,
London, UK
e-mail: kawal.rhode@kcl.ac.uk

G.F. Greil, MD, PhD
Consultant Paediatric Cardiologist/ Senior Clinical Lecturer,
Division of Imaging Sciences & Biomedical Engineering,
The Rayne Institute, King's College London, St. Thomas' Hospital, London, UK

© Springer International Publishing 2015
S. Plein et al. (eds.), *Cardiovascular MR Manual*,
DOI 10.1007/978-3-319-20940-1_33

Introduction

Rapid advances in the field of CMR have developed this modality to the extent that it can now be used to guide interventions. CMR provides exceptional 2D and 3D structural delineation for visualization and measurements. For these reasons, clinical programs using MRI guidance for cardiac catheterization have started and are showing promising results (Razavi et al. 2003).

Interventional MRI Systems

Currently there are no dedicated safe MR compatible catheters and devices for cardiovascular intervention commercially available. Therefore, it is still not possible to perform the complete procedure within the MR scanner. The immediate future of interventional MRI lies in exploiting multi-modality imaging. A good example of this is the XMR system, which combines X-ray and MRI by having both these modalities in the same room (Fig. 33.1).

XMR Facility Design

There are many design features that make this room different from standard MRI facilities. The XMR suite is designed so that half of the room is outside the 5-gauss line of the magnet, permitting use of traditional instruments and devices in this area (including echocardiography and radiofrequency ablation equipment). A movable tabletop allows the patient to be moved between modalities easily. The paramount factor in the design, build, and operation of an XMR facility is safety and a comprehensive safety protocol needs to be drawn up to minimize possible hazards (Table 33.1).

MR Visualization Strategies

Crucial to the success of interventional MRI is real-time tracking and visualization of catheters, guide-wires and devices in the MR environment.

Several approaches have been proposed in terms of catheter tracking. They can be separated into *passive, active* and *hybrid tracking* strategies (Henk et al. 2005).

Passive techniques are comparable to x-ray fluoroscopy, whereby the device itself is imaged without the need of additional hardware. This method has been successfully employed to guide catheters in patients under MR. The main challenge of all passive catheter tracking techniques is the concern regarding sufficient contrast between the instrument and its surrounding anatomy. Furthermore, real-time tracking limits the imaging to single-slice imaging with a limited field of view. *Active* tracking techniques employ small receiver coils, incorporated in the catheter device for signal reception and/or transmission, which necessitates hardware modification.

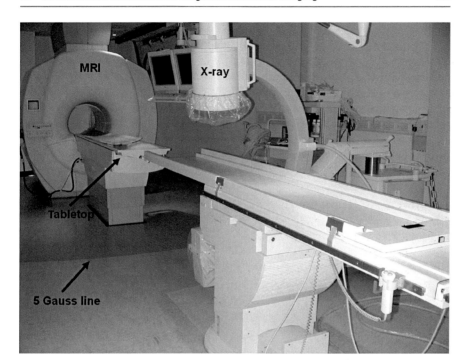

Fig. 33.1 A XMR system combines x-ray and MRI by having both modalities in the same room with a tabletop design that allows patients to be moved from one modality to the other in a very short time. The table position is stored within the system allowing image fusion between the MRI and x-ray system (XMRI) or even other imaging modalities (e.g. echocardiography). This system additionally allows the safe use of electronic devices, such as echocardiography machines and computer equipment, in the scanner room beyond the five gauss line

Table 33.1 XMR facility-safety features

1. Compulsory safety training of all MR interventional staff
2. Specially designed clothes without pockets
3. Safety entry restrictions during XMR intervention
4. Clear demarcation of ferromagnetic safe areas within the room
5. MR compatible anesthetic and monitoring equipment
6. Noise proof headphone systems for all staff within the room
7. X-ray and RF shielded room
8. Positive pressure air handling and filtration system
9. Tethering of all ferromagnetic equipment to the wall/floor
10. Safety checks whenever patient is transferred between X-ray and MRI to ensure that metallic instruments used for catheterization are not taken across to the MRI end of the room
11. Written log of all safety infringements and regular review of safety procedures

In addition, the main disadvantage is the concern regarding safety because these devices use intra-vascular coils as radio-frequency antennae and this makes the induction of an electric current and heating possible. The main advantage is that the tracking step can be performed independently to the imaging and so more detailed imaging (including 3D imaging) can be achieved.

Some approaches share both passive and active characteristics and are called *hybrid* techniques. Hybrid catheters can be tracked easily when compared to passive catheters and have a relatively better safety profile when compared to some of the active catheter designs.

Performing XMR Procedures

In general terms, there are two ways in which the XMR laboratory can be used.

X-Ray Imaging as a Backup During MRI Cardiac Catheterization

The cardiac catheterization procedure is performed in the MR scanner after adequate arterial and/ or central venous access has been obtained in the MR safe area (Fig. 33.1). The patient is then placed in the MR scanner after safety checks, including an operating theatre-style check of all metallic objects used in the MR safe area. With real-time imaging, the end-hole or side-hole balloon angiographic catheter (4–7 F) is passively visualized with the balloon inflated with CO_2. It then can be tracked to the appropriate location for pressure measurement or deployment of a device. If catheter manipulation into a particular heart chamber or vessel using MR guidance alone is difficult, the patient is transferred back to the x-ray end of the room, where the catheterization can be continued under x-ray fluoroscopy (e.g. to use a guidewire or a braided catheter). The patient can be transferred back to the MR scanner for further MR measurements once the catheter is satisfactorily positioned to continue the procedure.

Performing X-Ray Fused MR-Guided Interventions

Interventional procedures and radiofrequency ablation of arrhythmias necessitate part of the procedure to be performed under x-ray fluoroscopy because the ablation catheters and delivery devices are not MR compatible. Therefore, MR imaging is performed at the beginning of the procedure for planning, during the procedure for guidance and at the end of the procedure for evaluation.

Recently image fusion technology has been developed for image fusion between high resolution MR imaging and electrophysiological models (Fig. 33.2). Several systems are on the market and are currently being evaluated for clinical utility.

Image fusion can be used for several different indications:

1. It can provide anatomical road-mapping by overlaying of 3D MRI-derived anatomy onto live x-ray fluoroscopy
2. It can provide functional information overlay. Examples are motion from tagged MRI, or ablation lesion/ myocardial scar visualization from late enhancement MRI

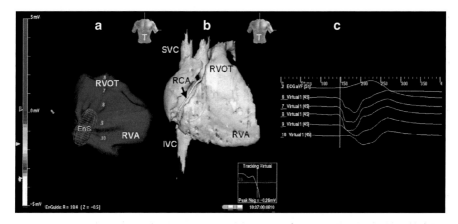

Fig. 33.2 A 13 year old patient was invasively treated for right ventricular outflow tract tachycardia. The geometric model, based on electrophysiology data (**a**) and the high resolution 3D magnetic resonance (MR) surface-rendered model (**b**), are presented side by side. Their spatial orientation within the thorax are shown by the thorax model (T). Their spatial coordinates are connected and movement of the electrophysiology model (**a**) results in the appropriate motion of the corresponding anatomic MR model (B). The 3D MR model (**b**) shows better anatomical details of the superior vena cava (*SVC*), inferior vena cava (*IVC*), right ventricular apex (*RVA*) and the right ventricular outflow tract (*RVOT*). The right coronary artery (*RCA*) can be seen in the 3D MR surface-rendered model (**b**), but not on the geometric model based on the electrophysiology data (**a**). The surface (Henk et al. 2005) and virtual (6–10) ECG signal generated from the Ensite Array® catheter (EnSite System St. Jude Medical) are displayed (**c**)

Table 33.2 Interventional XMR cardiovascular procedures	Radiofrequency ablation for tachyarrhythmias and pacemaker implants
	Interventional Procedures in Congenital Heart Disease
	Guided cardiac biopsy

3. It can provide 3D localization of devices within an MR images.
4. It can provide integration of data for biomechanical modeling.

Using these techniques a number of clinical cardiac applications are listed (Table 33.2).

Physiological Information

Traditional cardiac catheterization involves invasive pressures and blood gas measurements to calculate systemic and pulmonary blood flow and resistance using the Fick principle. However, this is dependent on multiple measurements and this can be a considerable source of inaccuracy. In addition, in patients with large intracardiac shunts or high pulmonary blood flow, the accuracy is further reduced. However, velocity encoded phase contrast magnetic resonance (MR) enables non-invasive quantification of blood flow in major vessels. Cardiac output and the pulmonary to systemic flow ratio (Qp:Qs) measured using this technique have been shown to be more accurate. In addition, phase contrast MR has been validated in numerous phantom experiments. This allows for a more accurate method of quantification of pulmonary vascular resistance (PVR) in patients with pulmonary hypertension by using invasive pressure measurements and MR flow data (Muthurangu et al. 2004).

Assessment of global and regional ventricular function can also be carried out much more accurately with 2D cine SSFP or time resolved 3D SSFP cardiac MR than with x-ray angiography. This is particularly important when assessing right ventricular function, volume and regional wall motion. Additional information can be obtained from myocardial tagging, delayed enhancement or spectroscopy and this can be combined with invasive pressure measurements or real time volumes from conductance catheter measurements.

Finally, combining invasive pressure measurement with MR derived blood flow and ventricular volumes also opens up interesting new ways of looking at pathophysiology. It allows the study of pulmonary vascular compliance, the derivation of ventricular pressure-volume loops and the assessment of load independent ventricular function.

Early Experiences

In our centre, MR is used to assess PVR in patients as it offers a more accurate quantification of the PVR in humans and reduced exposure to ionizing radiation. XMR fusion technology is also being used to carry out interventional procedures in congenital heart disease such as stent implantation in patients with coarctation of the aorta (Fig. 33.3) as well as positioning of RF ablation devices within the heart (Fig. 33.4).

Another very promising area for clinical applications, is the area of newly developed methods of scar imaging after electrophysiological ablation procedures. This allows assessment of the effectiveness of the ablation procedure. This can be combined with the results of the electrophysiological mapping systems and 3D anatomic MRI imaging results. Using this unique XMR technology, we have carried out radio-frequency ablation in pulmonary veins, atria and ventricles to successfully treat arrhythmias. This MR to x-ray registration method also allows us to relate the position of measured electrophysiology data to cardiac motion data from 3D MR images (Figs. 33.5 and 33.6).

Future Perspectives

Several groups have demonstrated the immense potential of interventional CMR in animal models. The interventions have been shown to be feasible with passive and active catheter techniques range from balloon angioplasty of arterial stenoses and

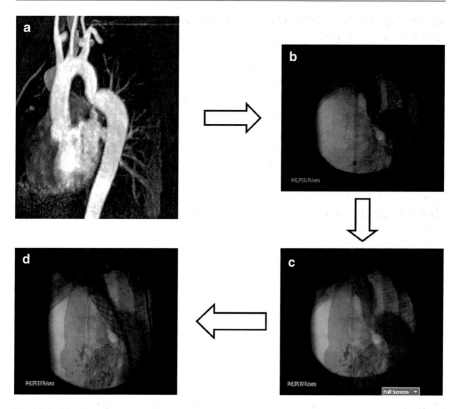

Fig. 33.3 The three dimensional (3D) contrast-enhanced magnetic resonance angiography (*MRA*) dataset of the aorta (**a**) is fused with the 2D angiography dataset (**b**) after injection of contrast agent (**c**). The high temporal resolution x-ray angiography 2D dataset (**b**) is used for implantation of a stent in the area of the coarctation. The 3D MRA/ 2D x-ray angiography fused dataset (**c**) is ideal for assessment of correct placement of the stent in the very complex 3D shape of the coarctation (**d**)

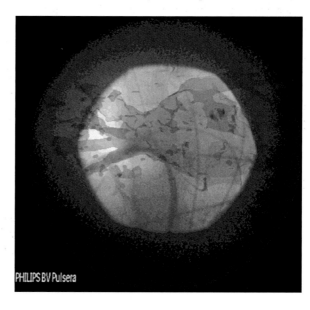

Fig. 33.4 A 3D contrast-enhanced MRA dataset (*red*) of the left atrium is fused with 2D live x-ray fluoroscopy images (*greyscale*) during a radio-frequency ablation procedure to treat a patient with paroxysmal atrial fibrillation. Contrast injection into the lower branch of the right lower pulmonary vein shows good agreement with the MR overlay

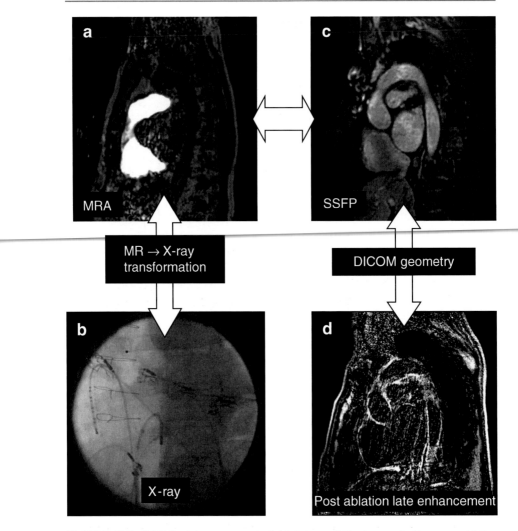

Fig. 33.5 Using MRI for the measurement of ablation scar following a radio-frequency ablation for right atrial flutter. (**a**) A 3D MRA scan showing the right heart which is used to construct a 3D surface model of the right atrium; (**b**) an x-ray image showing the catheters present in the right heart; (**c**) a 3D SSFP whole heart post-contrast agent MR data set; and (**d**) a delayed enhancement image showing marked enhancement in the region of the right atrial floor. All the different types if image data were related by using image registration

stenting of vessels to atrial septal puncture and atrial septostomy. Device closure of atrial septal defects is another application that has been explored. MRI guided percutaneous pulmonary and aortic valve stent implantation has also been successfully carried out.

More complex interventions such as percutaneous coronary catheterization and intervention have also been demonstrated in healthy animals using MR. Balloon

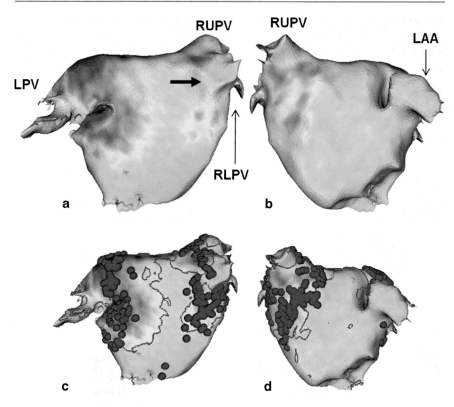

Fig. 33.6 Mapping the late enhancement information from MRI to the 3D surface model for patient who underwent radio-frequency ablation for paroxysmal atrial fibrillation. (**a** posterior view & **b** anterior view) Enhancing regions are shown in red (most enhancing) and yellow (moderately enhancing) and non-enhancing regions are shown in *green*. The encirclement patterns around both left- and right-side veins are apparent. (**c** posterior view & **d** anterior view) The addition of the ablation points from NavX to show the good correlation between these points and the enhancing regions from the MRI data

dilation of aortic coarctation in patients under MR guidance has also been performed. Recently, new MR compatible guidewires and catheters have become available and interventions in patients with congenital heart disease under MR guidance should be possible in the near future.

Further development of novel catheters and guidewires have been made possible by groups using targeted intra-myocardial injection of progenitor stem cells in myocardial infarction in animal models (Dick et al. 2003). Also, using real-time MRI and direct apical access in porcine hearts, prosthetic aortic valves have been implanted in the beating heart. This breakthrough application may allow MR guidance of minimally invasive extra-anatomic bypass and beating-heart valve repair. MR guidance of intramyocardial gene therapy is another exciting field. Finally, three-dimensional electromechanical models of the heart have also been created which allow simulation of cardiovascular pathologies in order to test therapeutic strategies and to plan interventions.

Acknowledgements We wish to thank in particular Reza Razavi and Carsten Shirra for their contribution to this work. Some of the work described in this chapter was performed at Guy's Hospital, London, UK, by a team of academic and clinical staff: Tobias Schaeffter, Sanjeet Hegde, Vivek Muthurangu, Marc Miquel, Redha Boubertakh, Andrew Taylor, Aaron Bell, Victoria Parish, Maxime Sermesant, Derek Hill, Stephen Keevil, David Hawkes, Jas Gill, Shakeel Qureshi, Eric Rosenthal and Edward Baker in the Departments of Imaging Sciences, Pediatric and Adult Cardiology. We would also like to acknowledge the support of the anesthetic department as well as John Spence, Stephen Sinclair, Rebecca Lund, John Totman and other staff from the Radiology Department who have provided considerable support.

References

Dick AJ, Guttman MA, Raman VK, Peters DC, Pessanha BS, Hill JM, Smith S, Scott G, McVeigh ER, Lederman RJ. Magnetic resonance fluoroscopy allows targeted delivery of mesenchymal stem cells to infarct borders in Swine. Circulation. 2003;108:2899–904.

Henk CB, Higgins CB, Saeed M. Endovascular interventional MRI. J Magn Reson Imaging. 2005;22:451–60.

Muthurangu V, Taylor A, Andriantsimiavona R, Hegde S, Miquel ME, Tulloh R, Baker E, Hill DL, Razavi RS. Novel method of quantifying pulmonary vascular resistance by use of simultaneous invasive pressure monitoring and phase-contrast magnetic resonance flow. Circulation. 2004;110:826–34.

Razavi R, Hill DL, Keevil SF, Miquel ME, Muthurangu V, Hegde S, Rhode K, Barnett M, van Vaals J, Hawkes DJ, Baker E. Cardiac catheterisation guided by MRI in children and adults with congenital heart disease. Lancet. 2003;362:1877–82.

Incidental Extra-Cardiac Findings in CMR

34

Pankaj Garg and Sven Plein

Abstract

Incidental extra-cardiac findings (IEF) are common during routine clinical cardiac magnetic resonance studies and are found in up to one quarter of patients. The majority of these findings is minor and of low clinical relevance, but it is essential that all incidental extra-cardiac findings are detected and adequately reported. The aim of this chapter is to provide the reader with a systematic approach to look for and report routine incidental extra-cardiac findings.

Keywords

Magnetic resonance imaging • Cardiovascular • Incidental finding • Tumour • Mass • Infection • Haematopoiesis • Goitre • Azygos lobe • Liver cyst • Hepatosplenomegaly • Ascites • Polycystic kidney • Metastasis

Key Points

1. IEF are common (20-26 %)
2. Systematic approach should be applied to look for and report IEF in routine clinical practice
3. Major IEFs are rare (~1 %)
4. Report should mention follow-up, appropriate referral and possible route to confirm diagnosis (Computed Tomography, Ultrasound etc.)

P. Garg, MD (✉)
Leeds Institute of Cardiovascular and Metabolic Medicine (LICAMM),
University of Leeds, 8.001 Worsley Building, Leeds LS2 9JT, UK
e-mail: p.garg@leeds.ac.uk; panakjvic@gmail.com

S. Plein, MD, PhD
Division of Biomedical Imaging, Leeds Institute of Cardiovascular and Metabolic Medicine,
University of Leeds & Leeds Teaching Hospitals, Leeds, UK

© Springer International Publishing 2015
S. Plein et al. (eds.), *Cardiovascular MR Manual*,
DOI 10.1007/978-3-319-20940-1_34

Introduction

Cardiac magnetic resonance (CMR) is a cross-sectional imaging modality and although studies are focuses on the heart, the scans cover a large part of the thorax and often other structures. Hence, physicians reporting CMR studies need to be able to detect and adequately interpret extra-cardiac pathology.

Incidence and Classification

Incidental extra-cardiac findings (IEF) are common and the reported prevalence of IEF is in the range of 20–26 %. IEFs can broadly be divided into two groups depending on clinical significance – minor and major (Table 34.1). Minor IEFs are mainly benign findings which are of no clinical importance and do not necessarily require further imaging or follow-up. These findings include anatomical variants like azygos lobes but also minor lymphadenopathy and solitary hepatic or renal cysts. Major IEFs are those, which are of clinical significance and require further clinical assessment, referral, follow-up or investigation by either a non-invasive or invasive strategy, for example suspected mass lesions and major lymphadenopathy. Anatomically, IEF's are often divided into two groups - supra-diaphragmatic or infra-diaphragmatic (Table 34.1).

Detection of IEF

Reliably detecting IEF's requires a structured approach to reviewing all available CMR images. In many centres co-reporting between cardiologists and radiologists is undertaken to ensure that both cardiac and extracardiac findings are comprehensively detected and described. With appropriate training, reporting of both cardiac and extracardiac findings by either a cardiologist or radiologist alone is however also considered feasible in many institutions.

IEF are commonly picked up on the initial scout or survey CMR images as these cover the largest field of view. A systematic review of these images, paying attention to all imaged body areas, is therefore essential. However, as the spatial resolution of scout imaging sequences used in CMR tends to be low and they are often acquired during free breathing, it is generally not possible to make a definitive diagnosis of IEF. Also, the slice thickness of these sequences tends to be high and small pathologies may be overlooked. Any suspected abnormalities should be confirmed by reviewing all other images of the CMR study and also by putting the CMR study in the context of other available clinical and imaging information. Where significant pathologies are detected during scan acquisition, the acquisition of additional images should be considered if logistically feasible.

Table 34.1 Classification of incidental extra-cardiac findings

Type	Minor	Major
Supra-diaphragmatic		
Lung	Minor atelectasis	Major parenchymal lung abnormality
	Bronchogenic cyst	Pleural thickening and effusion with unknown case
	Azygous lobe	Lung mass or nodule
	Tracheal bronchus	Multiple lung metastasis
	Small solitary lymphadenopathy (<1 cm in the short axis)	Major lymphadenopathy
Gastro-oesophageal	Hiatus hernia	
	Patulous oesophagus	
Thyroid	Solitary cyst	Thyroid mass
	Goitre	
Musculo-skeletal	Solitary vertebral haemangioma	
	Chest wall deformity	
	Vertebral kyphosis/scoliosis	
Others	Vascular anomaly (benign)	Scarring around defective breast implant
	Lipomas (epicardial, pleural, mediastinal)	Breast lesion/mass
	Breast impants Subcutaneous cyst	
	Foreign body	
Infra-diaphragmatic		
Gastro-intestinal	Chilaiditi Syndrome	Pancreatic mass/lesion
	Gall bladder (solitary) cyst/stone	Dilated gall bladder with possible obstruction
Liver	Solitary hepatic cyst	Hepatomegaly
	Solitary haemangioma	Multiple hepatic cysts
		Chronic liver disease
Spleen		Splenomegaly
		Spleen lesion
		Accessory spleen
Renal	Small solitary cyst	Irregular kidney
		Multiple complex cysts
		Renal mass
		Polycystic kidney disease
		Adrenal mass
		Hydrocalycosis
Others	Foreign body	Ascites

Case Examples
Supra-Diaphragmatic Incidental Extra-Cardiac Findings

Supra-diaphragmatic IEFs are predominantly located in the lungs, gastro-oesophageal tract, thyroid and musculo-skeletal system. Figure 34.1 shows four examples of IEF's related to these organ systems.

Infra-Diaphragmatic Incidental Extra-Cardiac Findings

Infra-diaphragmatic IEFs are predominantly located in the liver, gastro-instestinal tract, spleen, pancreas, kidneys and the peritoneum. Figure 34.2 shows four examples of few IEF related to these organ systems during routine clinical CMR list.

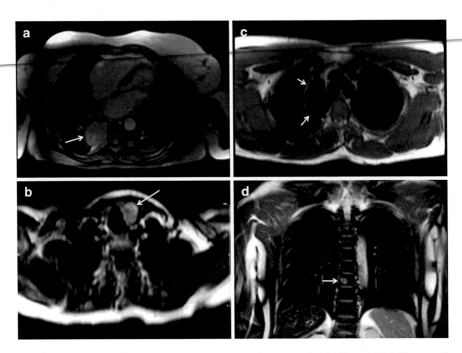

Fig. 34.1 Examples of supra-diaphragmatic incidental extra-cardiac findings – (**a**) A 55-year-old lady with a history of Thalassemia Intermedia, splenectomy underwent CMR for evaluation of cardiac function. On surveys, a large right-sided para-spinal mass measuring 44mmx63mm (*white arrow*) was found incidentally. On further investigations, the lesion was found to be extra-medullary hillar haematopoiesis. (**b**) A 44-year-old gentleman presented for a stress CMR study with a history of chest pain. On axial surveys, an irregular solitary left-sided mass in the thyroid glands was noted (*white arrows*). The final diagnosis was goitre. (**c**) A 35-year-old gentleman who had features of cardiomyopathy on echocardiography underwent CMR for clarification of aetiology. On black-blood imaging in a band can be seen dividing the right-sided upper lobes (*2 small arrows*). This was reported as a benign finding of azygous lobe for which no further imaging was recommended. (**d**) A 60-year-old gentleman had stress CMR study for evaluation of coronary artery disease. On coronal view of his surveys, a solitary small vertebral body lesion was noted. This was subsequently confirmed as a small haemangioma (*white arrow*)

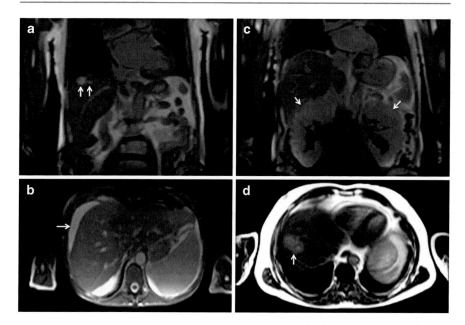

Fig. 34.2 Examples of infra-diaphragmatic incidental extra-cardiac findings – (**a**) A 45-year-old lady with cardiomyopathy had CMR study to clarify the aetiology. On coronal and axial surveys, two-rounded bright homogenous masses with smooth borders were identified (*white arrows*) in the liver. These were considered to being benign cystic lesions of the liver, which was confirmed on further investigation. (**b**) A 44-year-old lady with know history of liver failure and Hepatitis C infection presented with acute chest pain. Stress CMR was performed to evaluate for the presence of coronary artery disease and cardiac function. On axial surveys, hepatosplenomegaly was noted. Also, there was evidence of ascites (*white arrow*) in the peritoneum. Further abdominal imaging and haematology review were recommended. (**c**) A 35-year-old gentleman with hypertension presented with shortness of breath and had CMR for evaluation of cardiac function. On the coronal surveys, irregular kidney borders were identified. Multiple small cystic lesions were noted in both kidneys (*white arrows*). These findings were reported as suggestive of adult polycystic kidney disease with further assessment and imaging recommended. (**d**) A 77-year-old gentleman with history of colorectal cancer had stress CMR study for evaluation of coronary artery disease. On axial survey images, an irregular heterogeneous liver mass was noted (*white arrow*). These were reported as possible liver metastases with urgent further imaging recommended. No other pathologies were found on the CMR study

Reporting

A comprehensive CMR report, as described in Chap. 22, should describe the IEF in the 'General findings' subsection of the main text.

IEFs should be reported with clear description of size, location, characteristics, relationship to surrounding structures and invasion of other structures. Given that CMR studies are focussed on the heart or vasculature, it is often not possible to derive a definite diagnosis of an observed IEF. However, the report should seek to provide an overall assessment whether an IEF is likely to be a major clinical diagnosis and should suggest appropriate additional investigations. Sometimes, IEF may be part of a cardiac syndrome, for example, association of ascites, bilateral pleural effusion in a patient with poor bi-ventricular function. This clinical association should also be mentioned where applicable in the report.

Further Reading

Greulich S, Backes M, Schumm J, Grün S, Steubing H, Sechtem U, et al. Extra cardiac findings in cardiovascular MR: why cardiologists and radiologists should read together. Int J Cardiovasc Imaging. 2014;30(3):609–17.
Irwin RB, Newton T, Peebles C, Borg A, Clark D, Miller C, et al. Incidental extra-cardiac findings on clinical CMR. Eur Heart J Cardiovasc Imaging. 2013;14(2):158–66.
McKenna DA, Laxpati M, Colletti PM. The prevalence of incidental findings at cardiac MRI. Open Cardiovasc Med J. 2008;2:20–5.
Wyttenbach R, Médioni N, Santini P, Vock P, Szucs-Farkas Z. Extracardiac findings detected by cardiac magnetic resonance imaging. Eur Radiol. 2012;22(6):1295–302.

Index

© Springer International Publishing 2015
S. Plein et al. (eds.), *Cardiovascular MR Manual*,
DOI 10.1007/978-3-319-20940-1

Printed in the United States
By Bookmasters